BAYESIAN INFERENCE FOR GENE EXPRESSION AND PROTEOMICS

The interdisciplinary nature of bioinformatics presents a research challenge in integrating concepts, methods, software, and multiplatform data. Although there have been rapid developments in new technology and an inundation of statistical methodology and software for the analysis of microarray gene expression arrays, there exist few rigorous statistical methods for addressing other types of high-throughput data, such as proteomic profiles that arise from mass spectrometry experiments. This book discusses the development and application of Bayesian methods in the analysis of high-throughput bioinformatics data that arise from medical, in particular cancer, research, as well as molecular and structural biology. The Bayesian approach has the advantage that evidence can be easily and flexibly incorporated into statistical models.

A basic overview of the biological and technical principles behind multi-platform high-throughput experimentation is followed by expert reviews of Bayesian methodology, tools, and software for single group inference, group comparisons, classification and clustering, motif discovery and regulatory networks, and Bayesian networks and gene interactions.

Kim-Anh Do is a professor in the Department of Biostatistics and Applied Mathematics and the University of Texas M.D. Anderson Cancer Center. Her research interests are in computer-intensive statistical methods with recent focus in the development of methodology and software to analyze data produced from high-throughput technologies.

Peter Müller is also a professor in the Department of Biostatistics and Applied Mathematics and the University of Texas M.D. Anderson Cancer Center. His research interests and contributions are in the areas of Markov chain Monte Carlo posterior simulation, nonparametric Bayesian inference, hierarchical models, mixture models, and Bayesian decision problems.

Marina Vannucci is a professor of Statistics at Texas A&M University. Her research focuses on the theory and practice of Bayesian variable selection techniques and on the development of wavelet-based statistical models and their applications. Her work is often motivated by real problems that need to be addressed with suitable statistical methods.

BAYESIAN INFERENCE FOR GENE EXPRESSION AND PROTEOMICS

Edited by

KIM-ANH DO
University of Texas M.D. Anderson Cancer Center

PETER MÜLLER
University of Texas M.D. Anderson Cancer Center

MARINA VANNUCCI
Texas A&M University

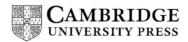
CAMBRIDGE
UNIVERSITY PRESS

CAMBRIDGE
UNIVERSITY PRESS

University Printing House, Cambridge CB2 8BS, United Kingdom

One Liberty Plaza, 20th Floor, New York, NY 10006, USA

477 Williamstown Road, Port Melbourne, VIC 3207, Australia

314-321, 3rd Floor, Plot 3, Splendor Forum, Jasola District Centre, New Delhi - 110025, India

103 Penang Road, #05-06/07, Visioncrest Commercial, Singapore 238467

Cambridge University Press is part of the University of Cambridge.

It furthers the University's mission by disseminating knowledge in the pursuit of education, learning and research at the highest international levels of excellence.

www.cambridge.org
Information on this title: www.cambridge.org/9781107636989

First published 2006

A catalogue record for this publication is available from the British Library

Library of Congress Cataloging in Publication data
Bayesian inference for gene expression and proteomics /
edited by Kim-Anh Do, Peter Müller, Marina Vannucci.
p.   cm.
Includes bibliographical references.
ISBN-13: 978-0-521-86092-5 (hardback)
ISBN-10: 0-521-86092-X (hardback)
1. Gene expression – Statistical methods.   2. Proteomics –
Statistical methods.   I. Do, Kim-Anh, 1960–   II. Müller, Peter, 1963–
III. Vannucci, Marina, 1966–   IV. Title.
QH450.B39   2006
572.8´6501519542 – dc22   2006005635

ISBN 978-0-521-86092-5 Hardback
ISBN 978-1-107-63698-9 Paperback

Contents

Contributors

Keith A. Baggerly, *Department of Biostatistics & Applied Mathematics, University of Texas M.D. Anderson Cancer Center, 1515 Holcombe Blvd., Houston, TX 77030-4075*

Veerabhadran Baladandayuthapani, *Department of Biostatistics & Applied Mathematics, University of Texas M.D. Anderson Cancer Center, 1515 Holcombe Blvd., Houston, TX 77030-4075*

Ghislain Bidaut, *Department of Genetics, The University of Pennsylvania School of Medicine, 1423 Blockley Hall, 423 Guardian Drive, Philadelphia, PA 19104-6021*

Andrea Bild, *Institute for Genome Sciences and Policy, Duke University, Durham, NC 27710*

Linda L. Breeden, *Fred Hutchinson Cancer Research Center, 1100 Fairview Ave. N., Mailstop A2-168, P.O. Box 19024, Seattle, WA 98109-1024*

Bradley M. Broom, *Department of Biostatistics & Applied Mathematics, University of Texas M.D. Anderson Cancer Center, 1515 Holcombe Blvd., Houston, TX 77030-4075*

Philip J. Brown, *Institute of Mathematics, Statistics and Actuarial Science, Room E218, Cornwallis Building, University of Kent, Canterbury, Kent CT2 7NF, UK*

Raymond J. Carroll, *Department of Statistics, Texas A&M University, 3143 TAMU, College Station, TX 77843-3143*

Carlos Carvalho, *Institute of Statistics and Decision Sciences, Box 90251, Duke University, Durham, NC 27708-0251*

Meng Chen, *Department of Statistics, The University of Wisconsin-Madison, 1220 Medical Sciences Center, 1300 University Ave., Madison, WI 53703*

Merlise A. Clyde, *Institute of Statistics and Decision Sciences, Box 90251, Duke University, Durham, NC 27708-0251*

Kevin R. Coombes, *Department of Biostatistics & Applied Mathematics, University of Texas M.D. Anderson Cancer Center, 1515 Holcombe Blvd., Houston, TX 77030-4075*

David B. Dahl, *Department of Statistics, Texas A&M University, 3143 TAMU, College Station, TX 77843-3143*

Kim-Anh Do, *Department of Biostatistics & Applied Mathematics, University of Texas M.D. Anderson Cancer Center, 1515 Holcombe Blvd., Houston, TX 77030-4075*

Arnoldo Frigessi, *Department of Biostatistics, University of Oslo, P.O. Box 1122, Blindern, 0317 Oslo, Norway*

Elizabeth Garrett-Mayer, *Johns Hopkins Kimmel Cancer Center, Johns Hopkins University, Suite 1103, 550 N. Broadway, Baltimore, MD 21205*

Ingrid K. Glad, *Department of Mathematics, University of Oslo, P.O. Box 1053, Blindern, 0316 Oslo, Norway*

Michele Guindani, *Department of Biostatistics & Applied Mathematics, University of Texas M.D. Anderson Cancer Center, 1515 Holcombe Blvd., Houston, TX 77030-4075*

Mayetri Gupta, *Department of Biostatistics, University of North Carolina at Chapel Hill, McGavran, Greenberg Hall B CB#7420, Chapel Hill, NC 27599-7420*

Alexander J. Hartemink, *Department of Computer Science, Duke University, Box 90129, Durham, NC 27708-0129*

Anne-Mette K. Hein, *Department of Epidemiology and Public Health, Imperial School of Medicine, St. Mary's Campus, Norfolk Place, London W2 1PG, UK*

Marit Holden, *Norwegian Computing Center, P.O. Box 114, Blindern, 0314 Oslo, Norway*

Chris C. Holmes, *Department of Statistics, University of Oxford, 1 South Parks Road, Oxford OX1 3TG, UK*

Leanna L. House, *Institute of Statistics and Decision Sciences, Box 90251, Duke University, Durham, NC 27708-0251*

Christina Kendziorski, *Department of Biostatistics and Medical Informatics, 6785 Medical Sciences Center, 1300 University Ave., Madison, WI 53703*

Sinae Kim, *Department of Biostatistics, School of Public Health, University of Michigan, 1420 Washington Heights, Ann Arbor, MI 48109-2029*

Andrew V. Kossenkov, *Division of Population Science, Fox Chase Cancer Center, 333 Cottman Ave., Philadelphia, PA 19111-2497*

Deukwoo Kwon, *Radiation Epidemiology Branch, National Cancer Institute, 6120 Executive Blvd, MSC 7238, Executive Plaza South, Room 7045, Bethesda, MD 20892-7238*

Alex Lewin, *Department of Epidemiology and Public Health, Imperial School of Medicine, St. Mary's Campus, Norfolk Place, London W2 1PG, UK*

Jun S. Liu, *Statistics Department, Harvard University, Science Center, One Oxford Street, Cambridge, MA 02138-2901*

Joseph Lucas, *Institute of Statistics and Decision Sciences, Box 90251, Duke University, Durham, NC 27708-0251*

Heidi Lyng, *Department of Biophysics, The Norwegian Radium Hospital, Montebello, 0310 Oslo, Norway*

Bani K. Mallick, *Department of Statistics, Texas A&M University, 3143 TAMU, College Station, TX 77843-3143*

Jeffrey S. Morris, *Department of Biostatistics & Applied Mathematics, University of Texas M.D. Anderson Cancer Center, 1515 Holcombe Blvd., Houston, TX 77030-4075*

Peter Müller, *Department of Biostatistics & Applied Mathematics, University of Texas M.D. Anderson Cancer Center, 1515 Holcombe Blvd., Houston, TX 77030-4075*

Michael A. Newton, *Department of Statistics, University of Wisconsin-Madison, Medical Sciences Center, RM 1245A, 1300 University Ave., Madison, WI 53706-1532*

Joseph R. Nevins, *Institute for Genome Sciences and Policy, Duke University, Durham, NC 27710*

Michael F. Ochs, *Division of Population Science, Fox Chase Cancer Center, 333 Cottman Ave., Philadelphia, PA 19111-2497*

Sylvia Richardson, *Department of Epidemiology and Public Health, Imperial School of Medicine, St. Mary's Campus, Norfolk Place, London W2 1PG, UK*

Christian Robert, *Ceremade – Université Paris-Dauphine, Bureau C638, Place du Maréchal de Lattre de Tassigny, 75775 Paris Cedex 16, France*

Judith Rousseau, *Ceremade – Université Paris-Dauphine Bureau B638, Place du Maréchal de Lattre de Tassigny, 75775 Paris Cedex 16, France*

Robert Scharpf, *Department of Biostatistics, Bloomberg School of Public Health, Johns Hopkins University, E3034 615 N. Wolfe Street, Baltimore, MD 21205-2179*

Naijun Sha, *Department of Mathematical Science, University of Texas at El Paso, Bell Hall 203, El Paso, TX 79968-0514*

Devika Subramanian, *Department of Computer Science, Rice University, 6100 Main Street, Houston, TX 77005*

Ning Sun, *Division of Biostatistics, Department of Epidemiology and Public Health, Yale University School of Medicine, 60 College Street, P.O. Box 208034, New Haven, CT 06520-8034*

Michael Swartz, *Department of Statistics, Texas A&M University, 3143 TAMU, College Station, TX 77843-3143* and *Department of Biostatistics & Applied Mathematics, University of Texas M.D. Anderson Cancer Center, 1515 Holcombe Blvd., Houston, TX 77030-4075*

Mahlet G. Tadesse, *Department of Epidemiology & Biostatistics, University of Pennsylvania School of Medicine, 918 Blockley Hall, 423 Guardian Drive, Philadelphia, PA 19104-6021*

Mark A. van de Wiel, *Department of Mathematics, Vrije Universiteit, De Boelelaan 1081a, 1081 HV Amsterdam, The Netherlands*

Marina Vannucci, *Department of Statistics, Texas A&M University, 3143 TAMU, College Station, TX 77843-3143*

Jon C. Wakefield, *University of Washington, Department of Biostatistics, Box 357232, Seattle, WA 98195-7232* and *Department of Statistics, Box 354322, Seattle, WA 98195-4322*

Ping Wang, *Department of Statistics, The University of Wisconsin-Madison, B248 Medical Sciences Center, 1300 University Ave., Madison, WI 53703*

Quanli Wang, *Institute for Genome Sciences & Policy, Duke University, Durham, NC 27710* and *Institute of Statistics & Decision Sciences, Duke University, Durham, NC 27708-0251*

Mike West, *Institute of Statistics and Decision Sciences, Box 90251, Duke University, Durham, NC 27708-0251*

Robert L. Wolpert, *Institute of Statistics and Decision Sciences, Box 90251, Duke University, Durham, NC 27708-0251*

Hongyu Zhao, *Division of Biostatistics, Department of Epidemiology and Public Health, Yale University School of Medicine, 60 College Street, P.O. Box 208034, New Haven, CT 06520-8034*

Chuan Zhou, *Department of Biostatistics, Vanderbilt University, S-2323 Medical Center North, Nashville, TN 37232-2158*

Preface

Recent rapid technical advances in genome sequencing (genomics) and protein identification (proteomics) have given rise to research problems that require combined expertise from statistics, biology, computer science, and other fields. The interdisciplinary nature of bioinformatics presents many research challenges related to integrating concepts, methods, software, and multiplatform data. In addition to new tools for investigating biological systems via high-throughput genomic and proteomic measurements, statisticians face many novel methodological research questions generated by such data. The work in this book is dedicated to the development and application of Bayesian statistical methods in the analysis of high-throughput bioinformatics data that arise from problems in medical research, in particular cancer research, and molecular and structural biology. This book does not aim to be comprehensive in all areas of bioinformatics. Rather, it presents a broad overview of statistical inference problems related to three main high-throughput platforms: microarray gene expression, serial analysis gene expression (SAGE), and mass spectrometry proteomic profiles. The book's main focus is on the design, statistical inference, and data analysis, from a Bayesian perspective, of data sets arising from such high-throughput experiments.

Chapter 1 provides a detailed introduction to the three main data platforms and sets the scene for subsequent methodology chapters. This chapter is mainly aimed at nonbiologists and covers elementary biological concepts, details the unique measurement technology with associated idiosyncrasies for the different platforms, and generates an overall outline of issues that statistical methodology can address.

Subsequent chapters focus on specific methodology developments and are grouped approximately by the main bioinformatics platform, with several chapters discussing the integration of at least two platforms. The central statistical topics addressed include experimental design, single group inference, group comparisons, classification and clustering, motif discovery and regulatory networks, and Bayesian networks and gene interactions. The general theme of each chapter is to review existing methods, followed by a specific novel method developed by the author(s). Results are often demonstrated on simulated data and/or a real application data set. Additionally, relevant software may be discussed.

Chapters 2 through 11 are concerned with Bayesian inference for gene expression, focusing on microarray data. Chapter 2 discusses inference about differential expression based on hierarchical mixture models, including a discussion of more than two patterns of differential expression. Inference is based on conjugate parametric models, with empirical Bayes estimation of hyperparameters. Chapter 3 explores the use of Bayesian hierarchical models for an integrated approach to the analysis of microarray data that includes flexible model-based normalization. The chapter defines a Bayesian gene expression (BGE) index as a gene-specific mean parameter in a hierarchical model. In Chapter 4, a model that mimics the detailed experimental process, from gene preparation to image analysis, is developed. The detailed process-based model allows to estimate absolute and relative mRNA concentrations. The use of Bayesian variable selection methods for biomarker selection in classification and clustering problems is reviewed in Chapter 5. The model for classification includes a mixture prior that specifies a positive probability of a given gene not being included in the model. In the clustering setting, the group structure of the data is uncovered by specifying mixture models where the random inclusion of genes can be interpreted as an attribute selection. Chapter 6 applies multivariate adaptive regression splines (MARS) to define a flexible model for the relationship between gene expression and disease status. For a binary classification problem the MARS model is defined on the logistic transformation of the class probability. The resulting classification boundaries are highly nonlinear and account for gene interactions. Chapter 7 reviews the popular probability of expression (POE) model for differential gene expression. The model postulates a mixture of a uniform submodel for under- and overexpression, and a central normal for typical expression. Posterior probabilities of mixture indicators in this model define the POE scale. Chapter 8 explores the use of sparsity priors in multivariate regression and latent factor regression, applied to inference for gene expression. The sparsity prior is a variation of a mixture prior on regression coefficients, with a positive point mass at zero- and a second-level mixture allowing for gene- and covariate-specific relative weights in the mixture. Chapter 9 develops a model for cell cycle gene expression, using a first-order Fourier model. The set of all genes is partitioned into subsets of different frequency and time-dependent amplitude, including a zero class of not-cycle-dependent genes. The prior on the random partitioning is defined as a Dirichlet distribution for cluster membership indicators. Chapter 10 defines a semiparametric Bayesian model for gene expression. The model exploits the clustering that is implicitly defined by the Dirichlet process prior to define subsets of genes based on gene-specific mean and sampling precision. Chapter 11 reviews the expression quantitative trait (eQTL) mapping problem and commonly used approaches. A new method is proposed to facilitate eQTL interval mapping that can account for multiplicities across transcripts. The problem is to match microarray gene expression (phenotype) with a set of genetic markers (genetic map). The mixture over markers (MOM) model defines a mixture model for gene expression, with the mixture being defined over submodels corresponding to the transcript mapping to one of the considered markers. An extension to interval mapping is discussed.

Chapters 12 through 15 discuss statistical inference for protein spectrometry. Chapter 12 reviews the use of semiparametric mixture models for inference on differential gene expression, for protein mass/charge spectra, and for SAGE data. The underlying models are Dirichlet process mixtures of normals, mixtures of beta kernels, and Dirichlet process mixtures of Poissons, respectively. Specific focus on SAGE data alone is detailed in Chapter 13, highlighting the two main characteristics of such data: skewness in the distribution of relative abundances, and small sample size relative to the dimension. A new Bayesian procedure based on the mixture Dirichlet prior is reviewed and specific properties depicted in terms of efficiency advantages over existing methods. Chapters 14 and 15 present two different Bayesian approaches of analyzing MALDI-TOF mass spectrometry. Chapter 14 generalizes the linear mixed model to the case of functional data by using a wavelet-based functional mixed model. In contrast, Chapter 15 presents model-based inference by focusing on nonparametric Bayesian models; a sum of kernel functions is chosen as basis functions for modeling spectral peaks.

Chapters 16 through 21 review motif discovery and regulatory networks. During the process of gene transcription, proteins (transcription factors) interact with control points of DNA sequences known as cis-acting regulatory sequences, called motifs. Chapter 16 focuses on the problem of locating these short sequence patterns in the DNA. The chapter provides an extensive explanation of the biological background and then describes a Bayesian framework for gene regulatory binding site discovery. Alternative models are also reviewed. Recent efforts in the development of methods that aid the detection of transcription factor binding sites have attempted to integrate sequence data with gene expression. In Chapter 17 the authors describe a regression model and a Bayesian variable selection formulation that helps refine the search for candidate motifs by selecting those that correlate with the gene expression. The authors also propose a model extension that includes gene regulators. Data integration is also the focus of Chapter 18, where gene expression and protein–DNA binding information, obtained from ChIP-Chip data, are integrated via a linear classification model to aid the reconstruction of gene regulatory networks. Chapter 19 deals with models that exploit the links between transcription factors and signaling pathways via gene ontologies and annotation databases. Bayesian decomposition models allow the extraction of overlapping transcriptional signatures. Popular approaches to infer gene regulatory networks are those that utilize probabilistic network models. Bayesian networks, in particular, have received much attention. Chapter 20 provides an extensive survey of computational techniques for learning Bayesian networks from gene expression data. State-of-the art and open questions are also addressed. Chapter 21 discusses the developments of Bayesian networks and dynamic networks. Additional data are used to derive informative prior structures, in particular combining gene expression data with protein–DNA binding information.

The final chapter, Chapter 22, addresses the choice of the sample size for microarray experiments. The authors take a decision theory point of view that attempts to minimize a conditional expected loss. The method is exemplified using a mixture Gamma/Gamma model.

We thank our friends and collaborators for contributing their ideas and insights toward this collection. We are excited by the continuing opportunities for statistical challenges in the area of high-throughput bioinformatics data. We hope our readers will join us in being engaged with changing technologies and statistical development.

Kim-Anh Do
Peter Müller
Marina Vannucci

1

An Introduction to High-Throughput Bioinformatics Data

KEITH A. BAGGERLY, KEVIN R. COOMBES,
AND JEFFREY S. MORRIS

University of Texas M.D. Anderson Cancer Center

Abstract

High throughput biological assays supply thousands of measurements per sample, and the sheer amount of related data increases the need for better models to enhance inference. Such models, however, are more effective if they take into account the idiosyncracies associated with the specific methods of measurement: where the numbers come from. We illustrate this point by describing three different measurement platforms: microarrays, serial analysis of gene expression (SAGE), and proteomic mass spectrometry.

1.1 Introduction

In our view, high-throughput biological experiments involve three phases: experimental design, measurement and preprocessing, and postprocessing. These phases are otherwise known as deciding what you want to measure, getting the right numbers and assembling them in a matrix, and mining the matrix for information. Of these, it is primarily the middle step that is unique to the particular measurement technology employed, and it is there that we shall focus our attention. This is not meant to imply that the other steps are less important! It is still a truism that the best analysis may not be able to save you if your experimental design is poor.

We simply wish to emphasize that each type of data has its own quirks associated with the methods of measurement, and understanding these quirks allows us to craft ever more sophisticated probability models to improve our analyses. These probability models should ideally also let us exploit information across measurements made in parallel, and across samples. Crafting these models leads to the development of brand-new statistical methods, many of which are discussed in this volume.

In this chapter, we address the importance of measurement-specific methodology by discussing several approaches in detail. We cannot be all-inclusive, so we shall focus on three. First, we discuss microarrays, which are perhaps the most common high-throughput assays in use today. The common variants of Affymetrix Gene Chips and spotted cDNA arrays are discussed separately. Second, we discuss serial analysis of gene expression (SAGE). As with microarrays, SAGE makes measurements at the mRNA level, and thus provides a picture of the expression profile of a set of cells, but the mechanics are different and the data may give us a different way of looking at the biology. Third, we discuss the use of mass spectrometry for profiling the proteomic complement of a set of cells.

Our goal in this chapter is not to provide detailed analysis methods, but rather to place the numbers we work with in context.

1.2 Microarrays

Microarrays let us measure expression levels for thousands of genes in a single sample all at once. Such high-throughput assays allow us to ask novel biological questions, and require new methods for data analysis.

In thinking about the biological context of a microarray, we start with our underlying genomic structure [4]. Your genome consists of pairs of DNA molecules (chromosomes) held together by complementary nucleotide base pairs (in total, about 3×10^9 base pairs). The structure of DNA provides an explanation for heredity, by copying individual strands and maintaining complementarity.

All of your cells contain the same genetic information, but your skin cells are different from liver cells or kidney cells or brain cells. These differences come about because different genes are expressed at high levels in different tissues. So, how are genes "expressed"?

The "central dogma" of molecular biology asserts that "DNA makes RNA makes protein." In order to direct actions within the cell, parts of the DNA will uncoil and partially decouple to expose the piece of the single strand of DNA on which a given gene resides. Within the nucleus, a complementary copy of the gene sequence (not the entire chromosome) is assembled out of RNA. This process of RNA synthesis is called transcription: copying the message. The initial DNA sequence containing a gene may also contain bits of sequence that will not be used – one feature of gene structure is that genes can have both "coding" regions (exons) and "noncoding" regions (introns). After the initial RNA copy of the gene is made, processing within the nucleus removes the introns and "splices" the remaining pieces together into the final messenger

RNA (mRNA) that will be sent out to the rest of the cell. Once the mRNA leaves the nucleus, the external machinery (ribosomes) will read the code and assemble proteins out of corresponding sequences of amino acids. This process of assembling proteins from mRNA is called translation: mapping from one type of sequence (nucleotides) to another (amino acids). The proteins then fold into 3d configurations that in large part drive their final function. If different genes are copied into RNA (expressed) in different cells, different proteins will be produced and different types of cells will emerge. Microarrays measure mRNA expression.

In thinking about the informational content of these various stages for understanding cellular function, we need to know different things. For DNA, we need to know sequence. For mRNA, we need both sequence and abundance; many copies can be made of a single gene. Gene expression typically refers to the number of mRNA copies of that gene. For protein, we need sequence, abundance, and shape (the 3d configuration).

If we could count the number of mRNA molecules from each gene in a single cell at a particular time, we could assemble a barchart linking each gene with its expression level. But how do we make these measurements? As suggested, we exploit complementarity: sequences of DNA or RNA containing complementary base pairs have a natural tendency to bind together:

$$...\texttt{AAAAAGCTAGTCGATGCTAG}...$$
$$...\texttt{TTTTTCGATCAGCTACGATC}...$$

If we know the mRNA sequence (which we typically do these days, since we can look it up in a database), we can build a probe for it using the complementary sequence. By printing the probe at a specific spot on the array, the probe location tells us the identity of the gene being measured.

There are two common variants of microarrays:

- Oligonucleotide (oligo) arrays, where short subsequences of the gene are deposited on a silicon wafer using photolithography (primarily Affymetrix).
- Full-length (entire gene) arrays, where probes are spotted onto a glass slide using a robotic arrayer. These generally involve two samples run at the same time with different labels.

1.2.1 Affymetrix Gene Chips

In looking at the structure of Affymetrix data, there are several in-depth resources [2, 3, 39] that serve as major sources for what follows, including the company's Web site, `www.affymetrix.com`.

In general, genes will be hundreds or thousands of bases in length, and the probes are shorter by an order of magnitude. This is driven in part by the manufacturing process, as the cost of synthesis increases with the number of bases deposited. Thus, choosing probes to print requires finding sequences that will be unique to the gene of interest (for specific binding) while still being short enough to be affordable. The final length decided on was 25 bases, and all Affymetrix probes are this length. It is important to note that different probes for the same gene have different binding affinities, and these affinities are unknown a priori. Thus, it's difficult to tell whether "gene A beats gene B," as opposed to "there's more gene A here than there." Microarrays only produce relative measurements of gene expression.

Given that the affinities are unknown, we can guard against problems with any specific probe by using several different probes for each gene. The optimal number of probes is not clear. Subsequent generations of Affymetrix chips have used 20 (e.g., HuGeneFL, aka Hu6800), 16 (U95 series), and 11 (U133 series) probes. There are some further difficulties with choosing probes:

- Some genes are short, so multiple subsequences will overlap.
- Genes have an orientation, and RNA degradation begins preferentially at one end (3' bias).
- The gene may not be what we think it is, as our databases are still evolving.
- Probes can "cross-hybridize," binding the wrong targets.

Overlapping, we can live with. Orientation can be addressed by choosing the probes to be more tightly concentrated at one end. Database evolution we simply cannot do anything about. Cross-hybridization, however, we may be able to address more explicitly.

Affymetrix tries to control for cross-hybridization by pairing probes that should work with probes that should not. These are known as the Perfect Match (PM) and Mismatch (MM) probes, and constitute "probe pairs." The PM probe is perfectly complementary to the sequence of interest. The MM probe is the same as the PM probe for all bases except the middle one (position 13), where the PM base is replaced by its Watson–Crick complement.

```
PM :    GCTAGTCGATGCTAGCTTACTAGTC
MM :    GCTAGTCGATGCAAGCTTACTAGTC
```

Ideally, the MM value can be used as a rough assessment of the amount of cross-hybridization associated with a given PM probe.

Affymetrix groups probe pairs associated with a given gene into "probe sets"; a given gene would be represented on a U133A chip by a probe set containing 11 probe pairs, or 22 probes with distinct sequences. The probes within a probe set are ordered according to the position of the specific PM sequence within the gene itself. We have described the ideal case above, but in practice the correspondence between genes and probe sets is not 1-to-1, so some genes are represented by several probe sets.

Having printed the probes, we now need to attach the target mRNA in such a way that we can measure the amounts bound. When we extract mRNA from a sample of cells, we do not measure this mRNA directly. Rather, we make copies. Copies are produced of the complementary sequence out of RNA (cRNA). Some of the nucleotides used to assemble these copies have been modified to incorporate a small molecule called biotin. Biotin has a strong affinity for another molecule called streptavadin; their binding affinity is the strongest known noncovalent biological interaction. After the biotin-labeled cRNA molecules are hybridized to the array, they are stained with a conjugate of streptavadin and phycoerythrin; phycoerythrin is one of the brightest available fluorescent dyes. The final complex of printed probe, biotinylated target, and streptavadin-phycoerythrin indirect label is then scanned, producing an image file. For our purposes, this image constitutes bedrock: *The image is the data.*

All Affymetrix Gene Chips are scanned in an Affymetrix scanner, and the initial quantification of features is performed using Affymetrix software. The software involves numerous files. The file types are

[EXP] Contains basic information about the experiment
[DAT] Contains the raw image
[CEL] Contains feature quantifications
[CDF] Maps between features, probes, probe sets, and genes
[CHP] Contains gene expression levels, as assessed by the Affy software

Most frequently, we start with a DAT file, derive a CEL file, and then make extensive use of the CEL and CDF files. We make no further use of the EXP and CHP files here.

To illustrate the procedure, we begin by looking at the contents of a DAT file from a U95Av2 chip (the raw image), shown in Figure 1.1A.

The array has 409,600 probes (features) arranged in a 640×640 grid. There is actually some structure that can be seen by eye, as we can see if we zoom in on the upper left corner: Figure 1.1B. The pixelated features have been combined with positive controls to spell out the chip type – this helps ensure that the image is correctly oriented. We note the border lattice of alternating dark and bright QC probes, making image alignment and feature detection easier.

If we zoom in further on a single PM/MM pair or feature, shown in Figure 1.2A and B, we can see that features are square. The horizontal and vertical

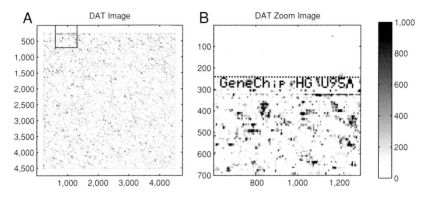

Fig. 1.1. An Affymetrix image (.DAT) file. (A) The entire image, 4,733 pixels on a side, containing 409,600 features. (B) A zoom on the upper left corner of the image. Controls are used in a checkerboard pattern to indicate the print region border, and to designate the chip type. This is a U95Av2 chip; on v2 chips the "A" is filled in.

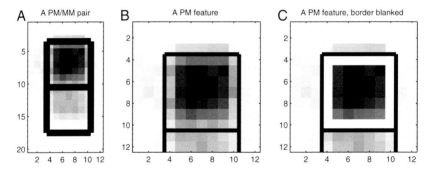

Fig. 1.2. Sets of Affymetrix image features. (A) A PM/MM pair. Note that the PM pixel readings are higher than the MM readings. (B) A zoom on the PM feature. (C) The PM feature after trimming the outer boundary. Only the remaining pixels are used in deriving a summary quantification (the 75th percentile).

alignment with the edges of the image is pretty good, but feature boundaries can be rather blurry.

Each feature on this chip is approximately 20 μm on a side. The scanner used for this scan had a resolution of 3 μm/pixel, so the feature is about 7 pixels on a side (more recent scanners have higher resolution). In general, Affymetrix features are far smaller than the round spots in the images of other types of microarrays.

The DAT file structure consists of a 512-byte header followed by the raw image data. The image shown above involved a 4733×4733 grid of pixels, so the total file size is $2 \times 4733^2 + 512 = 44,803,090$ bytes (45 MB). This is big.

File size is a nontrivial issue with Affy data; earlier versions of the software could only work with a limited number of chips (say 30). Given this size, our first processing step is to produce a single quantification for each feature, keeping in mind that the edges are blurry and that the features may not be perfectly uniform in intensity.

The CEL file contains the feature quantifications, achieved as follows. First, the four corners of the entire feature grid (here 640 × 640) are located within the DAT file, and a bilinear mapping is used to determine the pixel boundaries for individual features. Given the pixels for a single feature, the outermost boundary pixels are trimmed off, as shown in Figure 1.2C. Finally, the 75th percentile of the remaining pixel values is stored as the feature summary. Trimming is understandable, as this accounts for blurred edges in a moderately robust way. Similarly, using a quantile makes sense, but the choice of the 75th percentile as opposed to the median is arbitrary.

When Affymetrix data is posted to the Web, CEL files are far more often supplied than DAT files. Over time, there have been various versions of the CEL format. Through version 3 of the CEL file format, this was a plain text file. In version 4, the format changed to binary to permit more compact storage of the data. Affymetrix provides a free tool to convert between the file formats.

In the plain text version, sections are demarcated by headers in brackets, as in the example below. The header tells us which DAT file it came from, the feature geometry (e.g., 640 × 640), the pixel locations of the grid corners in the DAT file, and the quantification algorithm used. This is followed by the actual measurements, consisting of the X and Y feature locations (integers from 0 to 639 here), the mean (actually the 75th percentile) and standard deviation (this, conversely, *is* the standard deviation), and the number of pixels in the feature used for quantification after trimming the border. An example of a CEL file header is given below.

```
[CEL]
Version=3
[HEADER]
Cols=640
Rows=640
TotalX=640
TotalY=640
OffsetX=0
OffsetY=0
GridCornerUL=219 235
GridCornerUR=4484 253
GridCornerLR=4469 4518
```

```
GridCornerLL=205 4501
Axis-invertX=0
AxisInvertY=0
swapXY=0
DatHeader=[0..19412]  U95Av2_CDD0_12_14_01: CLS=4733
RWS=4733 XIN=3  YIN=3  VE=17 2.0 12/14/01 12:23:30
HG_U95Av2.1sq  6 Algorithm=Percentile
AlgorithmParameters=Percentile:75;CellMargin:2;
OutlierHigh:1.500;OutlierLow:1.004
[INTENSITY]
NumberCells=409600
CellHeader=X Y MEAN STDV NPIXELS
  0    0 133.0 16.6   25
  1    0 8150.0 1301.3   20
```

A version 3 CEL file reduces the space required to about 12 MB from 45 MB for a DAT file, but we could do better. The X and Y fields are not necessary, as these can be inferred from position within the CEL file. Keeping 1 decimal place of accuracy for the mean and standard deviation doubles the storage space required (moving from a 16-bit integer to a float in each case) and supplies only marginally more information. Finally, most people do not use the STDV and NPIXELS fields. Keeping only the mean values and storing them as 16-bit integers, storage can be reduced to $2 \times 640^2 = 819,200$ bytes. This type of compression is becoming more important as the image files get even bigger.

The above description covered Affymetrix version 3.0 files. In version 4.0, in binary format, each row is stored as a MEAN-STDV-NPIXEL or float-float-short triplet, which cuts space, but not enough. Most recently, Affymetrix has introduced a CCEL (compact CEL) format, which just stores the integer mean values as discussed above.

The above problem, going from the image to the feature quantification, is a major part of the discussion for quantification of other types of arrays because there, we get only one spot per gene. For Affymetrix data, the company's quantification has become the de facto standard. It may not be perfect, but it is reasonable. The real challenge with Affymetrix data lies in reducing the many measurements of a probe set to a single number.

In summarizing a probe set, we first need to know where its component probes are physically located on the chip. With any set of microarray experiments, one of the major challenges is keeping track of how the feature quantifications map back to information about genes, probes, and probe sets. The CDF file specifies what probes are in each probe set, and where the probes are. There is one CDF

file for each type of GeneChip. The header is partially informative, as shown
in the example below.

```
[CDF]
Version=GC3.0
[Chip]
Name=HG_U95Av2
Rows=640
Cols=640
NumberOfUnits=12625
MaxUnit=102119
NumQCUnits=13
ChipReference=

[Unit250_Block1]
Name=31457_at
BlockNumber=1
NumAtoms=16
NumCells=32
StartPosition=0
StopPosition=15
```

CellHeader=X	Y	PROBE	FEAT	QUAL	EXPOS	
	POS	CBASE	PBASE	TBASE	ATOM	INDEX
	CODONIND	CODON	REGIONTYPE	REGION		
Cell1=517	568	N	control	31457_at	0	
	13	A	A	A	0	364037
	-1	-1	99			
Cell2=517	567	N	control	31457_at	0	
	13	A	T	A	0	363397
	-1	-1	99			
Cell3=78	343	N	control	31457_at	1	
	13	T	A	T	1	219598

For this probe set, 31457_at, there are 16 "atoms" corresponding to probe
pairs (this is the standard number for this vintage chip) and 32 "cells" corresponding to individual probes or features. The first probe pair (index 0), with
the PM sequence closest to one end of the gene, is located on the chip in the
518th column (the X offset is 517) and in the 568th and 569th rows. The index values for these probes are $(567 \times 640) + 517 = 363397$ and 364037. The
feature in Cell 2 is the PM probe, as (a) it has a smaller Y index value, and (b)
the probe base (PBASE) in the central base position (POS) 13 is a T, which
is complementary to the corresponding target base (TBASE). The remaining
values in a given row are less important. The CDF files do not contain the actual

probe sequences, but all CDF files and probe sequences are now downloadable from `www.affymetrix.com`.

On early Affymetrix chips, all probes in a probe set were plotted next to each other. This was soon realized to be imperfect, as any artifact on a chip could corrupt the measurements for an entire gene. On more recent chips, probes within a probe set are spatially scattered, though PM/MM pairs are always together (the PM probe is always closer to the edge on which the chip id is spelled out).

Given quantifications for individual chips, we turn next to quantifying a data set, relating probe set values across chips.

Before we quantify individual probe sets, however, we need to address the problem of *normalization*: Is the image data roughly comparable in intensity across chips? Adding twice as much sample may make the resultant image brighter, but it does not tell us anything new about the underlying biology. In most microarray experiments, we are comparing samples of a single tissue type (e.g., diseased brain to normal brain), and in such cases we *assume* that "most genes do not change." Typically, we enforce this by matching quantiles of the feature intensity distributions. Given that the chips have been normalized, we still need to find a way of summarizing the intensities in a probe set. The PM and MM features for an example probe set are shown in Figure 1.3A and B.

The earliest widely applied method was supplied by Affymetrix in version 4 of their Microarray Analysis Suite package, and is commonly referred to as MAS 4.0 ("Mass 4") or AvDiff [2]. AvDiff works with the set of PM−MM differences in a probe set one array at a time. These differences are sorted in magnitude, the minimum and maximum values are excluded, and the mean and standard deviation of the remaining differences are computed. Using this mean and standard deviation, an "acceptance band" for the differences is defined as ± 3 s.d. about the mean. All of the differences falling within this band are then averaged to produce the final AvDiff value. This is illustrated in Figure 1.3C. In the case illustrated here, the minimum value was excluded at the first step, but fell into the acceptance band and was thus included in the final average, moving the value down slightly.

AvDiff does have some nice features. It combines measurements across probes, trying to exploit redundancy, and it attempts to insert some robustness. However, there are some questionable aspects. AvDiff weights the contributions from all probes equally, even though some may not bind well. It works on the PM−MM differences in an additive fashion, but some of the effects may be multiplicative in nature. It can give negative values, which are hard to interpret. In some cases, where all of the signals for a probe set are concentrated in a very small number of probes, these may be omitted altogether if they fall outside

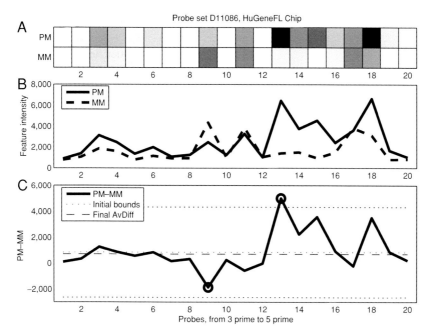

Fig. 1.3. A single probe set from a Hu6800 chip, containing 20 PM/MM pairs. (A) A heatmap of the feature intensities extracted from the CEL file. (B) Plots of the PM (solid) and MM (dashed) values shown in (A). Feature values are not uniform across the probe set, and MM values occasionally exceed PM. (C) A plot of the PM−MM differences, showing the computation of AvDiff. The extreme values (circled) are initially excluded, and the mean and ±3 s.d. bounds (dotted) are imposed. All points within this band are then averaged to produce AvDiff (dashed).

the band. All of these drawbacks, in our view, can be tied to the fact that AvDiff works one chip at a time, and does not "learn" with the addition of more chips.

Learning from multiple chips requires an underlying model with parameters that can be estimated. In 2001, Cheng Li and Wing Wong introduced a new method of summarizing probe set intensities as "model-based expression indices," or MBEI [35, 36, 59]. At the crux of their argument was a very simple observation – the relative expression values of probes within a probe set were very stable across multiple arrays.

Looking at the PM and MM profiles for the same probe set in 10 chips from a single experiment, as shown in Figure 1.4, we can see that the overall shape of the profile is fairly consistent. It is the amplitude of this profile which changes, and which contains the summary information about the level of gene expression.

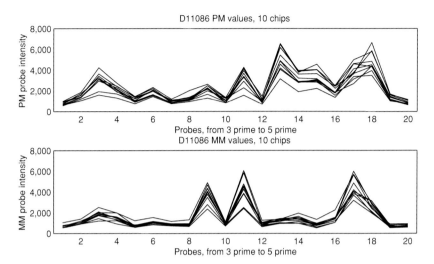

Fig. 1.4. Plots of PM and MM intensities for the same probe set on 10 different chips. The overall profile shapes are fairly consistent across chips, with changes in gene expression linked to amplitude. Modeling the shapes can improve inferences about expression levels.

In order to exploit this stability, Li and Wong fit a model for each probe set: for sample i and probe pair j, they posit that

$$PM_{ij} = \nu_j + \theta_i\alpha_j + \theta_i\phi_j + \epsilon,$$
$$MM_{ij} = \nu_j + \theta_i\alpha_j + \epsilon,$$

where ν_i and $\theta_i\alpha_j$ are intended to capture nonspecific binding, and ϵ is Gaussian noise. Focusing on the PM−MM differences, this model condenses to one with two sets of unknowns: θ_i and ϕ_j. The ϕ_j terms correspond to the individual probe affinities, and give the shape of the profile. The θ_i values give the amplitudes.

The MBEI approach caught on fairly quickly, in part because the numerical approach made sense, but also due to the fact that it was imbedded in the freeware "DNA Chip Analyzer" (dChip) package, available at www.dchip.org. This package has a very friendly user interface, and addresses many of the most common questions (which genes are different? how should I cluster them?) in a straightforward fashion. Further, by encoding the contents of CEL and CDF files in a binary format using analogs of the data structures outlined above, the program could handle lots of chips at once, and it could handle them quickly.

Using a model has several benefits. By using multiple chips, it can keep all of the probes; there is no tossing of the most informative ones. By checking the residuals from the model, it is possible to identify outliers due to artifacts. Using the hypothesized error model, confidence bands for the fold change can be computed. Probe profiles can be computed in one experiment and used in another.

The downside of most models is that they require several chips in order to estimate the underlying model parameters. It is not a good idea to trust the fits too much if they are based on just one or two chips; 10 or more is better. However, we are not convinced that it is a bad thing to require a larger minimum number of chips for drawing inferences.

The dChip model captures effects that are multiplicative, and inherits the other good features of a model. However, the probability model is too simplistic, as larger intensity probes typically also have larger variances.

In the wake of dChip, several other quantification methods have been suggested, with many (but not all) using model-based approaches. A partial list includes MAS 5.0, RMA, and PDNN.

The next algorithm from Affymetrix, MAS 5.0 [3], still produces quantifications one chip at a time, but replaces the MM values with a rather intricate change threshold (CT) to avoid negative values. The differences are then combined using a robust measure:

$$\text{Tukey Biweight}(\log(\text{PM}_j - \text{CT}_j)).$$

The robust multichip analysis (RMA) method of Irizarry et al. [27, 28] also uses a model for fitting the data, but the model differs from dChip's in some key ways. First, the authors elected to ignore the MM values, contending that any gains in accuracy were more than offset by losses in precision, in a classic bias-variance tradeoff. Second, since the MM values were not on hand, "background" levels were estimated from the distribution of PM probe intensities and subtracted off in such a way as to avoid negative values [13]. Third, the model introduced stochastic errors on the log scale as opposed to the raw intensity scale. The final model is of the form

$$\log(PM_{ij} - BG) = \mu_i + \alpha_j + \epsilon_{ij}.$$

The above approaches use the probe intensities, but there is additional biological structure that can be exploited. In particular, Affymetrix now makes the actual probe sequences available, though it did not when it first started selling chips. Using the sequences, it is possible to build models describing the default binding efficiencies for individual probes, and to decouple this from binding due to gene abundance. This approach was first exploited in the Position-Dependent Nearest Neighbor (PDNN) approach introduced by Zhang et al. [76]. The RMA method has since been extended to incorporate sequence information in its modeling, giving GCRMA [73].

Given the proliferation of models, we need some means of deciding which ones are "better." In order to make such assessments, we need to have some datasets for which "truth" can be known a priori, and some set of defined metrics that measure proximity to truth. The most widely used truth-known data set is a Latin Square experiment supplied by Affymetrix, in which 14 genes were spiked into a common mixture according to a twofold dilution series, which was then cyclicly permuted so that each gene was assessed at each dilution level. In this case, only the spiked-in genes should be changing in expression, and the amount of change is potentially known. In order to quantify truth, Cope et al. [20] introduced a suite of metrics for putting each method through its paces on the canonical data sets. The results for many different methods have been assembled and posted at `http://affycomp.biostat.jhsph.edu/`, and new submissions are welcome.

In addition to dChip, there are now several software packages available for analyzing Affymetrix data, but the most widely used in the statistical community are probably those implemented in R and freely available from Bioconductor. R packages exist for implementing all of the approaches discussed here, and most methods are sufficiently modular that different background correction, normalization, and quantification methods can be juggled to suit. The book by Gentleman et al. [25] provides an excellent introduction to this resource. Not all of the methods available are equally fast; however, so for the analysis of large data sets dChip and "justRMA" or "justGCRMA" in R are the ones that we would suggest.

The models for Affymetrix data are now reasonably good, but dozens of questions remain. Combining results of Affymetrix experiments across different labs and different chip types is still difficult, and integrating these results with those from glass arrays is still harder. Eventual combination of results at the RNA level with those from the DNA and protein levels is tantalizing.

1.2.2 Spotted cDNA Arrays

We now shift from Affymetrix oligonucleotide arrays to spotted cDNA arrays. Here, a good set of overview articles (from 1999) is available as a special supplement to *Nature Genetics*, "The Chipping Forecast" [47]; see also [60, 61]. While the biological questions of interest are similar, the probes used are quite different. On most cDNA arrays, the probes used correspond to full-length copies of the gene of interest (sans introns), though there has been recent interest in long-oligo arrays that use probes that are 60 or 70 bases in length

(60-mers or 70-mers). Typically, each gene will be represented by one probe, not a set. The other major distinction is that two samples, not one, are typically hybridized to each array. The samples are prepared using different incorporated dyes, mixed, and the mixture is then hybridized to the array.

The method of dye incorporation is different for spotted arrays than for Affymetrix Gene Chips. On a gene chip (as noted), the fluorescent dye is applied after hybridization has taken place (indirect labeling), but this strategy does not work if multiple samples need to be labeled with different dyes. Rather, when copies of mRNA are made for spotted arrays, they are made of cDNA, and some of the bases used in the assembly of these copies have had molecules of fluorescent dye attached. Thus, the dye is incorporated into the copies before hybridization (direct labeling). These labeled copies are then hybridized to the array, binding molecules of dye in specific positions.

The most commonly reported gene summary is the log ratio of two intensity measurements, corresponding to the two dyes with which the two types of cells being compared have been respectively tagged. The most commonly used dyes are Cy5 (red) and Cy3 (green). Thus, the single number quoted is derived from the two intensity values. The intensity values are also derived quantities; they are derived from images. Again, for our purposes these images represent bedrock. Images are our raw data.

These images are scans of slides with lots of dots on them, each dot corresponding to the location of a DNA probe to which labeled cDNA derived from the cells of interest has been bound. In some early experiments from M.D. Anderson, there were approximately 4,800 dots on a slide, arranged in a 4 by 12 grid of patches, with each patch containing a 10 by 10 grid of dots. When the images of the slide were produced, we got 3248 by 1248 arrays of grayscale pixel values. The scans from one such slide are shown in Figure 1.5A and B. The patch structure is quite apparent. This structure is linked to the method of depositing the probes. In printing, a robotic arrayer takes an array of print tips (similar to needles), dips them in wells of the DNA to be printed, moves the coated print tips over to the slide, taps lightly to transfer probes, and takes the print tips over to a wash solution before repeating the process. The arrayer we used had a 4 by 12 array of print tips; each visible patch has been applied by a single print tip.

Returning to consideration of the images, each pixel is a 16-bit intensity measurement, so values range from 0 to 65,535. There is no color inherently associated with these images, which is why we have presented them in grayscale; other colormaps are externally applied to enhance contrast. Each image is about 8 MB in size, which is large enough to make manipulation and transmission somewhat unwieldy at times. As more genes are spotted on the

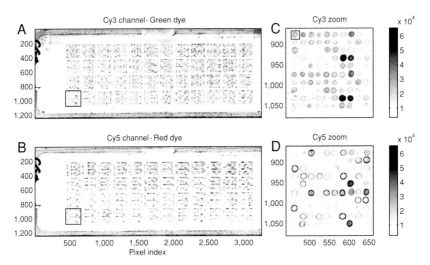

Fig. 1.5. Cy3 and Cy5 image scans from a spotted cDNA microarray. (A) The full Cy3 image. (B) The full Cy5 image. In both A and B, the patch structure (one per print-tip on the arrayer) is apparent. (C) A zoom on a Cy3 patch. (D) A zoom on the corresponding Cy5 patch. The top half of each patch is replicated in the bottom half, and this structure is visible. Imperfections in both the spotting and the image can also be seen, most clearly in the zooms.

arrays, and the scanner resolutions are improved so that smaller objects can be seen, these images will increase in size. It should be noted that the 16-bit nature of the images can make things difficult to work with in ways not having to do with file size. Some image viewing software assumes that the values are 8-bit, ranging from 0 to 255, and consequently either fails to show the large image or shows it as full white (all values set to 255). The values can be converted to 8-bit fairly simply, as 8-bit = floor(16-bit/256), but we lose gradation information. As the dynamic range of these images is quite large, this loss can be damaging for the purposes of analysis.

To make things more concrete in getting down to the actual spot level, we focus on a single 10 by 10 patch, marked in the bottom left of the large images. The corresponding regions from the two image files are shown in Figure 1.5C and D. These arrays were printed with replicate spottings of the same genes: within each patch, the top half of the patch is replicated in the bottom half. This replicate structure is visible – the brightest Cy3 spots are in rows 4 and 9 of column 7 of the patch, a replicate pair – giving us some confidence in the assay.

A few other things are immediately apparent. First, the "dots" are not really "dot-like" in most cases. Rather, there are rings of high intensity about

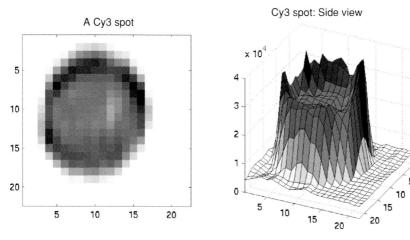

Fig. 1.6. Zoom on a single Cy3 spot. The ring shape is visible, indicating uneven hybridization. Further, the side view shows that readings outside the spot are not at zero intensity. (See color plate 1.6.)

lower-level centers. This is true across both channels, indicating that the ring pattern matches the amount of cDNA on the slide. The most likely explanation is that surface tension on the drop as it dries may cause clumping at the edges. In any event, how does morphology affect our measurements? Second, the dots are not of equal size. This may make it difficult for an automatic procedure to find the appropriate placement of a dot-shaped target ring. Third, there is some mottling in the lower left corner (most visible in the Green channel). How does this affect our assessment of how intense the dots in that region are?

Before considering these questions further, let us take a closer look at a single spot, highlighted in Figure 1.5C. An expanded view of this spot is shown in Figure 1.6. The ring shape is visible, indicating uneven hybridization. Further, the side view shows that readings outside the spot are not at zero intensity, indicating the need for some type of background subtraction so that we have moderately good estimates of where zero should be.

All of these issues point out the need for good image quantification algorithms for summarizing the spots. Some more detailed descriptions of algorithms for image segmentation, background estimation, and spot summaries are given in Yang et al. [74]. There are several software packages (mostly commercial) now available for quantifying array images.

Given the metrics, however, a more basic question is why two samples are used per array as opposed to one. The main reason is to guard against artifacts. Some spots are bigger than others, and thus bind more material. The slide can be tilted while hybridization is proceeding, resulting in more binding at one edge than another. Ideally, such artifacts will affect both channels similarly, and taking ratios will cancel them out. If there are replicate spots printed on the arrays, the importance of ratios can be checked by plotting the variance of the replicate log intensities as a function of the mean, first for each individual channel and then for the ratios. The variability of the ratios is typically less (often much so).

While the use of two samples does protect against some large-scale biases, it can also introduce new ones. The dyes used have different physical shapes, and thus can have different binding efficiencies for given genes. In recognition of this fact, many studies use one of two approaches for comparing two groups of samples. The first approach involves direct comparison of a sample of type A with a sample of type B on the same array. In this case, "dye swaps" are used so that the A samples are labeled with Cy3 on some arrays and with Cy5 on others, so that dye biases can be factored out. The second approach is to use the same dye to label the samples from both groups of interest, and to contrast these with some common reference material labeled with the other dye. Some of the design issues raised by this natural paired blocking structure are discussed in [33, 63].

Even with these balancing features, normalization remains an issue, both within and across arrays. Again, most methods make the simplifying assumption that most genes do not change. Given this assumption, a common means of correction is to plot the difference in channel log intensities as a function of the average log intensity, and to fit a loess curve to the dot cloud. These plots were introduced by Bland and Altman [12], but are more commonly referred to as "MA" plots in the microarray context [22]. Subtracting the loess curve ideally normalizes expression values within the array. A further extension of this approach is to apply a separate loess fit for the spots associated with each print tip. This makes stronger assumptions about which groups of genes are not expected to change, but smooths things more evenly. While we have seen cases where print-tip loess has produced more stable values (and better agreement between replicate spots), in many of these cases we are correcting for spatial trends that are visible on the array images, as opposed to discrepancies that are ascribable to the pins. Print-tip loess works in part because it is a surrogate for spatial position. Once the individual arrays have been normalized, quantile normalization can be used to match log ratio values across arrays [75].

Given the spot quantifications, and knowledge of what samples are bound on which arrays, there are freeware tools available for most basic analyses. Again, the book by Gentleman et al. [25] provides a nice survey of the suite of R tools available with Bioconductor.

One last concern with glass arrays relative to Affymetrix chips is simply that the number of different array configurations and gene spotting patterns is legion. This means that annotation and gene information must be checked carefully keeping the gene to spot mappings clear. It also means that comparisons across different array platforms may yield different measures of the "same" gene if different cDNAs are used.

1.3 SAGE

Microarrays work by exploiting hybridization to assess amounts of dye aggregating to specific probes printed on the arrays. There are, however, some potential downsides to microarrays. First, a microarray is a closed system, in the sense that you will only be able to measure an mRNA if you have printed a probe for it. Unexpected transcripts will not be seen. Second, the quantitative nature of the data is somewhat questionable, as dye response is a nonlinear phenomenon. Third, differences in protocols or preparations have made comparison of array results across labs difficult.

We would like to have some mechanism for more directly counting all of the mRNA transcripts of a given type. Failing that, if we could take a random sample of all of the mRNA transcripts available and count those, then this would still provide an unbiased and quantitative profile of mRNA expression. This idea of sampling and counting underlies the serial analysis of gene expression (SAGE) technique. Some case studies are given in [50–52, 56, 57, 64, 67–69, 77].

As before, we still need to know both sequence (identity) and abundance to characterize the expression profile. With microarrays, the unknown sequence of the transcript is inferred from the known sequence of the printed probe. With SAGE, a part of the transcript itself is sequenced. Restricting attention to only a part of the transcript is deliberate. While sequencing the entire transcript would identify it unambiguously, sequencing is time-consuming and costly enough that the expense would be prohibitive. We want to sequence just enough of the transcript to identify it, and then move on. The question now becomes one of how to biologically extract an identifying subsequence.

An identifying subsequence need not be long. Current estimates of the number of genes in the human genome are around 25,000–30,000. While alternative splicing of the exons within the gene may allow the same gene to produce several distinct transcripts, the total number of distinct transcripts is unlikely to be more than a few hundred thousand. Considering the 4-letter DNA alphabet, there are $4^{10} = 1,048,576$ distinct 10-letter "words," suggesting that a 10 bp (base pair) subsequence may be enough for unique identification. This rough calculation implicitly assumes that the 10 bp are in a specific location; it is considerably harder to find unique subsequences if these are allowed to occur anywhere within the gene. We are going to first specify position, and then extract sequence. This process is rather intricate. The steps are illustrated in Figure 1.7, and discussed in detail below.

We begin by harvesting the mRNA from a biological sample. The mRNA is single-stranded and has a poly-A tail (Figure 1.7A). The mRNA is difficult to work with, as it is prone to degradation, but DNA is more stable. We would thus like to map the mRNA to cDNA. To get to DNA, we introduce a biotin-labeled dT primer (Figure 1.7B) and use reverse transcriptase to synthesize more stable double-stranded complementary DNA (cDNA; Figure 1.7C). Like the initial mRNA, there is something special about one end (the biotin label), and we can use this to "anchor" the cDNAs.

We anchor the cDNAs by binding the biotin to streptavidin-coated beads. To focus on specific sites within the sequences, we introduce a restriction enzyme, known in the SAGE context as the "anchoring enzyme" (AE), which will cut the cDNA whenever a specific DNA "motif" occurs. We will only measure genes that contain at least one occurrence of the motif, so we want the motif to be fairly common; this in turn implies that the motif should be fairly short. Conversely, we do not want the motif to be too short, or it will reduce the number of distinct subsequences available afterwards. The most commonly used such enzyme is NlaIII, which searches for the motif "CATG." When this enzyme cleaves the cDNA, it produces an "overhang" (an unmatched single strand) at the cleavage site (Figure 1.7D). Cleaving produces a number of substrands, most of which are "loose" – unconnected to the streptavidin bead (Figure 1.7E). These loose fragments are washed away before the next step. At this point, we have zoomed in on a particular site on each cDNA: the occurrence of the AE motif closest to the bead (the mRNA poly-A tail).

As noted, cleaving typically produces an "overhang." We can use this overhang to bind new "linker sequences" at the end. As it turns out, we are going to bind *two distinct linkers* (Figure 1.7F). The two distinct linkers will be exploited in a PCR amplification step described below. So, we divide the material into two pools, and add the two linkers. The linkers are different only at one end; at the other they have an overhang (to match the bound sequence) and another short motif, which will guide yet another enzyme. Within each pool, the linker sequences will bind to the bound cDNAs due to base pairing – and the sequences are ligated (Figure 1.7G).

Next, we introduce a "type IIS" restriction enzyme (called the "tagging enzyme," TE) which looks for the motif we introduced with the linker sequence. Type IIS restriction endonucleases cleave not at the motif itself, but rather a

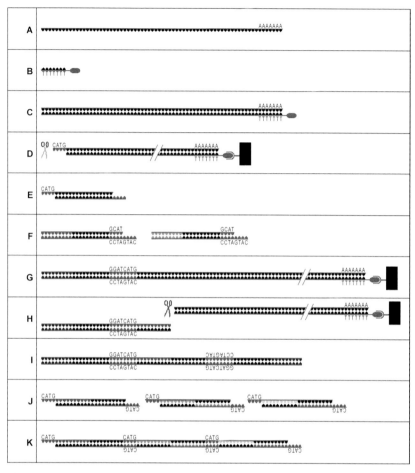

Fig. 1.7. Steps in the preparation of a SAGE library. (A) Extract mRNA. (B) Add a biotin-labeled primer. (C) Synthesize cDNA. (D) Cleave with an anchoring enzyme (AE). (E) Discard loose segments. (F) Split cDNA into two pools, and introduce a linker for each. (G) Ligate linker to bound cDNA fragments. (H) Cleave the product with a tagging enzyme, and discard the bound parts. In addition to the linker, the piece remaining contains a 10-base "tag" that can be used to identify the initial mRNA. (I) Ligate the fragments, and use PCR starting from the primers attached to the linkers to amplify. (J) Cleave with the AE again, and discard the pieces bound to the linker. The remaining fragments contain pairs of tags, or "ditags," bracketed by the motif recognized by the AE. (K) Ligate the ditags and sequence the product. (See color plate 1.7.)

specific number of base pairs (say 20) away from it. Unlike the motif for the anchoring enzyme, the motif for the tagging enzyme is asymmetric, so there is a direction for placing the cut site. This cut is "blunt," producing no overhang (Figure 1.7H).

At this point, the loose double strands in a pool have, in order, the linker, the TE motif, the AE motif, and *the 10 bp from the cDNA next to the anchoring enzyme motif closest to the poly-A tail.* This 10 bp subsequence is the "tag" that we shall use to identify the parent gene.

To focus on the tags, we now remove the beaded ends, leaving just the loose double strands. We then combine the two resultant pools, so that we have loose strands with two different linkers. We then induce ligation amongst the strands (Figure 1.7I).

The sequence geometry is now

Linker A – TE AE (motifs) – ditag – AE TE – Linker B,

where the central region, or "ditag," contains the identifying information for two distinct transcripts. Ideally, this ditag is bounded by linker A on one side, and linker B on the other. However, since the ligation is not targeted, it is possible to get linker A (or B) on both sides.

We now have a pool of DNA, but not necessarily a large amount. Since it is easier to work with large amounts of DNA, we amplify what we have using PCR. PCR requires primers at *both ends* of the target amplification sequence, and we can choose primers to match the two distinct linkers (this is why we divided things into two pools). Thus, the resultant products will be overwhelmingly of the form shown above, with linker A at one end and linker B at the other.

An amplified ditag with linkers has a fairly well-defined mass, so filtering of unwanted amplification products can be achieved using a gel. At this point, the information containing part of the data has been compressed (the length of the linker is less than the length of the gene, on average), but the linkers and enzyme motifs are still extraneous and we would prefer not to sequence them. Fortunately, if we reintroduce the AE, the linkers and the TE motifs will be cleaved off from the ditags. To isolate the ditags (Figure 1.7J), we use another gel to select for the appropriate target mass.

After the above selection and cleaving, the information content of a short piece of DNA (ditag plus overhangs) is quite high, but short reads are inefficient with respect to sequencing. Thus, we ligate the ditags together (Figure 1.7K). We then sequence the concatenated product. A typical sequencing read involves 500 bp, or about 20 ditags and motifs. The AE motif actually provides a useful bit of "punctuation" for quality control purposes.

Within the read, we locate a bracketing pair of motifs and extract the ditag (this can be between 20 and 26 bp). The 10 bp closest to the left end give one tag, and the 10 bp closest to the right end are reversed and complemented

Table 1.1. *Part of a SAGE Library*

Tag	Count	Tag	Count	Tag	Count
CCCATCGTCC	1286	CCTGTAATCC	448	TGATTTCACT	358
CCTCCAGCTA	715	TTCATACACC	400	ACCCTTGGCC	344
CTAAGACTTC	559	ACATTGGGTG	377	ATTTGAGAAG	320
GCCCAGGTCA	519	GTGAAACCCC	359	GTGACCACGG	294
CACCTAATTG	469	CCACTGCACT	359	–	–

to give the other. The tabulated results from a set of reads comprise a SAGE "library." Part of a typical SAGE library is shown in Table 1.1.

Given the data, what questions can we ask? The most common goal is (as with microarray experiments) to find genes that show expression levels that vary with phenotype. There are, however, complexities associated with the methods of measurement.

The first question is whether we see all the data. There are some sequences that we should not see. If we see the AE motif within a tag, we know that that is an artifact and should be excluded. In many cases, sequences corresponding to mitochondrial DNA will also be excluded. If there are multiple occurrences of a given ditag, typically only one is recorded, to preclude biases associated with PCR amplification. If there are genes that do not contain an occurrence of the cleavage site, these will not be seen. Similarly, if a cleavage site is too close to the poly-A tail, the true identity may be obscured. Conversely, if the RNA is of poor quality, sequence degradation can remove the cleavage site altogether.

There are other issues related to whether the tags we do see are "correct." Mappings of tags to genes are not always unique; the math suggesting that 10 bp should be "enough" relies on independence assumptions that likely do not hold. At present, our genomic information is still a draft, so annotations are not fixed. At the processing level, there are sequencing errors. Published rates are about 0.7% per base pair, so to a first approximation 7% of the tags will be so affected [66]. This can produce small "shadow" counts for tags that are "similar" to abundant tags. This renders estimation with rare counts difficult, and somewhat limits the dynamic range.

Interim fixes have been suggested for some of the above problems, but there is still room for improvement. "Long SAGE" [58], where the tags are 14 bp or more in length, has been introduced to address the issue of identification ambiguity. Many of the issues with identification could also potentially be resolved by using multiple restriction enzymes to produce "coupled libraries," but in practical terms this rarely happens (see, however, [72]). Errors in sequencing can be addressed by deconvolution, pulling shadows back to their source, given definitions of a local neighborhood in the sequencing space [18]. Alternatively, information about the tag quality could be acquired at the time of sequencing and used to suggest the most likely fixes; sequences can produce quality "phred" scores associated with each base read [11, 23].

Once the table of counts has been "finalized," there is still the question of choosing a good test statistic for assessing differential expression. Many statistics have been proposed, most focusing on comparing one library with another and dealing primarily with the Poisson sampling variability associated with extracting a count [5, 17, 30, 34, 40, 42, 44, 55, 77]. Some papers have looked at more than two groups [46, 52, 57, 77], and some analogs of ANOVA have been suggested [26, 65]. However, each library supplies a vector of proportions for an individual. Even under ideal conditions, estimates of the true level of a proportion in a group of individuals are subject to two sources of error: binomial variation associated with the count nature of the data, and variation in proportions between individuals within a group [6, 7]. Better methods for combining these proportions to estimate contrasts are still under development.

At present, SAGE is not as widely used as microarrays, due primarily to the higher costs of assembling libraries. However, these costs are also linked to the costs of sequencing, and the approach may become more viable as sequencing gets easier. The sequencing and counting approach, however, still has many open questions associated with it. Given estimated rates of sequencing errors, what is the realistic dynamic range of this approach? Given this dynamic range, how big does a library need to be to catch the measurable changes stably? Given the relative sizes of the between and within library variance components, should we assemble more small libraries or a small number of big ones? Massively parallel signature sequencing (MPSS) [16] enables the assembly of huge libraries, but the costs are still high. If we compare SAGE and microarray results, how should we measure agreement?

There are some software packages available for analyzing SAGE data, and some large repositories of SAGE data. We recommend SAGE Genie [14] as a source of data for further exploration.

1.4 Mass Spectrometry

Microarrays and SAGE let us measure the relative abundance levels of thousands of mRNA transcripts all at once, giving us some picture of the dynamic activity within the cell. However, much of the action is happening at the protein level, and we would really like to have the equivalent of a microarray for proteins as well. Some progress has been made on this front, but there are several limitations here.

- The number of distinct proteins is larger than the number of genes.
- Many proteins undergo posttranslational modifications (e.g., phosphorylation), and it is the amount of modification that can affect things.

Thus, it can be hard to get abundance and identity at the same time. However, we can make substantial progress if we relax one of these constraints, getting only partial identification. One tool for getting such information, letting us measure hundreds of proteins at once, is mass spectrometry. (More extensive descriptions are given in [38, 62].)

Mass spectrometry works by taking a sample and sequentially adding a charge to the substances to be measured (ionizing proteins, protein fragments, or peptides), using electromagnetic manipulation to separate the ionized peptides on the basis of their mass to charge (m/z) ratios, and using a detector to count the abundance of ions with a given m/z ratio. Plotting abundance as a function of m/z gives a mass spectrum. There are many variants of mass spectrometry, corresponding to different modular configurations of ionization, separation, and detection tools (not all combinations are possible), with much greater emphasis on the methods of ionization and separation than detection.

Mass spectrometry has been around for a long time; it was first introduced by J.J. Thomson around 1900, but it is only in recent decades that it has generated great excitement as a tool for exploring the proteome. This delay was due to limitations of the first few ionization methods available; charges were attached or broken off with sufficient force that larger molecules (including proteins) were torn apart into much smaller chunks. The late 1980s saw the introduction of two "soft" ionization methods, matrix-assisted laser desorption and ionization (MALDI) [31, 32] and electrospray ionization (ESI) [24] that allowed measurements to extend to the tens and hundreds of kiloDaltons (kDa, 1 Da = the mass of a hydrogen atom).

Recently, mass spectra have begun to be explored for their potential diagnostic utility – can peaks in the spectra serve as biomarkers of the early stages of diseases such as cancer? See, for example, [1, 37, 48, 49, 53, 71, 78]. While similar questions have been asked with respect to microarrays, a key difference has been that many explorations with mass spectra have focused on spectra obtainable from readily available biological fluids such as blood, urine, or saliva. In this context, the most common mass spectrometry methods used have been variants of MALDI coupled with a time-of-flight (TOF) ion separator (MALDI-TOF). This is the only method that we discuss in detail here.

In MALDI-TOF, the sample of interest (e.g., serum) is combined with one of several matrix compounds, and this mixture is applied to a stainless steel plate. As the mixture dries, the matrix forms a crystal structure holding the proteins in place. Many samples are typically spotted on the same plate; one MALDI plate we have (square, and about 7 cm on a side) has 100 deposition sites indicated. After the samples have been spotted, the plate is inserted into a receiving chamber connected to the main measurement instrument. The chamber is then pumped out to near vacuum conditions. A robotic arm is used to position the plate so that the spot of interest is in a desired target area, and a laser is then fired at the spot. Most of the laser energy goes into breaking the crystal structure of the matrix apart, and less to shaking the peptides apart. The physics of exactly how this works is not well understood. As a result of the matrix fragmentation, many peptides break free into the gas phase. Most matrix compounds are slightly acidic, and thus are willing to donate spare protons to nearby molecules during fragmentation – the peptides going into gas phase are ionized by capturing a small number of protons (typically 1–3 in the data we have seen). In the receiving chamber, a strong electric field propels the ions toward a flight tube. This electric field is typically set up by raising the potential of the plate itself (to V) before the laser is fired; the flight tube entrance is at zero. The flight tube itself is field-free, so the ions drift with the velocity imparted by the electric field until they reach a detector at the far end of the tube. The detector attempts to record the number of ions hitting it as a function of time of flight, assembling an initial form of the spectrum. Typically, several ($\sim$100) laser shots are made and the resulting spectra are summed to produce the final spectrum examined. To first order, the ions all cover the same potential difference and thus the kinetic energy imparted is proportional to the number of unbalanced charges, z (spare protons), the ion is carrying. The flight tube itself is typically much longer than the region over which the potential difference exists, and so the time spent in the acceleration region is typically discounted and the ion is treated as moving at a fixed velocity down the flight tube. Equating expressions for kinetic energy, we get

$$\frac{1}{2}mv^2 = zV.$$

As the velocity is fixed in the drift tube, $v = L/t$ where L is the length of the tube and t is the time of flight. Substituting and rearranging the above equation, we get

$$m/z = t^2(2V/L^2) = kt^2,$$

showing how the m/z ratio can be inferred from the time of flight.

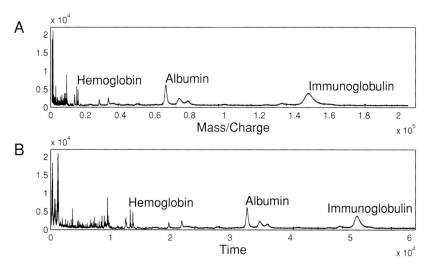

Fig. 1.8. Two views of the same MALDI-TOF spectrum. (A) Intensity plotted as a function of m/z, which is the standard display option. (B) Intensity plotted against time of flight, which is directly recorded by the instrument; m/z is a derived quantity. There are two natural scales on which to look at this data, as the time to m/z mapping is not linear.

MALDI spectra are commonly supplied as comma-separated value (CSV) files with two columns, containing the m/z value and spectrum intensity for each digitizer sample. Ignoring the m/z values, the rows give intensities that are equally spaced in time. An example of a MALDI spectrum is shown in Figure 1.8. The same spectrum is plotted against m/z in the panel A (the most common display option), and against file row in the panel B. This dual presentation is to emphasize that there is more than one natural scale on which to examine this type of data. This spectrum was derived from a serum sample, and peaks at 66 kDa and 150 kDa correspond to albumin and immunoglobulin, known serum proteins. Most of the interest in the biomarker papers published to date has been focused at somewhat lower m/z values; the identities of many of the peaks seen here are not known, and we want to find some that are present in patients with disease and not present in those without, or vice versa.

It is important to realize that not all of the peptides present in the sample will be seen in a spectrum. Different types of matrix can cause different groups of peptides to ionize more readily, so choosing a specific matrix amounts to choosing a subset of the peptides to be examined. It is common to further subset the peptides by "fractionating" the samples in a variety of ways; some separation axes include pH (acidity) and hydrophobicity (greasiness). Fractionation yields two clear benefits. First, it can allow for more precise identification of a peptide of interest. Several peptides may share a common (or very similar) m/z value, and thus be "aliased" if the entire sample is used. Fractionation introduces a second axis of separation for dealiasing. Second, it can remove (or split off) some of the most abundant peptides. This is an issue because our present instruments have a limited dynamic range, so if an abundant peptide is present at a level of 100, a trace peptide present at a level less than 1 will simply not be seen. The dynamic range of protein expression is thought to cover 9 or so orders of magnitude, which means that truly scarce peptides will be difficult to detect even with extensive fractionation [21]. The downside of fractionation is that it requires more time, effort, and amount of starting material. One variant of MALDI, known as surface-enhanced laser desorption and ionization (SELDI), works by depositing the sample/matrix mixture on a chemically precoated surface, where different surface coatings allow us to bind different subsets of peptides with high efficiency. SELDI has been commercialized by the company Ciphergen, which sells chips with different coatings preapplied, so some fractionation is done for you. Ciphergen also sells their own instruments and software, but there has been some experimentation with reading Ciphergen chips with other instruments.

Having introduced the structure of the data, we now turn to processing issues: Given a set of spectra, what do we have to do to it before analyzing an expression matrix? A partial list of important steps includes

- Spectral calibration
- Correcting for matrix noise
- Spectral denoising
- Baseline estimation and subtraction
- Peak detection and quantification
- Normalization
- Looking for common patterns and modifications (harmonics)

and we will address each in turn.

Earlier, we derived the relationship $m/z = kt^2$. In theory, physical parameters such as the potential difference, tube length, and digitizer rate of the detector are known and a value for k can be derived. In practice, the same peak may drift slightly over time due to changes in the instrument. One common way of addressing this problem is to run a "calibration sample" consisting of only a small number of proteins whose identities are known a priori, producing a spectrum with a small number of clearly defined peaks, as illustrated in Figure 1.9. The masses of the peptides are known, the flight times are empirically observed, and a set of (mass, time) pairs is used to fit a quadratic model

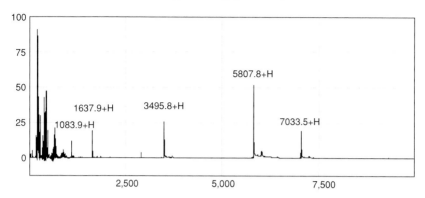

Fig. 1.9. A SELDI calibration spectrum. The sample was composed of a small number of known peptides, and the associated peaks are clearly seen. The known masses and the observed times of flight are then used to fit a quadratic calibration equation.

of the form

$$m/z = at^2 + bt + c$$

by least squares. The model parameters found are then assumed to hold for several samples. These parameters can change over time, so it is often useful to check that some of the biggest peaks seen "line up" across samples [29].

Matrix noise is a problem unique to MALDI. When a sample is blasted with a laser, many things break free, not just the peptides of interest. This other, unwanted stuff is colloquially referred to as "matrix noise," and it is predominantly present at the very low m/z end of the spectrum. Matrix noise can often saturate the detector, and detectors do not immediately recover after saturation. This effect is quite unstable [41]. Empirically, this has largely been addressed by excluding values below some chosen m/z cutoff. Exactly where this cutoff should go is not clear, and it can be affected by other machine settings such as the laser intensity. Higher intensity settings can blast loose heavier ions, allowing higher m/z regions to be explored, but these same settings kick up more noise and distort a larger low m/z region with noise. Conversely, low m/z regions can be probed with lower laser settings.

Mathematically, we tend to think of spectra as being composed of three pieces – the signals we want to extract, which are present as peaks, a smooth underlying baseline, and some high-frequency noise. In short,

$$Y_i(t) = k_i S_i(t) + B_i(t) + \epsilon_{it},$$

where $Y_i(j)$ is the intensity of spectrum i at time index t, k_i is a normalization factor, S_i is the protein signal of interest (a set of peaks), B_i is baseline, and

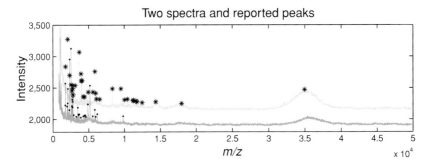

Fig. 1.10. Two raw MALDI spectra, with the peaks and intensities automatically flagged by software superimposed. There are differences in baseline and scaling visible in the raw spectra. These differences should be corrected for, but this was not done for the peaks found. Baseline cannot be estimated from the peaks alone.

$\epsilon \sim N(0, \sigma^2(t))$. We would like to remove the noise, subtract the baseline, estimate the peaks, and scale the spectra. There is a natural order to these steps, and performing them out of sequence (or omitting some) can make the downstream analysis more difficult.

Many mass spectrometry instruments are sold with associated software that will perform peak detection and quantification automatically, but these may not address all of the steps. For one data set we examined, we were supplied with both raw spectra and associated lists of peak locations and intensities. Two spectra from this set are plotted as curves in Figure 1.10, with the peaks supplied plotted as asterisks. The two spectra obviously have different baseline levels, still have additive white noise present, and may involve different normalization factors. However, the peak lists supplied use the intensities from the peaks before adjusting for baseline or normalization, and baseline cannot be reliably estimated from the peaks alone. We also note that one of the larger peaks, near m/z 36,000, is missed in one spectrum because it was not "sharp enough." Matrix noise is present at the very lowest m/z values, where the spectra jump out of view [10].

One problem with both denoising and peak detection is simply that peaks can have different shapes in different parts of the m/z range; higher m/z peaks are broader. Some factors that can contribute to this broadening are uncertainty in the initial velocity of the peptide, isotopic spread, and the nonlinearity of the clock tick to m/z mapping. The last of these was mentioned earlier, so we expand only on the former two. When peptides are blasted loose from the matrix crystal, all peptides of the same type do not break out with the same initial velocity. Rather, there is a velocity distribution, causing the peak to be spread out. This spread becomes more pronounced the longer the peptide drifts down the tube, and is thus bigger at higher m/z values. For higher m/z peptides, the definition of "mass" can actually be somewhat ambiguous. Carbon, for example, exists 99% as ^{12}C and 1% as ^{13}C. If a peptide contains 100 carbon atoms, the mass contribution from these atoms will be roughly 1,200 plus a small integer; this integer will have a Poisson distribution with mean $100 * 1\% = 1$. Similar effects are associated with other elements. The overall isotopic spread widens as mass increases, so that it is common to refer to both the monoisotopic mass (assuming all carbons have mass 12) and the average mass (incorporating the isotopic effects). It is possible to devise an approximate isotopic spread for a peptide given either mass estimate, using the general abundances of carbon and other elements in the population of amino acids. This can be used to sharpen the peaks through deconvolution.

There are a number of denoising filters that exist for spectra (e.g., Savitzky-Golay), but we admit a preference for wavelet-based methods that adapt naturally to the multiscale nature of the data. Here, we map to the wavelet domain, zero out the small coefficients (hard thresholding), and map back before looking for peaks [19].

Once the spectra have been smoothed, we attempt to estimate baseline. At present, we do not use very sophisticated algorithms for this purpose, generally sticking with a local minimum fit so that negative intensities will not be produced by subtraction. Again, the "local" neighborhood used needs to be altered as m/z increases. Even with basic algorithms, the effects can be rather dramatic. In Figure 1.11, we show spectra derived from 20 pH fractions for a single patient both before and after denoising and baseline subtraction (panels A and B, respectively). In this case, baseline subtraction causes the more dramatic effect, giving all of the base levels the same hue. As an aside, we note that this display also points out that fractionation is an imperfect procedure, and that signal from the same peptide can be found in several adjacent fractions.

After subtracting baseline from smoothed spectra, we still need to identify peaks and get summary values for them. A first pass approach can use a simple maximum finder. We could attempt to use peak areas instead, but we do not pursue this here. We note, however, that locating the peaks can be aided by considering a set of spectra rather than a single spectrum. Assuming the spectra have been roughly aligned, we have found it useful to average spectra within a group and perform peak detection on the average spectrum [45]. Averaging may even be useful before doing wavelet denoising, as small peaks can be reinforced as the noise level drops, and they can be retained. Values for individual spectra can be extracted as local maxima in small windows about the central peak location. The width of this window can be linked to the nominal precision of the instrument. For a low-resolution instrument, the uncertainty can be on the

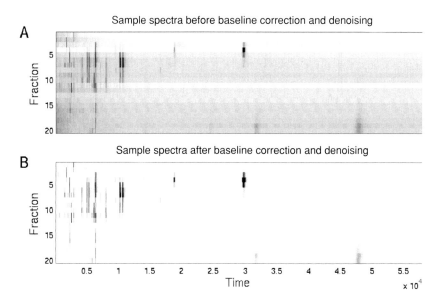

Fig. 1.11. Spectra derived from 20 pH fractions of the serum from a single patient. (A) Raw spectra. There are clear differences in baseline, seen as different shadings for the rows. There is also some unwanted noise, visible as periodic ripples in the spectra. (B) The same spectra after correcting for baseline and denoising. Peaks stand out more clearly against a flat "surface." In both cases, peaks can extend across neighboring fractions, as the separation process is imperfect.

order of 0.1% of the nominal *m/z*; higher-resolution instruments will attain mass accuracies expressed in parts per million (ppm).

Before comparing peak intensities across spectra, we need to normalize the spectra to make them comparable. One common method is to use the total ion current, or summed intensities for the entire spectrum. This is done after excluding the matrix noise region and subtracting baseline. This step is where we feel there is the most room for improvement, as there may be local scaling factors that are more appropriate than a single factor throughout. Even if a single scaling is to be used, it may be better to identify a small number of key peaks that appear to be relatively stable and to target the median log ratio for the set of peaks.

Having identified some peaks as being of potential interest, it also makes sense to look at other peaks that may be related (as assessed by correlation) or that should be related. The idea of "should be related" is different for mass spectrometry data than for microarray data in that there is a natural ordering to the peaks in a spectrum. In Figure 1.12, we show zooms on two distinct regions of averaged spectra from a higher-resolution (Qstar) instrument. The patterns

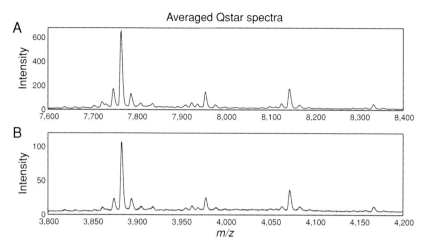

Fig. 1.12. Two regions derived from the average of several high-resolution Qstar spectra. (A) The *m/z* range from 7,600 to 8,400. (B) The *m/z* range from 3,800 to 4,200 [values exactly half those in (A)]. The peak patterns in the two panels are perfectly aligned, as we are seeing the same peptides. In (A), the peptides are singly charged ($z = 1$), and in (B) they are doubly charged ($z = 2$). Other regularities [offsets of 189 in (A)] are due to further identifiable phenomena (matrix adducts).

of peaks look the same, though the *m/z* range in the bottom panel is half that of the top panel, and the intensities are dramatically reduced. In this case, the parallel structure is due to the fact that the two panels are showing singly and doubly charged versions of the same peptides; finding the appropriate harmonic patterns on the *m/z* scale can tell us the charge state of the peptide (and thus its mass) and provide some reassurance that we have identified it correctly. (With higher-resolution data, the charge state can also be inferred from the spacing between isotopic peaks, which should be 1 Da apart.) Looking at the top panel, we can also see that there are groups of peaks offset from each other by 189 Da. This offset mass matches that of a single molecule of the matrix used here: α-cyano-4-hydroxycinnamic acid. These peaks are referred to as matrix adducts. Similarly, there are smaller peaks close to the biggest one, with the largest ones 18 Da below the main peak and 22 Da above. These correspond to loss of a water molecule or replacing an ionized hydrogen atom with one of sodium, respectively. Viewing the ensemble, we can see that almost all of the peaks visible here are differently modified forms of the same major peptide.

Graphically, we have found it useful to construct heat maps of the spectral regions surrounding peaks identified as potentially useful markers in a few different ways. First, in a very localized region (say 20 Da on either side) simply to check that the peak is reasonably clear. Second, in a larger window going out to either side by 250 Da or so, which is wide enough to capture most matrix adducts and common modifications such as phosphorlyation (a mass offset of 80 Da). Third, by checking heatmaps at half and twice the nominal m/z value to check the charge state.

Finally, a note of caution. The use of mass spectrometry data for biomarker discovery is more recent than the use of microarrays, and there are a number of external factors that can introduce unwanted biases. Some of these are discussed in Baggerly et al. [8, 9] and Villanueva et al. [70]. These tools are incredibly sensitive, which they need to be if they are to pick up new biomarkers. This very sensitivity, however, means that they will also pick up changes in experimental conditions quite well. In terms of keeping track of and reporting on your data, we recommend Ransohoff [54] for a discussion of some of the issues, and McShane et al. [43] for a more specific set of guidelines.

1.5 Finding Data

Simply discussing the features of various types of data is no substitute for diving in and working with raw data. If possible, we recommend visiting labs as the data is being collected or trying to collect some yourself. (Our colleagues have been willing to work with us on test cases.) Even without that, raw data of the types discussed are readily available on the Web.

Lots of microarray data has been on the web for a while, and much more has been posted since the advent of the minimum information about a microarray experiment (MIAME) standards [15]. Several major journals now require that the raw data be made available at the time of publication. For Affymetrix data, the first place to go is simply the company's web site, www.affymetrix.com. Sample data sets for several different chip types are available, as are all of the CDF files, probe sequences, and the latest annotation for what the probes on the chips actually correspond to. Registration is required, but free. For cDNA microarray data (and Affymetrix data), we also recommend the Gene Expression Omnibus (GEO) maintained by the NCBI, at http://www.ncbi.nlm.nih.gov/geo.

For SAGE data, we recommend SAGE Genie [14], maintained as part of the Cancer Genome Anatomy Project (CGAP), at http://cgap.nci.nih.gov/SAGE.

The data repositories for mass spectrometry data are not yet as extensive, but several proteomics journals are getting set to require raw data in a fashion akin to MIAME, so we hope this will change shortly. In the meantime, there are a few sites that have data of various types. The best known is probably the Clinical

Proteomics program jointly run by the NCI and FDA [48]. The databank is currently located at http://home.ccr.cancer.gov/ncifdaproteomics/ and has various SELDI and Qstar data sets. Questions have been raised about the quality of some of this data, and we strongly recommend reading Baggerly et al. [8] for a more detailed discussion of some of the issues involved. There is some SELDI data available from M.D. Anderson, at http://bioinformatics.mdanderson.org, together with Matlab scripts for processing and analysis.

Acknowledgment

This work was partially supported by NCI grant CA-107304.

Bibliography

[1] B.-L. ADAM, Y. QU, J. W. DAVIS, ET AL., Serum protein fingerprinting coupled with a pattern-matching algorithm distinguishes prostate cancer from benign prostate hyperplasia and healthy men, *Cancer Res*, 62 (2002), 3609–3614.

[2] AFFYMETRIX, *Affymetrix Microarray Suite Users Guide, Version 4.0*, Affymetrix, 1999.

[3] AFFYMETRIX, *Affymetrix Microarray Suite Users Guide, Version 5.0*, Affymetrix, 2001.

[4] B. ALBERTS, A. JOHNSON, J. LEWIS, ET AL., *Molecular Biology of the Cell*, 4th ed., Garland Publishing, New York, 2002.

[5] S. AUDIC AND J.-M. CLAVIRE, The significance of digital gene expression profiles, *Genome Res*, 7 (1997), 986–995.

[6] K. A. BAGGERLY, L. DENG, J. S. MORRIS, ET AL., Differential expression in SAGE: Accounting for normal between-library variation, *Bioinformatics*, 19(12) (2003), 1477–1483.

[7] K. A. BAGGERLY, L. DENG, J. S. MORRIS, ET AL., Overdispersed logistic regression for SAGE: Modelling multiple groups and covariates, *BMC Bioinformatics*, 5 (2004), 144.

[8] K. A. BAGGERLY, J. S. MORRIS, AND K. R. COOMBES, Reproducibility of SELDI-TOF protein patterns in serum: Comparing datasets from different experiments, *Bioinformatics*, 20(5) (2004), 777–785.

[9] K. A. BAGGERLY, J. S. MORRIS, S. R. EDMONSON, ET AL., Signal in noise: Evaluating reported reproducibility of serum proteomic tests for ovarian cancer, *J Natl Cancer Inst*, 97(4) (2005), 307–309.

[10] K. A. BAGGERLY, J. S. MORRIS, J. WANG, ET AL., A comprehensive approach to the analysis of MALDI-TOF proteomics spectra from serum samples, *Proteomics*, 3(9) (2003), 1667–1672.

[11] T. BEISSBARTH, L. HYDE, G. K. SMYTH, ET AL., Statistical modeling of sequencing errors in SAGE libraries, *Bioinformatics*, 20 (2004), i31–i39.

[12] J. M. BLAND AND D. G. ALTMAN, Statistical method for assessing agreement between two methods of clinical measurement, *Lancet*, i (1986), 307–310.

[13] B. M. BOLSTAD, R. A. IRIZARRY, M. ÅSTRAND, ET AL., A comparison of normalization methods for high density oligonucleotide array data based on variance and bias, *Bioinformatics*, 19 (2003), 185–193.

[14] K. Boon, E. C. Osorio, S. F. Greenhut, et al., An anatomy of normal and malignant gene expression, *Proc Natl Acad Sci USA*, 99(17) (2002), 11287–11292.

[15] A. Brazma, P. Hingamp, J. Quackenbush, et al., Minimum information about a microarray experiment (MIAME): Toward standards for microarray data, *Nat Genet*, 29 (2001), 365–371.

[16] S. Brenner, M. Johnson, J. Bridgham, et al., Gene expression analysis by massively parallel signature sequencing (MPSS) on microbead arrays, *Nat Biotechnol*, 18(6) (2000), 630–634.

[17] H. Chen, M. Centola, S. F. Altschul, et al., Characterization of gene expression in resting and activated mast cells, *J Exp Med*, 188(9) (1998), 1657–1668.

[18] J. Colinge and G. Feger, Detecting the impact of sequencing errors on SAGE data, *Bioinformatics*, 17(9) (2001), 840–842.

[19] K. R. Coombes, S. Tsavachidis, J. S. Morris, et al., Improved peak detection and quantification of mass spectrometry data acquired from surface-enhanced laser desorption and ionization by denoising spectra with the undecimated discrete wavelet transform, *Proteomics*, 5(16) (2005), 4107–4117.

[20] L. M. Cope, R. A. Irizarry, H. A. Jaffee, et al., A benchmark for Affymetrix genechip expression measures, *Bioinformatics*, 20 (2004), 323–331.

[21] E. P. Diamandis, Analysis of serum proteomic patterns for early cancer diagnosis: Drawing attention to potential problems, *J Natl Cancer Inst*, 96 (2004), 353–356.

[22] S. Dudoit, Y. H. Yang, M. J. Callow, et al., Statistical methods for identifying differentially expressed genes in replicated cDNA microarray experiments, *Statistica Sinica*, 12(1) (2002), 111–139.

[23] B. Ewing, L. Hillier, M. C. Wendl, et al., Base-calling of automated sequencer traces using Phred. I. Accuracy assessment, *Genome Res*, 8 (1998), 175–185.

[24] J. B. Fenn, M. Mann, C. K. Meng, et al., Electrospray ionization for mass spectrometry of large biomolecules, *Science*, 246 (1989), 64–71.

[25] R. Gentleman, V. J. Carey, W. Huber, et al., eds., *Bioinformatics and Computational Biology Solutions Using R and Bioconductor*, Springer-Verlag, New York, 2005.

[26] L. D. Greller and F. L. Tobin, Detecting selective expression of genes and proteins, *Genome Res*, 9 (1999), 282–296.

[27] R. A. Irizarry, B. M. Bolstad, F. Collin, et al., Summaries of Affymetrix genechip probe level data, *Nucleic Acids Res*, 31 (2003), e15.

[28] R. A. Irizarry, B. Hobbs, F. Collin, et al., Exploration, normalization, and summaries of high density oligonucleotide array probe level data, *Biostatistics*, 4 (2003), 249–264.

[29] N. Jeffries, Algorithms for alignment of mass spectrometry proteomic data, *Bioinformatics*, 21 (2005), 3066–3073.

[30] A. J. Kal, A. J. van Zonneveld, V. Benes, et al., Dynamics of gene expression revealed by comparison of serial analysis of gene expression transcript profiles from yeast grown on two different carbon sources, *Mol Biol Cell*, 10 (1999), 1859–1872.

[31] M. Karas, D. Bachmann, U. Bahr, et al., Matrix-assisted ultraviolet laser desorption of non-volatile compounds, *Intl J Mass Spectrometry Ion Processes*, 78 (1987), 53–68.

[32] M. KARAS AND F. HILLENKAMP, Laser desorption ionization of proteins with molecular masses exceeding 10,000 Daltons, *Anal Chem*, 60(20) (1988), 2299–2301.

[33] M. K. KERR, M. MARTIN, AND G. A. CHURCHILL, Analysis of variance for gene expression microarray data, *J Comp Biol*, 7 (2000), 819–837.

[34] A. LAL, A. E. LASH, S. F. ALTSCHUL, ET AL., A public database for gene expression in human cancers, *Cancer Res*, 59 (1999), 5403–5407.

[35] C. LI AND W. H. WONG, Model-based analysis of oligonucleotide arrays: Expression index computation and outlier detection, *Proc Natl Acad Sci USA*, 98 (2001), 31–36.

[36] C. LI AND W. H. WONG, Model-based analysis of oligonucleotide arrays: Model validation, design issues and standard error application, *Genome Biol*, 2(8) (2001), RESEARCH0032.

[37] J. LI, Z. ZHANG, J. ROSENZWEIG, ET AL., Proteomics and bioinformatics approaches for identification of serum biomarkers to detect breast cancer, *Clin Chem*, 48(8) (2002), 1296–1304.

[38] D. LIEBLER, *Introduction to Proteomics: Tools for the New Biology*, Humana Press, Totowa, NJ, 2001.

[39] R. J. LIPSHUTZ, S. P. FODOR, T. R. GINGERAS, ET AL., High density synthetic oligonucleotide arrays, *Nat Genet*, 21 (1999), S20–S24.

[40] S. L. MADDEN, E. A. GALELLA, J. ZHU, ET AL., SAGE transcript profiles for p53-dependent growth regulation, *Oncogene*, 15 (1997), 1079–1085.

[41] D. I. MALYARENKO, W. E. COOKE, B.-L. ADAM, ET AL., Enhancement of sensitivity and resolution of surface-enhanced laser desorption/ionization time-of-flight mass spectrometric records for serum peptides using time-series analysis techniques, *Clin Chem*, 51 (2005), 65–74.

[42] M. Z. MAN, X. WANG, AND Y. WANG, POWER_SAGE: comparing statistical tests for SAGE experiments, *Bioinformatics*, 16(11) (2000), 953–959.

[43] L. M. McSHANE, D. G. ALTMAN, W. SAUERBREI, ET AL., Reporting recommendations for tumor marker prognostic studies (REMARK), *J Natl Cancer Inst*, 97 (2005), 1180–1184.

[44] E. M. C. MICHIELS, E. OUSSOREN, M. VAN GROENIGEN, ET AL., Genes differentially expressed in medulloblastoma and fetal brain, *Physiol Genomics*, 1 (1999), 83–91.

[45] J. S. MORRIS, K. R. COOMBES, J. KOOMEN, ET AL., Feature extraction and quantification for mass spectrometry data in biomedical applications using the mean spectrum, *Bioinformatics*, 21(9) (2005), 1764–1775.

[46] M. NACHT, T. DRACHEVA, Y. GAO, ET AL., Molecular characteristics of non-small cell lung cancer, *Proc Natl Acad Sci USA*, 98(26) (2001), 15203–15208.

[47] NATURE, *The chipping forecast*, Nature Genetics Supplement, 21 (1999).

[48] E. F. PETRICOIN, III, A. M. ARDEKANI, B. A. HITT, ET AL., Use of proteomic patterns in serum to identify ovarian cancer, *Lancet*, 359 (2002), 572–577.

[49] E. F. PETRICOIN, III, D. K. ORNSTEIN, C. P. PAWELETZ, ET AL., Serum proteomic patterns for detection of prostate cancer, *J Natl Cancer Inst*, 94(20) (2002), 1576–1578.

[50] K. POLYAK AND G. J. RIGGINS, Gene discovery using the serial analysis of gene expression technique: Implications for cancer research, *J Clin Oncol*, 19(11), (2001), 2948–2958.

[51] K. POLYAK, Y. XIA, J. L. ZWELER, ET AL., A model for p53-induced apoptosis, *Nature*, 389 (1997), 300–305.

[52] D. A. PORTER, I. E. KROP, S. NASSER, ET AL., A SAGE (serial analysis of gene expression) view of breast tumor progression, *Cancer Res*, 61 (2001), 5697–5702.

[53] A. J. RAI, Z. ZHANG, J. ROSENZWEIG, ET AL., Proteomic approaches to tumor marker discovery: Identification of biomarkers for ovarian cancer, *Arch Path Lab Med*, 126 (2002), 1518–1526.

[54] D. F. RANSOHOFF, Bias as a threat to the validity of cancer molecular-marker research, *Nat Rev Cancer*, 5(2) (2005), 142–149.

[55] J. M. RUIJTER, A. H. C. VAN KAMPEN, AND F. BAAS, Statistical evaluation of SAGE libraries: Consequences for experimental desing, *Physiol Genomics*, 11 (2002), 37–44.

[56] B. RYU, J. JONES, N. J. BLADES, ET AL., Relationships and differentially expressed genes among pancreatic cancers examined by large-scale serial analysis of gene expression. *Cancer Res*, 62 (2002), 819–826.

[57] B. RYU, J. JONES, M. A. HOLLINGSWORTH, ET AL., Invasion-specific genes in malignancy: Serial analysis of gene expression comparisons of primary and passaged cancers, *Cancer Res*, 61 (2001), 1833–1838.

[58] S. SAHA, A. B. SPARKS, C. RAGO, ET AL., Using the transcriptome to annotate the genome, *Nat Biotechnol*, 20 (2002), 508–512.

[59] E. E. SCHADT, C. LI, B. ELLIS, ET AL., Feature extraction and normalization algorithms for high-density oligonucleotide gene expression array data, *J Cell Bioc*, 37 (2001), S120–S125.

[60] M. SCHENA, ed., *Microarray Biochip Technology*, BioTechniques Books, Natick, MA, 2000.

[61] M. SCHENA, D. SHALON, R. W. DAVIS, ET AL., Quantitative monitoring of gene expression patterns with a complementary DNA microarray, *Science*, 270 (1995), 467–470.

[62] G. SIUZDAK, *The Expanding Role of Mass Specrometry in Biotechnology*, MCC Press, San Diego, CA, 2003.

[63] T. SPEED, ed., *Statistical Analysis of Gene Expression Microarray Data*, Chapman and Hall/CRC Press, Danvers, MA, 2003.

[64] B. ST. CROIX, C. RAGO, V. VELCULESCU, ET AL., Genes expressed in human tumor epithelium, *Science*, 289 (2000), 1197–1202.

[65] D. J. STEKEL, Y. GIT, AND F. FALCIANI, The comparison of gene expression from multiple cDNA libraries, *Genome Res*, 10 (2000), 2055–2061.

[66] J. STOLLBERG, J. URSCHITZ, Z. URBAN, ET AL., A quantitative evaluation of SAGE, *Genome Res*, 10 (2000), 1241–1248.

[67] V. E. VELCULESCU, S. L. MADDEN, L. ZHANG, ET AL., Analysis of human transcriptomes, *Nat Genet*, 23 (1999), 387–388.

[68] V. E. VELCULESCU, L. ZHANG, B. VOGELSTEIN, ET AL., Serial analysis of gene expression, *Science*, 270 (1995), 484–487.

[69] V. E. VELCULESCU, L. ZHANG, W. ZHOU, ET AL. Characterization of the yeast transcriptome, *Cell*, 88 (1997), 243–251.

[70] J. VILLANUEVA, J. PHILIP, C. A. CHAPARRO, ET AL., Correcting common errors in identifying cancer-specific serum peptide signatures, *J Prot Res*, 4 (2005), 1060–1072.

[71] A. VLAHOU, P. F. SCHELLHAMMER, S. MENDRINOS, ET AL., Development of a novel proteomic approach for the detection of transitional cell carcinoma of the bladder in urine, *Am J Pathol*, 154 (2001), 1491–1502.

[72] C.-L. WEI, P. NG, K. P. CHIU, ET AL., 5' long serial analysis of gene expression (longSAGE) and 3' longSAGE for transcriptome characterization and genome annotation, *Proc Natl Acad Sci USA*, 101(32) (2004), 11701–11706.

[73] Z. WU, R. A. IRIZARRY, R. GENTLEMAN, ET AL., A model based background adjustment for oligonucleotide expression arrays, *J Am Statist Assoc*, 99 (2004), 909–917.

[74] Y. H. YANG, M. J. BUCKLEY, S. DUDOIT, ET AL., Comparison of methods for image analysis on cDNA microarray data, *J Comp Graph Statist*, 11 (2002), 108–136.

[75] Y. H. YANG, S. DUDOIT, P. LUU, ET AL., Normalization for cDNA microarray data: A robust composite method addressing single and multiple slide systematic variation, *Nucleic Acids Res*, 30 (2002), e15.

[76] L. ZHANG, M. F. MILES, AND K. D. ALDAPE, A model for interactions on short oligonucleotide microarrays: Implications for probe design and data analysis, *Nat Biotechnol*, 21(7) (2004), 818–821.

[77] L. ZHANG, W. ZHOU, V. E. VELCULESCU, ET AL., Gene expression profiles in normal and cancer cells, *Science*, 276 (1997), 1268–1272.

[78] Z. ZHANG, R. C. BAST JR., Y. YU, ET AL., Three biomarkers identified from serum proteomic analysis for the detection of early stage ovarian cancer, *Cancer Res*, 64 (2004), 5882–5890.

2
Hierarchical Mixture Models
for Expression Profiles

MICHAEL A. NEWTON, PING WANG,
AND CHRISTINA KENDZIORSKI
University of Wisconsin at Madison

Abstract

A class of probability models for inference about alterations in gene expression
is reviewed. The class entails discrete mixing over patterns of equivalent and
differential expression among different mRNA populations, continuous mixing
over latent mean expression values conditional on each pattern, and variation
of data conditional on latent means. An R package `EBarrays` implements inference calculations derived within this model class. The role of gene-specific
probabilities of differential expression in the formation of calibrated gene lists
is emphasized. In the context of the model class, differential expression is
shown to be not just a shift in expected expression levels, but also an assertion
about statistical independence of measurements from different mRNA populations. From this latter perspective, `EBarrays` is shown to be conservative in its
assessment of differential expression.

2.1 Introduction

Technological advances and resources created by genome sequencing projects
have enabled biomedical scientists to measure precisely and simultaneously
the abundance of thousands of molecular targets in living systems. The effect
has been dramatic, not only for biology, where now the cellular role for all
genes may be investigated, or for medicine, where new drug targets may be
found and new approaches discovered for characterizing and treating complex
diseases, the effect has also been dramatic for statistical science. Many statistical methods have been proposed to deal with problems caused by technical and
biological sources of variation, to address questions of coordinated expression
and differential expression, and to deal with the high dimension of expression
profiles compared to the number of profiles. Our interest is in the question of
differential expression. We do not attempt to review the considerable body of

statistical research that addresses this question; we focus here on methods for this problem that are related to a class of *hierarchical mixture models*.

A model is hierarchical if it describes observed variation using both latent random variables and the conditional variation of data given realizations of these latent quantities. In our work, the latent random variables include gene- and condition-specific expected values, these being the target quantities that one would measure in the absence of either biological or technical variation. Hierarchical models naturally incorporate multiple sources of variation, and they have an important role in the analysis of experiments with few microarrays because they can channel relevant information from other genes into gene-specific calculations, thus improving sensitivity.

The term mixture model can be used in a very broad sense to describe distributions; however, in expression work it has the following narrow interpretation: gene-specific hypotheses about differential expression are treated as latent discrete random variables. In comparing two mRNA populations, for example, it is as if a gene tosses a coin to decide whether or not it is differentially expressed, and then produces data distributed according to the particular outcome. Mixture models are convenient in structuring high-dimensional inference; genes become apportioned to different components of the mixture model. Often this modeling is done late in the data analysis stream: a mixture is fit to one-dimensional gene-specific summary measures (e.g., p values) rather than to the full data, and thus it may be unable to recover information lost by forming these summaries. Another problem is that some mixture methods rely on permutation to develop null distributions. This can be effective but it can fail when there is limited replication, as is often the case.

The first empirical Bayesian analysis of expression data was published in 2001. Focusing on preprocessed, two-channel microarray data, our group noted an inefficiency of the naive fold change estimator R/G, obtained from each gene's intensity measurements R and G in the two color channels on a spotted cDNA microarray (Newton et al. 2001). Our model-based estimate of fold change was $(R + c)/(G + c)$ for a statistic c which depends on sources of variation affecting the intensity measurements and which is computed from data on all genes. This modified fold-change estimator emerged as an intermediate between the posterior mode and posterior mean of the true fold change in the context of a specific Gamma-Gamma (GG) hierarchical model. We showed by simulation how this estimator has reduced mean squared error (log scale) and also how the gene ranking is improved. In addition, this 2001 *JCB* paper addressed the question of testing for differential expression in the context of a parametric hierarchical mixture model, and gave formulas for the posterior probability and odds of differential expression. The paper also noted a statistical curiosity of testing in this mixture model context, namely, that the number of genes that may be confidently declared to be differentially expressed may be much smaller than the estimated proportion of genes that are truly differentially expressed. This concept is helpful in formalizing power calculations. Further, in spite of improvements in statistical computing, we also recognized in this first paper the importance of computationally efficient methods in the domain of high-throughput data; our models were sufficiently simple that Markov chain Monte Carlo methods could be safely avoided.

The 2001 *JCB* paper concerned both testing and estimation for high-dimensional microarray data based on novel hierarchical and mixture-modeling structures. However, the delivered methodology remained rather limited; it handled single-slide spotted-array data comparing expression profiles in two conditions. There was nothing intrinsic to the model development that forced such restrictions, and so we pursued extensions that allowed replicate expression profiles in multiple mRNA populations (Kendziorski et al. 2003). There, we extended the GG calculations to this setting and we also developed parallel calculations based on a log-normal-normal (LNN) hierarchical specification. Emphasis was taken away from estimation of fold change and was transferred to computing posterior probabilities for various patterns of equality among gene- and condition-specific expected values. This has more relevance for inference with multiple mRNA populations. Tools to implement the multigroup inference calculations were offered in the Bioconductor package EBarrays.

Data analysts tend to favor methods that are simply structured and that have little reliance on modeling assumptions. A popular approach to differential expression, for example, is to apply *ordinary* statistical procedures (such as the *t*-test) separately to each gene, and then to paste the inferences together in some reasoned way (e.g., Dudoit et al. 2002). Although often effective, this approach usually rests on implicit assumptions about variation and it can suffer inefficiencies when shared properties of genes are not well accommodated. EBarrays, on the other hand, delivers inference summaries by attempting to capture the relevant sources of variation of the entire high-dimensional expression profile. It is explicit about the underlying assumptions:

(i) Parametric observation component (log-normal or Gamma)
(ii) Parametric mean component (conjugate to observation component)
(iii) Constant coefficient of variation
(iv) Only marginal information (rather than among-gene dependence) is relevant

Much experience with the package indicates good operating characteristics, especially when the number of replicate chips per condition is low. In examples where the parametric fit is poor it is beneficial to have more flexible methods. Work since Kendziorski et al. (2003) has investigated these assumptions, examined their significance, and generalized the methodology.

Adopting our proposed mixture structure, but not the hierarchical modeling elements, Efron et al. (2001) described a nonparametric empirical Bayesian analysis for assessing differential expression. The nonparametric nature of the analysis is appealing, since it seems to alleviate parametric constraints and may thus be favored in routine data analysis. However, the flexibility is somewhat illusory; it enters mainly in estimation of a one-dimensional distribution of gene-specific summary measures. The proposed method relies on permutation to assess a common null distribution (so it can fail when the number of replicate microarrays is low), and takes advantage of the large number of genes to develop the nonparametric density estimate. Further, assumptions about the suitability of the proposed gene-specific summary statistic are left implicit. Importantly, the Efron et al. (2001) paper may have been the first to relate gene-specific posterior probabilities of equivalent expression to rates of false detection in a reported list of genes. Much subsequent research on the control of the false discovery rate (FDR) seems to stem from this observation.

In the following sections we visit a few topics relevant to inference about expression alterations that seem to be notable developments since our first work in the area.

2.2 Dual Character of Posterior Probabilities

In the context of multiple simultaneous hypothesis testing, posterior probabilities have a curious dual character that other testing summaries lack. The duality is almost transparent once stated, but we think it is worth noting here because it simplifies the interpretation of gene lists.

Each gene j from a large set of J genes may or may not be differentially expressed between two mRNA populations. We say it is equivalently expressed, EE_j, if it is not differentially expressed; data are analyzed to assess this null hypothesis. A Bayesian (or empirical Bayesian) analysis yields the posterior probability $e_j = P(EE_j|\text{data})$; a non-Bayesian analysis might yield a p value or some other gene-specific summary statistic.

Genes exhibiting the strongest evidence for differential expression will be those with the smallest e_j, and one could naturally consider forming a list of *discoveries*, $\mathcal{D} = \{j : e_j \leq \tau\}$, for some threshold τ. The duality is this: gene j gets to be in $\mathcal{D}$ by virtue of the small magnitude of e_j. At the same time, e_j

is the probability (conditional on the data) that this assignment is a mistake. In other words, it is the probability of a type I error; that gene j should not have been placed on the list of differentially expressed genes. The magnitude e_j conveys both a decision about j and the conditional probability of a faulty decision. Other gene-specific summaries, like p values, do not have this dual character.

The property is useful for multiple simultaneous inference because the expected number of false discoveries (conditional on the data) is simply

$$cFD(\tau) = \sum_j \underbrace{e_j}_{\text{error rate}} \underbrace{1[e_j \leq \tau]}_{\text{discovery}} \qquad (2.1)$$

and the conditional false discovery rate is $cFDR(\tau) = cFD(\tau)/N(\tau)$, where $N(\tau) = \sum_j 1[e_j \leq \tau]$ is the size of the list. A list $\mathcal{D}$ formed from all genes for which $e_j < 5\%$, for example, has $cFDR$ less than 5%. A more refined usage tunes τ to set the conditional false discovery rate at some value like 5%, and has been called the *direct posterior probability approach* to controlling this rate (Newton et al. 2004).

In Efron et al. (2001), e_j was called the local FDR because it measured the conditional type I error rate for that specific gene. Storey (2002) criticized the unmodified use of e_j's for inference because they lack error rate control simultaneously for a list of discovered genes. Averages of e_j values over a short list of reported genes convey a more useful multiple-testing quantity. Storey (2002) introduced the q value as a gene-specific inference measure that carries a multiple-testing interpretation. In our notation, the q value for gene j is $q_j = cFDR(e_j)$. This is the expected proportion of type I errors among those genes k with e_k no larger than that of the input gene j. The procedure that rejects all null hypotheses EE_j for which $q_j \leq 5\%$ targets a *marginal* FDR of 5%. Literature on q values centers on the analysis not of raw data (or e_j's) but of p values derived from separate gene-specific hypothesis tests. Since p values do not have the dual character described above, their distribution needs to be modeled as a mixture in order that q values can be derived. In this way, modeling is transferred from the full data down to gene-specific p values. An advantage is that it is easier to be nonparametric with one-dimensional statistics; a disadvantage is that information may have been lost in first producing the gene-specific p values.

The dual character of posterior probabilities was pointed out in Newton et al. (2004), though the issue is understood in other work (Genovese and Wasserman 2002; Storey 2003; Müller et al. 2005). Notably, Müller et al. (2005) tackle the issue from a more formal Bayesian position, and study list-making inference as a general decision problem.

2.3 Differential Expression as Independence

Consider replicate profiles available from two mRNA populations, and allow that preprocessing has removed systematic sources of variation. Gene j provides measurements $x_j = (x_{j,1}, x_{j,2}, \ldots, x_{j,m})$ in one condition and $y_j = (y_{j,1}, y_{j,2}, \ldots, y_{j,n})$ in the second condition. The concept of equivalent expression, EE_j, and its counterpart differential expression, DE_j, are hypotheses that require some definition in terms of their effect on the probability density $p(x_j, y_j)$. Most studies focus modeling on the null hypothesis EE_j. One could state this in terms of a common expectation $\mu_j = E(x_{j,i}) = E(y_{j,k})$ (for any chips i, k) that the measurements are targeting, or one could state it in terms of exchangeability of all the measurements. Then under the null hypothesis, permutation of microarray labels would be valid, and this could be used to generate a null distribution of a test statistic (e.g., Dudoit et al. 2002). Such an approach can be effective when the number of microarrays is large, but notice that the approach avoids defining differential expression as anything more than the opposite of EE_j. The approach adopted in `EBarrays` does not require permutation and can be applied when there are very few replicate microarrays. In it, DE_j is defined as independence of x_j and y_j. This independence is marginal with respect to any gene level parameters and is conditional on genomic-level hyperparameters that are not specific to gene j. That is, gene j is differentially expressed if measurements from one condition are not useful predictors of measurements in the second condition. By contrast, all measurements x_j and y_j on a gene j that is equivalently expressed are correlated by virtue of having a shared, latent, random mean.

For the sake of demonstration, consider a comparison in which x_j and y_j are univariate ($m = n = 1$). The calculations embodied in the LNN model of `EBarrays` consider that these (log) expression values are conditionally independent normally distributed variables with means (μ_1, μ_2) and with a common variance σ^2. Further, the means (μ_1, μ_2) are random effects (suppressing the gene dependence); their marginal distribution is conjugate, being normal centered at a genomic mean μ_0 and having variance τ_0^2. Thus x_j and y_j have equal marginal distributions obtained after integrating the latent means: Normal($\mu_0, \sigma^2 + \tau_0^2$). The issue of EE_j or DE_j enters into the dependence between x_j and y_j. We assert that on EE_j, $\mu_1 = \mu_2$ with probability 1, and, further, that on DE_j, the component means are independent. Upon integrating the latent means, we have (1) exchangeability of gene-level measurements on the null EE_j, and (2) independence between x_j and y_j on the alternative DE_j. Mechanistically, we can imagine that on EE_j a single mean value is realized for the gene j, and then all the observations are generated as a random sample under that parameter setting. Alternatively, on DE_j, each mRNA population selects its mean value independently of the others, from the same distribution, and measurements arise conditionally on these different means.

A model is fully specified when in addition we consider the discrete mixing on EE_j (probability p_0) and DE_j (probability p_1). The marginal distribution of gene-level data is

$$p(x_j, y_j) = p_0 f(x_j, y_j) + p_1 f(x_j) f(y_j), \qquad (2.2)$$

where, conveniently, $f(\ )$ returns a marginal density of its argument treated as a conditional random sample given a common, latent, random mean. For instance in the case considered,

$$f(x_j, y_j) = p(x_j, y_j | EE_j) = \int p(x_j|\mu) \, p(y_j|\mu) \, \pi(\mu) \, d\mu,$$

where $\pi(\ )$ is a normal univariate conjugate prior, $p(x_j, y_j)$ is a normal density with common margins, as above, and with correlation $1/(1 + \sigma^2/\tau_0^2)$ between x_j and y_j owing to them having a common, latent mean. General formulas for this LNN case, and for the GG case, are presented in Kendziorski et al. (2003). Two-group comparisons in EBarrays are based on (2.2); the code allows other combinations and user input of the function $f(\ )$.

Gene-level inference is based on posterior probabilities, such as

$$e_j = P(EE_j | x_j, y_j) = p_0 f(x_j, y_j)/p(x_j, y_j).$$

Any decision about gene j is based on e_j; in this normal no-replicate case, for example, the odds favor differential expression if

$$\frac{1 - e_j}{e_j} > 1 \qquad \Leftrightarrow \qquad (x_j - y_j)^2 > C \qquad (2.3)$$

where, more precisely,

$$C = \frac{4\sigma^2(a - \mu_0)^2}{\sigma^2 + 2\tau_0^2} + \frac{4\sigma^2\left(\sigma^2 + \tau_0^2\right)}{\tau_0^2}\left[\log\frac{p_0}{p_1} + \frac{1}{2}\log\frac{\left(\sigma^2 + \tau_0^2\right)^2}{\sigma^2\left(\sigma^2 + 2\tau_0^2\right)}\right].$$

In other words, we favor DE_j if the measurements in the two conditions are sufficiently far apart, the necessary distance depending on overall expression $a = (x_j + y_j)/2$ and global parameters that delineate the different sources of variation. Ultimately, the analysis is *empirical* Bayes because these global parameters are estimated from the genomic data using an EM algorithm to maximize a marginal likelihood.

We have presented two views about differential expression. The rather direct view considers DE_j as a difference in expected expression measurements between the two mRNA populations, as revealed by a large difference in the observed expression values for gene j (the difference $x_j - y_j$ above, or the difference of averages in the case of replication). The alternative view holds that differential expression corresponds to independence of measurements between the two conditions; one sample is not a useful predictor of the other. This view, which is not so widely appreciated, has the advantage of supporting a specific alternative hypothesis to EE_j with which we can develop posterior inference. Conveniently, these two seemingly different views are two sides of the same coin.

There is an intermediate ground on which DE_j entails a shift in expected expression without marginal independence between x_j and y_j. However, this formulation is related to a nonidentifiability of the mixture model, and thus is difficult to work with (see Newton et al. 2004). It is possible to establish that inferences derived using the independence view of DE_j (i.e., using EBarrays) are conservative if some positive dependence happens to exist between x_j and y_j on DE_j. Wang and Newton (2005) show that when σ^2/τ_0^2 is sufficiently small, then the EBarrays even–odds threshold C [see (2.3)] is larger than the threshold C' one would have computed if one were supplied with the correct correlation between x_j and y_j. In other words EBarrays is conservative: DE_j is harder to declare using EBarrays than if you know the true distribution, and so you make fewer claims of differential expression. It is a rather realistic condition, furthermore, that σ^2/τ_0^2 is small, since we expect variation within a gene (certainly variation of an average in the case of replication) to be small compared to the variation between genes.

2.4 The Multigroup Mixture Model

Pairwise comparisons are the bread and butter of statistics, but they may not be suitable when analyzing data from more than two mRNA populations. Extending (2.2) to three groups by the inclusion of data z_j, we mix over $\nu = 4$ possible discrete patterns of differential expression and one pattern of equivalent expression:

$$p(x_j, y_j, z_j) = p_0 f(x_j, y_j, z_j) + p_1 f(x_j) f(y_j, z_j) \qquad (2.4)$$
$$+ p_2 f(x_j, z_j) f(y_j) + p_3 f(x_j, y_j) f(z_j)$$
$$+ p_4 f(x_j) f(y_j) f(z_j).$$

For instance, p_3 is the proportion of genes for which x_j and y_j are equivalently expressed while being differentially expressed from z_j, and p_4 is the proportion of genes that are differentially expressed among all three conditions. More generally, let $\mathbf{d}_j = (d_{j,1}, \ldots, d_{j,N})$ denote the vector holding all measurements on gene j taken across all conditions. We mix over equivalent expression and ν patterns of differential expression so that the joint distribution

$p(\mathbf{d}_j) = \sum_{k=0}^{\nu} p_k f_k(\mathbf{d}_j)$, where p_k is the overall proportion of genes governed by the kth pattern and f_k is the distribution of data conditional on that pattern. The patterns are hypotheses about possible clustering of the expected expression levels across the N measurements, and so, like the case above with $\nu = 4$, each f_k becomes a product of contributions from each component of the clustering. The null pattern $k = 0$ corresponds to $\mu_j = E(d_{j,s})$ being the same for all samples $s \in S = \{1, 2, \ldots, N\}$. Any pattern k partitions S into $r(k)$ mutually exclusive and exhaustive subsets $\{S_{k,i} : i = 1, 2, \ldots, r(k)\}$ on each of which the expected expression level is constant. To complete the specification, we write

$$f_k(\mathbf{d}_j) = \prod_{i=1}^{r(k)} f(\mathbf{d}_{j,S_{k,i}}) = \prod_{i=1}^{r(k)} \int \left(\prod_{s \in S_{k,i}} f_{\text{obs}}(\mathbf{d}_{j,s}|\mu) \right) \pi(\mu)\,d\mu, \quad (2.5)$$

where $\pi(\mu)$ is a random effects distribution governing the latent, gene-specific expression means and f_{obs} is the observation component of the hierarchical model. Model fitting amounts to estimating the mixing proportions p_k, parameters of the observation component, and parameters of the mean component $\pi(\mu)$.

As a brief illustration, we reconsider data on gene expression in mammary epithelial tissue from a rat model of breast cancer. Each of 10 pools of mRNA was probed with an Affymetrix U34 chip set having 26, 379 distinct probe sets; the 10 pools represent rats of four different genetic strains (1 Copenhagan; 5 Wistar Furth; 2 Congenic I; 2 Congenic II) where each congenic strain was genetically identical to the Wistar Furth parental strain except for a small genomic region in which the genome is homozygous for Copenhagan alleles, at least one of which confers resistance to the development of breast cancer (Shepel et al. 1998; Kendziorski et al. 2003). Expression alterations among these groups are relevant to understanding the Copenhagan strain's resistance to breast cancer.

Table 2.1 shows the $\nu = 14$ patterns of differential expression among the 4 mRNA populations (strains), and the overall equivalent expression pattern. Previous analysis of these data (Kendziorski et al. 2003) was restricted to a subset of four patterns, as code at that point was not sufficiently flexible to handle arbitrary sets of patterns. Figure 2.1 shows the proportions of genes satisfying each pattern based on fitting the LNN model in EBarrays.

Detectable differential expression is rather limited in this example, as an estimated 92.7% of genes are equivalently expressed among the four rat strains. DE pattern $k = 4$ represents one case of interest as it concerns genes that may be altered by the process of congenic formation. Filtering by gene-specific posterior probabilities of this pattern $P(\mu_{j,1} = \mu_{j,2} \neq \mu_{j,3} = \mu_{j,4}|\text{data}) =: 1 - e_j$,

Table 2.1. *Patterns of DE Among Four Rat Strains*

k	Mean pattern[a]	k	Mean pattern
0	$\mu_1 = \mu_2 = \mu_3 = \mu_4$	8	$\mu_1 = \mu_2 = \mu_4 \neq \mu_3$
1	$\mu_1 \neq \mu_2 = \mu_3 = \mu_4$	9	$\mu_1 = \mu_2 \neq \mu_3 \neq \mu_4$
2	$\mu_1 = \mu_4 \neq \mu_2 = \mu_3$	10	$\mu_1 = \mu_3 \neq \mu_2 \neq \mu_4$
3	$\mu_1 = \mu_3 = \mu_4 \neq \mu_2$	11	$\mu_1 = \mu_4 \neq \mu_2 \neq \mu_3$
4	$\mu_1 = \mu_2 \neq \mu_3 = \mu_4$	12	$\mu_1 \neq \mu_2 = \mu_4 \neq \mu_3$
5	$\mu_1 = \mu_2 = \mu_3 \neq \mu_4$	13	$\mu_1 \neq \mu_2 \neq \mu_3 = \mu_4$
6	$\mu_1 \neq \mu_2 = \mu_3 \neq \mu_4$	14	$\mu_1 \neq \mu_2 \neq \mu_3 \neq \mu_4$
7	$\mu_1 = \mu_3 \neq \mu_2 = \mu_4$		

[a] (1) Copenhagan, (2) Wistar Furth, (3) Congenic I, (4) Congenic II. Here, μ_i refers to the expected expression level for mRNA population i.

we can apply the direct posterior probability approach (2.1) to control FDR. We find that five probe sets constitute a 5% $cFDR$ short list of genes satisfying this DE pattern. These probe sets have $e_j \leq 0.013$. One of the interesting ones, rc_AI105022_at, corresponds to Cullin-3, a gene involved in the ubiquitin cycle and related to breast cancer tumor suppression (Fay et al. 2003). Investigating the biological significance of altered genes such as this is part of ongoing research; it is important to have tools like EBarrays which can efficiently sort and calibrate genes by alterations of interest.

2.5 Improving Flexibility

Utility of results from the hierarchical mixture model analysis, as obtained from EBarrays, is limited by the suitability of the four structural modeling assumptions described in the introduction. Each of these has been the subject of analysis, and we find that certain assumptions seem to be more important than others. For example, the use of a parametric observation component is often innocuous. Tools in EBarrays provide diagnostic qq-plots for this component; both Gamma and log-normal distributions often fit well, though a search for improved robust alternatives would be valuable. Calculations in Gottardo et al. (in press) allow log-t errors, and thus are less susceptible to heavy-tailed observations.

The diagnostic plots often indicate suitability of the observation component; however, marginal diagnostics can suggest an overall poor fit from EBarrays. This has to do with inflexibility of the distribution $\pi(\mu)$ of latent means. The issue was studied in Newton et al. (2004), and there a nonparametric mean component was proposed. A nonparametric version of the EM algorithm enabled model fit. Comparisons indicated improvements in terms of error rates

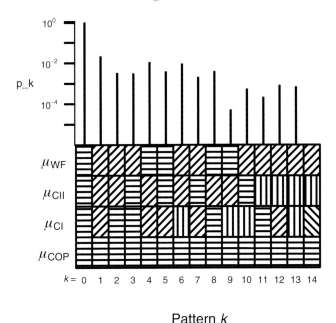

Pattern *k*

Fig. 2.1. Estimated mixing proportions for 15 patterns of mean expression among four mRNA populations in a rat breast cancer study: Equality of angles in a column stands for equality of the means. Above, height of lines indicates estimated proportion of genes in each pattern.

on short lists compared to the parametric model, gene-specific *t*-testing, and the method of Efron et al. (2001). That paper also showed how to formulate the mixture model in terms of directional alternatives, which can further improve flexibility, but it left unaddressed an extension beyond two-group comparisons to multigroup comparisons.

It may be that improvements obtainable by nonparametric analysis of the mean component are modest compared to improvements that would be possible through a more effective modeling of gene-specific variances. Advances in this direction by Lonnstedt and Speed (2002) and Smyth (2004) are significant, though their empirical Bayesian formulation is rather different than the one described here underlying EBarrays. In that work, expression shifts have to do with nonzero contributions in a linear model for expected expression, rather than separately realized mean values. The relative merits of the two forms of mean modeling remain to be worked out (e.g., the role played by discrete mixing proportions is present but less prominent in the linear-model formulation). With regard to variances, Lonnstedt and Speed (2002) and Smyth (2004) put a prior on gene-specific variances, and this provides some flexibility beyond the constant variance assumption in the LNN version of `EBarrays`. The idea was also used by Baldi and Long (2001) and also by Ibrahim et al. (2002). Kendziorski and Wang (2005) investigate flexible variance modeling in the context of `EBarrays`.

Among-gene dependence is an ever-present concern, though it is difficult to handle owing to the dimensions involved. Permutation-based methods are helpful in guarding against ill-effects of dependence, but they are not always effective. Note that FDR controlling procedures are popular in part because they are fairly robust to among-gene dependencies compared to other multiplicity-adjustment methods. Dahl (2004), generalizing Medvedovic and Sivaganesan (2002), investigates methodology that directly models dependence among genes using a Dirichlet process mixture (DPM) formulation. In the Bayesian effects model for microarrays (BEMMA), different genes share parameters in much the same way that different mRNA populations share mean parameters on a given gene in `EBarrays`. Thus, correlation among genes is explained in terms of shared, latent parameter values. The grouping of genes into clusters where sharing occurs is mediated by the discrete clustering distribution inherent in the DPM model, and is assessed by posterior sampling via Markov chain Monte Carlo. Dahl (2004) shows improvements in the assessment of differential expression when one accommodates coordinated expression by this BEMMA approach. We note that BEMMA uses DPMs in a different way than Do, Müller, and Tang (2005), which used them to improve nonparametric inference based on one-dimensional reductions of the gene-level data. Using a novel mixture formulation, Yuan and Kendziorski (in press) offer another approach for using between-gene dependencies to improve differential expression analysis.

In summary, we see rapid development of methodology for altered gene expression based on the flexible class of hierarchical mixture models reviewed here. As new data analysis and data integration problems emerge in genomics, there will be further demand for such modeling in order to organize variation and to provide effective analysis of data.

Bibliography

Baldi, P. and Long, A.D. (2001). A Bayesian framework for the analysis of microarray expression data: Regularized t-test and statistical inferences of gene changes. *Bioinformatics*, **17**, 1–11.

Dahl, D. Conjugate Dirichlet process mixture models: Gene expression, clustering, and efficient sampling, PhD thesis, University of Wisconsin, 2004.

Do, K., Müller, P. and Tang, F. (2005). A Bayesian mixture model for differential gene expression. *Journal of the Royal Statistical Society C*, **54**, 627–644.

Dudoit, S., Yang, Y.H., Speed, T.P., and Callow, M.J. (2002). Statistical methods for identifying differentially expressed genes in replicated cDNA microarray experiments. *Statistica Sinica*, **12**, 111–139.

Efron, B., Tibshirani, R., Storey, J.D., and Tusher, V. (2001). Empirical Bayes analysis of a micro array experiment. *Journal of the American Statistical Association*, **96**, 1151–1160.

Fay, M.J., Longo, K.A., Karathanasis, G.A., Shope, D.M., Mandernach, C.J., Leong, J.R., Hicks, A., Pherson, K., and Husain, A. (2003). Analysis of *CUL-5* expression in breast epithelial cells, breast cancer cell lines, normal tissues and tumor tissues. *Molecular Cancer*, **2**, 40.

Genovese, C. and Wasserman, L. (2002). Operating characteristics and extensions of the false discovery rate procedure. *Journal of the Royal Statistical Society B*, **64**, 499–518.

Gottardo, R., Raftery, A.E., Yeung, K.Y., Bumgarner, R. (2006). Bayesian robust inference for differential gene expressionin cDNA microarrays with multiple samples. *Biometrics*, **62**, pp. 10–18.

Ibrahim, J.G., Chen, M.-H., and Gray, R.J. (2002). Bayesian models for gene expression with DNA microarray data. *Journal of the American Statistical Association*, **97**, 88–99.

Kendziorski, C.M., Newton, M.A., Lan H., and Gould, M.N. (2003). On parametric empirical Bayes methods for comparing multiple groups using replicated gene expression profiles. *Statistics in Medicine*, **22**, 3899–3914.

Kendziorski, C.M. and Wang, P. (2005). Flexible variance modeling with EBarrays. Technical Report # 192, UW Department of Biostatistics and Medical Informatics.

Lonnstedt, I. and Speed, T.P. (2002). Replicated microarray data. *Statistica Sinica*, **12**, 31–46.

Medvedovic, M. and Sivaganesan, S. (2002). Bayesian infinite mixture model based clustering of gene expression profiles. *Bioinformatics*, **18**, 1194–1206.

Müller, P., Parmigiani, G., Robert, C., and Rousseau, J. (2005). Optimal sample size for multiple testing: The case of gene expression microarrays. *Journal of the American Statistical Association*, **99**, 990–1001.

Newton, M.A., Kendziorski, C.M., Richmond, C.S., Blattner, F.R., and Tsui, K.W. (2001). On differential variability of expression ratios: Improving statistical inference about gene expression changes from microarray data. *Journal of Computational Biology*, **8**, 37–52.

Newton, M.A., Noueiry, D., Sarkar, D., and Ahlquist, P. (2004). Detecting differential gene expression with a semiparametric hierarchical mixture method. *Biostatistics*, **5**, 155–176.

Shepel, L.A., Lan, H., Haag, J.D., Brasic, G.M., Gheen, M.E., Simon, J.S., Hoff, P., Newton, M.A., and Gould, M.N. (1998). Genetic identification of multiple loci that control breast cancer susceptibility in the rat. *Genetics*, **149**, 289–299.

Smyth, G.K. (2004). Linear models and empirical Bayes methods for assessing differential expression in microarray experiments. *Statistical Applications in Genetics and Molecular Biology*, **3**(1) 3.

Storey, J.D. (2002). A direct approach to false discovery rates. *Journal of the Royal Statistical Society, Series B*, **64**, 479–498.

Storey, J.D. (2003). The positive false discovery rate: A Bayesian interpretation and the q-value. *Annals of Statistics*, **31**, 2013–2035.

Wang, P. and Newton, M.A. (2005). Robustness of EBarrays to one form of dependence. Technical Report #1114, UW Department of Statistics. *Biometrics*, **62**, pp. xx–xx.

Yuan, M. and Kendziorski (2006). A unified approach for simultaneous gene clustering and differential expression. *Biometrics*, **62**, 19–27.

3

Bayesian Hierarchical Models for Inference in Microarray Data

ANNE-METTE K. HEIN, ALEX LEWIN, AND SYLVIA
RICHARDSON

Imperial College

Abstract

We review Bayesian hierarchical models for inference in microarray data. The chapter consists of two main parts that deal with use of Bayesian hierarchical models at different levels of analysis encountered in the context of microarrays. The first part reviews a Bayesian hierarchical model for the estimation of gene expression levels from Affymetrix GeneChip data, and for inference on differential expression. In the second part, an integrated model that incorporates expression-dependent normalization within an ANOVA model of differential expression is reviewed and compared to a model where normalization is preprocessed. The chapter concludes by discussing how predictive Bayesian model checking can be usefully included within the model inference.

3.1 Introduction

3.1.1 Background

Microarrays are one of the new technologies that have developed in line with genome sequencing and developments in miniaturization and robotics. The technology exploits the fact that single-stranded RNA (or DNA) molecules have a high affinity to form double-stranded structures. Pairing is specific and complementary strands have particularly high affinity for binding. On microarrays gene-specific sequences are attached in tiny specified locations. By hybridizing a cell sample of fragmented, fluorescently labeled RNA (or DNA) to the array and measuring the fluorescence at the defined locations, one can obtain measures of the amount of the different RNA or DNA transcripts present in the sample hybridized.

Arrays generally contain thousands of spots (or probes) at each of which a particular gene or sequence is represented. In effect, a microarray experiment thus represents data comparable to that obtained by performing tens of thousands of experiments of a similar type in parallel. The experiments on a given array will share certain characteristics related to the manufacturing process of the particular array used, the extraction and handling of the biological sample hybridized to the array, as well as the extraction and preparation for hybridization of the RNA (or DNA). The interest is in comparing expression levels between arrays with samples from different biological conditions of interest (e.g., cancerous against noncancerous cells) and the challenge is identifying differences that are related to the biology of the samples rather than to technical experimental variation.

Many of the characteristic features of experiments involving microarrays render them particularly well suited to the flexible modeling strategy of Bayesian hierarchical modelling (BHM). The aim of this chapter is to highlight this by discussing in detail the steps taken for modelling the variability in gene expression data at several levels that can be roughly qualified as variability of the signal, biological variability, and variability due to experimental contrasts. Beforehand, a brief summary of the key points of the BHM strategy is presented.

3.1.2 *Bayesian Hierarchical Modeling*

The framework of Bayesian hierarchical modelling (BHM) refers to a generic model building strategy in which unobserved quantities (e.g., latent effect size associated with experimental contrasts, statistical parameters, missing or mismeasured data, random effects, etc.) are organized into a small number of discrete levels with logically distinct and scientifically interpretable functions and probabilistic relationships between them that capture inherent features of the data. It has proved to be successful for analyzing many types of complex data sets arising in biology, genetics, and medicine as illustrated, for example, by the case studies detailed in Gilks et al. (1996) and Green et al. (2003). The general applicability of Bayesian hierarchical models has been enhanced by advances in computational algorithms, notably those belonging to the family of stochastic algorithms based on Markov chain Monte Carlo (MCMC) techniques. Nevertheless, the formidable dimension of many genomics data sets requires their use to be pertinent and efficient. It is clear that full-scale implementation of BHM for analyzing large microarray experiments will require exploitation of parallel processing as well as judicious approximations.

There are several related aspects that render BHM attractive for analyzing microarray data; what is particularly interesting is the ability to potentially build *all these aspects* in a common modelling scheme. Of course, before encompassing simultaneously several components into a global model, modularity is first exploited to study each aspect in turn. Key benefits of the BHM strategy are:

(i) *Accounting for diverse sources of variability:* Gene expression data arising from experimental protocols are naturally hierarchically structured along descending layers: Substantive question $\longrightarrow$ Experimental design $\longrightarrow$ Sample preparation $\longrightarrow$ Array design and manufacture $\longrightarrow$ Gene expression matrix $\longrightarrow$ Probe level data $\longrightarrow$ Image quantification.

Consequently, gene expression data are the end process of multiple sources of variability, systematic and random, biologically interpretable, or obscuring. We shall see in the next sections how the modelling translates these different sources of variability into fixed effects (possibly dependent on unknown quantities), random effects, and distributional assumptions.

(ii) *Modelling noise additively, multiplicatively or in a nonlinear fashion:* It has been noted that, empirically, gene expression data often exhibit a complex mean–variance relationship. Thus, data transformation functions with nonstandard forms that combine additive and multiplicative noise have been proposed (Durbin et al. 2002; Huber et al. 2002). In a BHM strategy, instead of an all-encompassing functional transformation, two latent variables can be introduced, the first to represent the true level of the data after additive background noise correction, the second to summarize signal information on the log scale. Each of these latent variables are interpretable and the associated distributional assumptions can be checked separately.

(iii) *Borrowing information:* Gene expression experiments are used by biologists to study fundamental processes of activation/suppression. Such protocols frequently involve genetically modified animals or specific cell lines and such experiments are typically carried out only with a small number of biological samples, as little as 3 or 4 in each experimental condition. It is clear that this amount of replication renders hazardous the estimation of gene-specific variability using empirical estimates and the use of standard tests for comparing conditions. As with many situations of sparse data, inference is strengthened by borrowing information from the comparable units through hierarchical modelling, here through the modelling of the "population" of gene variances. Thus, genes exhibiting by chance unusual small variability across the samples will not lead to artificially inflated test values as their empirical variance will be smoothed toward that of the group of genes. This regularization process is now widely used in the microarray context, often outside the Bayesian paradigm (e.g., Smyth 2004), but is best seen as an integral part of the BHM strategy, as will be illustrated below. Similarly, in Section 3.2 we shall see that by combining within a single model the information from the probe level *and* the biological replicates, inference on differential expression may be strengthened in comparison to analyses that treat these two steps separately.

(iv) *Propagation of uncertainty:* Gene expression data is usually processed through a series of steps that aim to correct the artefactual variations potentially introduced by the technical treatment of the samples. For example, array effects are estimated and subtracted in order to make the arrays overall comparable. The uncertainty associated with these adjustments is usually not taken into account in the final analysis. The situation is akin to that occurring in measurement error problems, when inference is carried out on corrected values without accounting for the uncertainty of the correction. In this case, it is known that suboptimal inference is achieved (Carroll et al. 1995). It is thus important to investigate whether BHM that include the preprocessing steps within the global model carry some benefit.

(v) *Model checking:* An additional benefit of BHM is that without much extra computational burden, predictive inference can be made. This aspect can be exploited to perform model checks, so long as care is taken to avoid the overconservativeness arising from using the data twice (Marshall and Spiegelhalter 2003; O'Hagan, 2003). Using the structure of the hierarchical models, predictive checks can be made at several levels to assess, for example, distributional choice made for latent parameters. This aspect will be illustrated in Section 3.4.

3.2 Bayesian Hierarchical Modeling of Probe Level GeneChip Data

In this section, we review a fully Bayesian integrated approach to the analysis of Affymetrix GeneChip data (Hein et al. 2005). In the approach, background correction for nonspecific hybridization, signal extraction, gene expression estimation, and assessment of differential expression are performed as one integrated analysis. We demonstrate how the Bayesian approach allows the parallel nature of the thousands of hybridizations with shared experimental characteristics to be exploited, e.g., by borrowing information between signals within probe sets, between genes within an array, or between the same genes on replicate arrays within a condition. The integrated treatment of the different steps in an analysis (e.g., gene expression level estimation and assessment of differential expression) allows propagation of the associated errors and is likely to lead to more realistic measures of uncertainty of parameters and other quantities of interest. We illustrate the difference between a stepwise approach and the integrated approach, in relation to estimation of uncertainty and differential expression, in analyses of a controlled data set.

3.2.1 Affymetrix GeneChip Arrays

Affymetrix is one of the leading manufacturers of microarrays. Their GeneChips differ from some of the other available array types in a number of important ways. They are oligonucleotide arrays and, in contrast to two-color arrays, rely on hybridization of a single, fluorescently labeled sample of mRNA, the intermediate product between the gene sequences and their products: the proteins. On a GeneChip array an oligonucleotide of length 25 is represented at each location. As genes cannot in general be uniquely identified by a single sequence of length 25, each gene is represented by a *probe set*, consisting of 11–20 *probe pairs*. Each probe pair contains a *perfect match* (PM) probe and a *mismatch* (MM) probe. At each PM probe an oligonucleotide that perfectly matches part of the sequence encoding the gene is represented. As nonspecific hybridization is known to occur, an identical oligonucleotide except for the middle nucleotide is represented at the accompanying MM probe. The intention is that since PM and MM probes are almost identical, equal amounts of nonspecific hybridization will occur at these probes, and excess hybridization to the PM probe, relative to the MM probe, will be due to *specific hybridization*, that is, the hybridization of the intended gene-specific sequences.

With the launch of the GeneChips, Affymetrix provided software that allowed gene expression values for each of the genes represented on the GeneChip arrays to be calculated from the scanned array images. Initially these measures were derived as a robust mean value of the set of background corrected PM–MM values obtained for the probes in the probe set representing each gene (Lockhart et al. 1996). A considerable effort has since been devoted to the further study of probe behavior and development of gene expression estimates with improved performance by Affymetrix and the wider scientific community (Li and Wong 2001; Hubbell, Liu and May 2002; Irizarry et al. 2003; Hein et al. 2005). Focus has mainly been on model-based methods that result in outlier robust and variance stable point estimates. The derived point estimates are subsequently used in the downstream gene expression analysis, as reviewed in a number of chapters throughout this book, typically with no reference to the gene expression estimation process that resulted in the point estimates.

3.2.2 Model Formulation

3.2.2.1 Single Array Setting

Bayesian gene expression (BGX) relies on the formulation of a Bayesian hierarchical model for the estimation of gene expression indices from Affymetrix GeneChip probe level data. In the BGX model the estimation of gene expression measures is dealt with in two (integrated) steps: a "signal extraction" level and a "signal summarization" level. In controlled experiments both PM and MM probes have been found to be subject to nonspecific hybridization, that is, even in the absence of transcripts for the gene, some fluorescence is observed at PM (and MM) probes representing the gene, due to the hybridization of short fragments and fragments that do not perfectly match the probes. Furthermore, contrary to the intention, the MM probes have been found to hybridize part of the fragments perfectly matching the PM probes. At the "signal extraction" level of the BGX model these features are modeled by assuming that the intensity observed at a PM probe is the result of hybridization partly of fragments that perfectly match the probe (specific hybridization: S_{gj}) and partly by fragments that do not perfectly match the probe (nonspecific hybridization: H_{gj}). A similar pattern is assumed for the MM probe, with only a fraction ϕ of the signal S_{gj} binding. Both specific and nonspecific hybridization is assumed to be gene- and probe-specific, hence the indexing by g (gene) and j (probe). To account for the common situation of the MM being bigger than the PM we assume an additive error on the normal scale, and hypothesize

$$\begin{aligned} \text{PM}_{gj} &\sim N(S_{gj} + H_{gj}, \tau^2) \\ \text{MM}_{gj} &\sim N(\phi S_{gj} + H_{gj}, \tau^2). \end{aligned} \tag{3.1}$$

We omit for simplicity in this and subsequent displays of distributions to state that these are conditional on variables appearing on the right-hand side, and are independent over all values of indexing suffixes.

At the "signal summarization" level we proceed on the log-scale, as is generally recommended in the microarray setting. We obtain a (log-scale) measure of gene expression for gene g from a simultaneous consideration of the set of signals, $\{S_{gj} \mid j = 1, \ldots, J_g\}$, by assuming gene-specific distributions for these. For the (log-scale) nonspecific hybridization parameters, H_{gj}, we assume an array-wide distribution intended to capture the common experiment's specific characteristics of the handling of the array and sample hybridized. To allow for zero signal and nonspecific hybridization terms while operating on the log-scale we shift by 1 before logging, and consequently consider truncated normal distributions TN (obtained from a normal distribution by conditioning the variable to be nonnegative),

$$
\begin{aligned}
\log(S_{gj} + 1) &\sim TN\left(\mu_g, \sigma_g^2\right), \\
\log(H_{gj} + 1) &\sim TN\left(\lambda, \eta^2\right).
\end{aligned}
\tag{3.2}
$$

In Hein et al. (2005) the medians of the truncated normal distributions, θ_g, were used as measures of gene expression. From experience there is little difference between θ_g and μ_g, and as μ_g is computationally advantageous we use μ_g here. We refer to μ_g as *Bayesian gene expression* or BGX index.

To stabilize the gene-specific variance parameters, we assume exchangeability

$$
\log\left(\sigma_g^2\right) \sim N(a, b^2),
\tag{3.3}
$$

with a and b^2 fixed at values obtained by an empirical procedure in the same spirit as Empirical Bayes approaches (for details see Hein et al. 2005). A full specification of the model is achieved by assuming a uniform prior, $U(0, 15)$, on μ_g, which comfortably covers the range of possible log-intensities, a $\mathcal{B}(1, 1)$ prior on ϕ, a flat normal prior on λ ($N(0, 1000)$), and flat gamma priors on the precisions $(\tau^2)^{-1}$ and $(\eta^2)^{-1}$ ($\Gamma(0.001, 0.001)$).

3.2.2.2 Multiple Array Setting

Extending the model to a situation with multiple conditions and replicate arrays under conditions is straightforward. We let $c = 1, \dots, C$ refer to the conditions, and $r = 1, \dots, R_c$ refer to the replicates under condition c. At the first level of the model, we allow for different additive errors on the arrays, $\tau_{cr}^2, c = 1, \dots, C$, $r = 1, \dots, R_c$. We assume gene-, probe-, condition-, and replicate-specific signals and nonspecific hybridization terms, and generalize (3.1) to

$$
\begin{aligned}
\text{PM}_{gjcr} &\sim N\left(S_{gjcr} + H_{gjcr}, \tau_{cr}^2\right) \\
\text{MM}_{gjcr} &\sim N\left(\phi S_{gjcr} + H_{gjcr}, \tau_{cr}^2\right).
\end{aligned}
\tag{3.4}
$$

We base the estimation of the expression of gene g under condition c on a joint consideration of the full set of signals represented by the replicate probe sets on the arrays for this gene: $\{S_{gjcr} \mid j = 1, \dots, J_g, r = 1, \dots, R_c\}$. We retain the assumption of distributions of nonspecific hybridization that are specific to each array and arrive at

$$
\begin{aligned}
\log(S_{gjcr} + 1) &\sim TN\left(\mu_{gc}, \sigma_{gc}^2\right) \\
\log(H_{gjcr} + 1) &\sim TN\left(\lambda_{cr}, \eta_{cr}^2\right).
\end{aligned}
\tag{3.5}
$$

As in the single array model we assume that the σ_{gc}^2, $g = 1, \ldots, G$, parameters are exchangeable, with condition-specific distributions

$$\log(\sigma_{gc}^2) \sim N(a_c, b_c^2). \qquad (3.6)$$

The hyperparameters and specification of priors are as in the single array setting, with priors specified independently for each g, c, and r (for details see Hein et al. 2005).

3.2.2.3 MCMC Implementation

The models have been implemented in WinBUGS and C++. In the C++ implementations a flat prior was used for ϕ in place of the Beta prior for computational convenience; since ϕ did not vary outside the $(0, 1)$ interval in any of the MCMC runs reported here, our results continue to be valid for the Beta prior.

The C++ implementation performs single-variable updating using Gibbs sampler steps for parameters ϕ and $\widetilde{\tau_{cr}}$. Simple random walk Metropolis updates were used for the remainder of the parameters. These were tuned using pilot runs so that acceptance rates fell in the range $(0.2, 0.3)$.

The sampler used by WinBUGS also relies on single-site updating, but with some more sophisticated individual updates, based on Neal's overrelaxation method. This gave improved performance by reducing the chain's autocorrelation on a sweep-by-sweep basis; however, sweeps were so much slower than those of the C++ code that this advantage was easily outweighed.

3.2.3 *Performance of the BGX Model*

3.2.3.1 *Single Array Setting*

A single array from the Choe et al. (2005) data set (condition C, replicate 1) was analyzed using the single array model. Probe intensity values for four example genes along with summaries of the posterior distributions of parameters related to the expression of the genes are given in Figure 3.1. Note that to allow the PM–MM values to be depicted for all probe pairs, the raw probe response is given on the normal scale (upper part of Figure 3.1). In the posterior distribution plots log-scale PM–MM values are indicated for probe pairs for which they exist, for the remaining probe pairs they are indicated as zero (the 1's in the lower part of Figure 3.1). The first gene, gene 1, illustrates the case of a gene with a probe set of intensity values that are consistently high. This is reflected in the spiky posterior distribution of μ_1. The second gene, gene 11, has a few outlying probe pair values of which two have MM>PM. By borrowing information

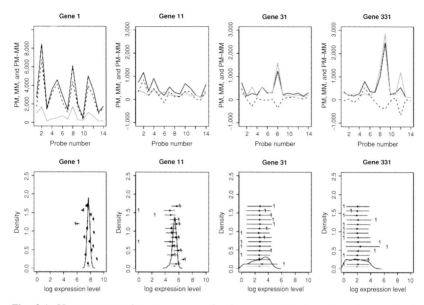

Fig. 3.1. Upper row: probe set response for four genes. Each probe set consists of 14 probe pairs. The solid lines show PM, the dotted lines plot MM, and the dashed lines plot PM–MM. Lower row: summaries of posterior distributions of parameters related to expression of the four genes. The 5–95% credibility intervals for the 14 log-scale signals for each gene are shown as black horizontal lines (shifted vertically) and should be read off the x-axis. The gray line is for the gene expression index μ_g. The 1's show the observed log(PM–MM) values (plotted at zero for PM–MM$<$0) for each probe pair.

from the rest of the probes in the set, the posterior signals corresponding to these are drawn upwards toward the remaining signals. In contrast, the last two genes have much less homogeneous probe set responses, with more probe pairs exhibiting MM$>$PM, and the rest having moderate to large PM–MM values. This is well reflected in the posterior gene expression distributions that are flatter for both genes and for gene 331 actually multimodal.

How information is borrowed within probe sets is summarized in Figure 3.2, left. Here mean posterior log-scale signals are plotted against their approximate empirical values: $\log(((PM–MM)\wedge 0) + 1)$. The stratified plots reveal that signals for probe pairs with large $\log((PM–MM) + 1)$ values but that belong to probe sets with overall low expression (Figure 3.2, middle) are drawn downwards. At the opposite end of the spectrum, log-scale signals for probe pairs with small or zero $\log((PM–MM) + 1)$ but that belong to probe sets with overall high level of expression are drawn upwards (Figure 3.2, right). The borrowing of information between probe sets is illustrated in Figure 3.3, left. The plot shows shrinkage of posterior mean σ_g values relative to the empirical standard

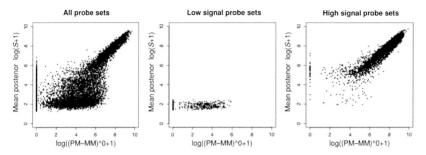

Fig. 3.2. Mean posterior $\log(S_{gj} + 1)$ values against $\log(\mathrm{PM}_{gj} - \mathrm{MM}_{gj}^{\wedge}0) + 1)$ for different probe set strata. Left: signals for all probe pairs; middle: signals for probe pairs that belong to probe sets with at least 10 probe pairs with MM>PM, and with a mean log(PM–MM) value of the remaining lower than 4, right: signals for probe pairs that belong to probe sets with at most 2 probe pairs with MM>PM.

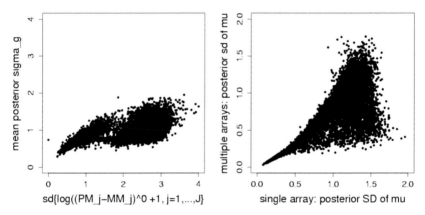

Fig. 3.3. Left: shrinkage of probe set signal standard deviation, right: posterior standard deviation of gene expression index using one against three arrays.

deviations (calculated over the set of $\log(((\mathrm{PM}-\mathrm{MM})^{\wedge}0) + 1)$ values for each probe set), resulting from the assumption of exchangeable variances (3.3).

3.2.3.2 Multiple Arrays Setting

We now consider a situation where we have a number of replicate arrays available to study the expression under an experimental condition. We focus on two aspects of the performance of the BGX multiple array model relative to standard analysis using point estimates of gene expression for each array: (1) borrowing information between replicate arrays and (2) how the signal extraction and gene expression level estimation are integrated. We use the three

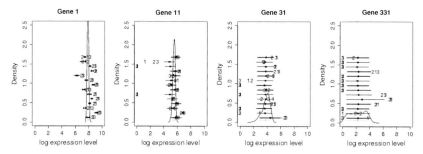

Fig. 3.4. Summaries of posterior distributions of parameters related to expression for four genes using three replicates. The numbers 1, 2, and 3 indicate the log(PM–MM) values for the probe pairs on array 1, 2, and 3, respectively.

replicate condition C arrays of the Choe data set (Choe et al. 2005) to illustrate the multiple array model performance.

Figure 3.4 shows summaries of posterior distributions related to the expression of the same genes as previously shown for the single array model in Figure 3.1 that are obtained for a multiple array model run on the three replicate condition 1 arrays in the Choe data ($c = 1$, $R_1 = 3$). Comparing the posterior distributions of the gene expression indices obtained in the single and triple array analyses (Figures 3.1 and 3.4), it is seen that for three of the genes (genes 1, 11, and 31) the posterior distribution is considerably tightened by the additional information available in the triple array setting, relative to that of a single array. This is particularly striking for gene 31, where the additional information results in the shape of the posterior becoming clearly unimodal. In contrast, the inconsistent probe set behavior of gene 331 is reiterated on the replicate arrays with half of the probe pairs indicating no expression (MM>PM) and the other half indicating moderate to high expression. The posterior distribution of the gene expression index for this gene remains dispersed, with the multimodality found in the analysis of the single array persisting in the triple array analysis. A summary of the effect of borrowing information over replicate arrays is given in Figure 3.3, right, for the full set of genes. In general, the posterior distributions of the gene expression indices are tighter for the triple array analysis than for the analysis of a single array.

A further illustration of the difference in the BGX multiple array approach and the point estimate approach is illustrated in Figure 3.5 (right). The plot shows that the standard deviations calculated over the three point estimates of gene expression (one for each replicate) are generally smaller than the standard deviations of gene expression indices obtained in a triple array analysis. This reflects that the posterior standard deviations from the integrated analysis

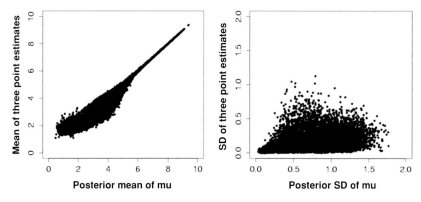

Fig. 3.5. Mean and standard deviation of three BGX point estimates plotted against posterior mean and standard deviation of gene expression index using multiple array model with three replicates.

incorporate uncertainty in the estimate of the expression level (stemming from the within probe set variability) as well as between replicated probe sets, whereas in the point estimate case the standard deviations reflect only the uncertainty between the three gene expression point estimates. Importantly, the difference is not just of scale – there is little correlation between the standard deviation of point estimates of gene expression levels and the standard deviation of posterior distributions of gene expression levels from the integrated analysis. In contrast, as expected, there is a high correlation in the means (Figure 3.5, left).

3.2.4 Differential Expression with the BGX Model

In the following we illustrate the difference between a two-step and an integrated approach in the context of differential expression analysis. We use the full Choe data set consisting of two conditions, C and S, each with three replicate arrays. The data set has the special virtue that it was generated by spiking in 3,870 gene fragments at known concentrations, with concentrations varying between conditions for a subset of 1,331 genes. Thus it is known which of the 14,010 genes represented on the arrays should be expressed and, importantly, which genes should be differentially expressed under the two conditions.

In a step-by-step approach one first obtains a point estimate of expression for each gene on each array, using a specific approach to process the probe level data, and then tests for differential expression between two groups of gene expression indices using a *t*-type statistic. In the microarray setting a particularly popular choice is SAM (Significance Analysis of Microarrays; Tusher et al. 2001), which uses a t-statistic with the denominator boosted by adding a "fudge

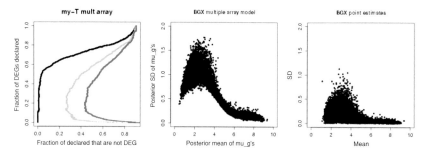

Fig. 3.6. Left: sensitivity (*y*-axis) vs. false positive rate (*x*-axis) for BGX multiple array model (left, black), BGX point estimates and exchangeable variances (middle, light gray), and with SAM (right, dark gray). Middle: posterior mean and standard deviation relationship for BGX gene expression indices in multiple array setting. Right: mean standard deviation relationship for BGX point estimates.

factor." This factor is chosen so that the coefficient of variation between the nominator and denominator is minimized. SAM produces a ranking of the genes according to these modified *t* values, and uses a permutation approach to assess significance.

Differential expression in the BGX multiple array setting may be assessed directly, for example, by examining the posterior distributions of the differences in log-expression levels under two conditions, $\mu_{g,1} - \mu_{g,2}$. In the following we obtain for each gene the ratio of the mean to standard deviation of the posterior sample of $\mu_{g,1} - \mu_{g,2}$, $g = 1, \ldots, G$, and rank the genes according to these values.

Figure 3.6. plots sensitivity (fraction of those genes that are classified as differentially expressed among all truly differentially expressed genes) against false discovery rate (fraction of truly non-differentially expressed genes among all those that are classified as differentially expressed) for the multiple array BGX model analysis and the BGX point estimate with SAM analysis. To produce the curves, we consider the ranked gene list for each method, and count for each possible cutoff in rank the number of true and false positives and negatives in the list above the cutoff. We also show results for an intermediate procedure between these two, which uses the model defined in Section 3.3 of exchangeable variances within each condition (e.g., Lewin et al. 2005), starting from the BGX point estimates of gene expression. This third approach is thus a two-step procedure (like the SAM approach) but allows borrowing of information between genes (like the BGX multiple array approach) through hierarchical modelling of the population of variances. As with the multiple array BGX model, the ratio of posterior mean to standard deviation of the difference in gene expression is used to rank the genes.

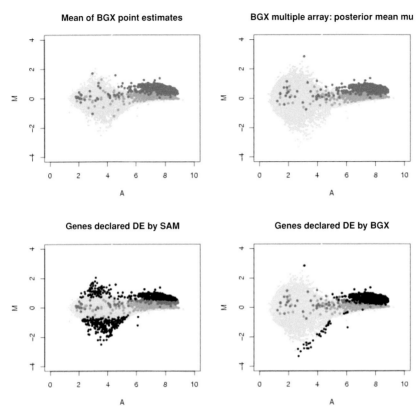

Fig. 3.7. Upper row: MA plot showing differences in expression levels against mean expression levels, using means of three point estimates to represent each condition (left) and using mean posterior value under each condition (right). Point for genes are color-coded according to fold change (FC). The darker the gray, the higher the fold change, light gray is FC = 1. Lower row: Same as upper row, with genes that are called differentially expressed by each method with a cutoff of 5% (700 genes) shown in black.

The ROC curves show that the BGX multiple array model performs markedly better than the other methods. Some improvement is achieved by assuming exchangeable variances on the point estimates (middle curve) relative to the one-common-fudge factor approach employed by SAM. The MA plots of Figure 3.7 illustrate the differences in performance: the SAM approach wrongly declares many genes with low average expression differentially expressed (the pattern for the intermediate approach is similar although weaker, not shown). This is likely to be due to unstable estimation caused by the limited number of available replicates, which, as shown by the illustration of the mean variance relationship of BGX point estimates in Figure 3.6 (right), is particularly pronounced at lower levels of expression, a feature that is not taken into account in the SAM approach. Hence the SAM approach is not suitable for analyzing BGX point estimates or any expression index with a strong mean variance relationship. The BGX multiple array model approach also exhibits a strong mean variance relationship on the posterior samples of gene expression values (Figure 3.6, middle), but this is implicitly accounted for in the global model that integrates the gene expression level estimation and the assessment of differential expression.

3.3 Bayesian Hierarchical Model for Normalization and Differential Expression

In the previous section, we have discussed the benefits of integrating within a single model the low-level signal extraction and the assessment of between condition contrasts. In this section, we again consider the way in which an integrated approach differs from the more usual step-by-step procedures, but this time our focus is on proposing model specifications that can also account for flexible normalization procedure. To be precise, we now consider a model for differential gene expression which incorporates expression-level-dependent array effects to normalize arrays.

3.3.1 The Model

We start with an ANOVA model for the log gene expression y_{gcr} for gene g, experimental condition $c = 1, 2$, and replicate r, as suggested by Kerr et al. (2000). Relating to the BGX model of the previous section, y_{gcr} corresponds to posterior mean of μ_{gcr}, from single array analyses. The model includes additive effects for gene and array:

$$y_{g1r} \sim N\left(\alpha_g - \frac{1}{2}\delta_g + \beta_{g1r}, \sigma_{g1}^2\right)$$
$$y_{g2r} \sim N\left(\alpha_g + \frac{1}{2}\delta_g + \beta_{g2r}, \sigma_{g2}^2\right), \qquad (3.7)$$

where α_g is the gene effect or overall expression level, β_{gcr} is the array effect (this normalizes the arrays) that depends on g through α_g (see below), and σ_{gc}^2 is the gene-specific variance for condition c. The differential effect between conditions is δ_g.

The array effect is a function of the expression level, $\beta_{gcr} = f_{cr}(\alpha_g)$. For flexibility, we choose f_{cr} to be a quadratic spline:

$$\beta_{gcr} = b_{cr0}^{(0)} + b_{cr0}^{(1)}(\alpha_g - a_0) + b_{cr0}^{(2)}(\alpha_g - a_0)^2$$

$$+ \sum_{k=1}^{K} b_{crk}^{(2)}(\alpha_g - a_{crk})^2 I[\alpha_g \geq a_{crk}], \qquad (3.8)$$

where the polynomial coefficients $b_{crk}^{(p)}$ and knots a_{crk} are unknown parameters that are estimated as part of the model. The number of knots K is fixed (but sensitivity to different choices of K can be investigated as part of model checking).

The equations (3.7) and (3.8) define the first level of the hierarchical model. At the second level, information is shared between genes to stabilize the variances. The variances are modeled as exchangeable within each condition, that is, the variances are assumed to come from a common distribution, chosen here to be log Normal:

$$\sigma_{gc}^2 \sim \text{logNorm}\left(\mu_c, \eta_c^2\right). \qquad (3.9)$$

The third level of the model specifies prior distributions for all the unknown parameters, which are intended to be noninformative. The gene effects α_g and knots a_{crk} are uniformly distributed on (a_0, a_{K+1}) where a_0 and a_{K+1} are fixed lower and upper limits (chosen to be wide enough not to affect the results). Polynomial coefficients $b_{crk}^{(p)}$ have independent $N(0, 10^2)$ priors and the hyperparameters μ_c and η_c^{-2} have $N(0, 10^3)$ and Gamma$(10^{-2}, 10^{-2})$ priors respectively. In this work, the differential effects δ_g are given independent $N(0, 10^4)$ priors.

The model is made identifiable by normalizing *within each condition* by setting $\bar{\beta}_{gc.} = 0 \; \forall \, g, c$, where the dot indicates that we are taking an average over the index r. This fully identifies the model. Normalizing using all genes within condition seems reasonable, as we do not expect systematic differences between genes on replicate arrays.

3.3.2 Comparison of Integrated and Nonintegrated Analyses

When covariates in a regression are not measured accurately but have some unknown variability, it is well known that ignoring this variability leads to a bias in estimates of regression coefficients (Carroll et al. 1995). Therefore, we would expect to obtain biased estimates of the array effects if they are estimated in a preprocessing step, which in turn will lead to worse estimates of the differential effects δ_g. To illustrate this, we compare the results from the full

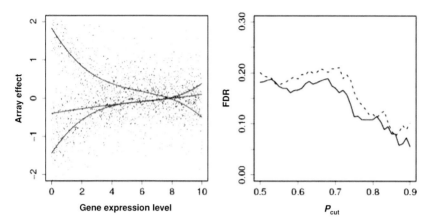

Fig. 3.8. Left panel: Array effects β_{gcr} (lines) used for three of the simulated arrays. The points on the plot are the simulated data points with the overall gene expression level subtracted for each gene. Right panel: Observed false discovery rate (FDR) versus probability cutoff p_{cut} for the simulated data set described in Section 3.3.2. The solid line is for the full, integrated model and the dashed line is for the prenormalized model. Curves are averages over five simulations.

model with those found by pre-normalizing the data using array effects from local regression smoothing (loess).

As in Lewin et al. (2005), we simulate a microarray data set with 1000 genes and three repeat arrays under two conditions. The gene effects α_g range uniformly between 0 and 10, and the array effects are cubic functions of the gene effects. The gene variances are simulated from the model we fit (equation (3.9)), with $\mu_1 = -1.8$, $\mu_2 = -2.2$, $\eta_c^2 = 1$ for $c = 1, 2$, giving a similar range of variances to those we have observed in real data. The differential effects δ_g are zero for 900 genes, $N(\log(3), 0.1^2)$ for 50 genes, and $N(-\log(3), 0.1^2)$ for the other 50, with the differentially expressed genes uniformly spread over the range of α_g. The left-hand panel of Figure 3.8 shows the array effects and data points for one set of three simulated arrays.

To calculate loess estimates of array effects, we use the R function "loess" with $y_{gcr} - \bar{y}_{gc.}$ as a function of $\bar{y}_{g..}$. The array effects $\hat{\beta}_{gcr}^{\text{loess}}$ are the values of the loess curve for sample c and array r predicted at $\bar{y}_{g..}$.

In order to assess the effect on the differential effects δ_g of using a preprocessing step, we fit a model where we prenormalize the data by subtracting point estimates of the array effects, $y'_{gcr} \equiv y_{gcr} - \hat{\beta}_{gcr}$, and run our model without array effects.

To assess the results, we need a decision rule to classify genes as differentially expressed or not. For the purposes of this chapter, we focus on the differential effects δ_g and use posterior probabilities to pick genes: if $\mathbb{P}(|\delta_g| > \delta_{cut}|$ data $) \geq p_{cut}$ then gene g is selected. The choice of δ_{cut} corresponds to a statement of biological interest. The choice of p_{cut} is determined by the evaluation of the false discovery rate and/or false nondiscovery rate (Benjamini and Hochberg 1995; Storey 2002).

Based on decision rules as above, we can calculate the number of false positives and negatives. The right panel of Figure 3.8 shows the observed false discovery rate (FDR: the number of false positives divided by the number of genes declared positive) for both the full and prenormalized models, as a function of the cutoff probability p_{cut}, for a choice of $\delta_{cut} = \log(3)$. Graphs shown are curves averaged over five simulations. The FDR is consistently lower for the integrated model than for the prenormalized model.

The difference shown here between the full and prenormalized models is fairly small, as the simulation is inspired by the data we use in this work, which has small array effects. In general, the larger the magnitude of array effects, the larger the difference between the prenormalized and integrated models.

Note that the differences found here are not due to difference between the loess and spline array effects. We have carried out the two-step analysis using array effects from the full model $\hat{\beta}_{gcr} = E(\beta_{gcr}|$ data$)$, and the results are closer to those of the two-step model using loess array effects than those of the full model.

3.4 Predictive Model Checking

The Bayesian setting allows us to criticize various aspects of the model from a predictive point of view. The idea is similar to cross-validation, in which observations are taken out of the model a unit at a time. Each time, the model is run to obtain a predictive distribution for the statistic of interest associated with the observational unit that has been removed, and this is compared to the observed statistic for that unit.

There are several choices to be made in order to carry out this procedure. The test statistic T must be chosen, along with a method of comparing its predicted distribution to the observed value. It is possible for T to be a function of both data and parameters; however, here we will only consider a function of data. In this case the natural method of comparison is the "p value", that is, the probability under the null of T being more extreme than the observed value.

In hierarchical models there is also a choice of how to calculate the predictive distribution, that is, which parameters of the model to condition on. Several choices are considered in Gelman et al. (1996) and Bayarri and Berger (2000). For our work we use the mixed predictive distribution proposed in Gelman et al. (1996) and Marshall and Spiegelhalter (2003), discussed below.

Under the null hypothesis of the model being "true," the distribution of cross-validation p values is uniform. This property provides a straightforward way to see if any observations do not agree with the rest. If the distribution of p values contains a small excess of small values, these observations can be declared outliers. If the distribution is far from uniform, the model can be said to be a bad fit to the data.

For large data sets cross-validation is computationally unfeasible, so full data predictive p values have been proposed as approximations to their cross-validatory equivalent. Here the predictive distributions are calculated for each unit simultaneously, without removing any data from the analysis. Since in this case the data from a particular unit influences its prediction, these p values are conservative (Bayarri and Berger 2000). Such sharing of information shrinks the p values toward 0.5.

In order to lessen the effect of using the data twice, another kind of predictive checking for hierarchical models has been proposed, known as mixed predictive checking (Gelman et al. 1996; Marshall and Spiegelhalter 2003). Here new model *parameters* are predicted for each unit, before new statistics are predicted. To illustrate this, consider a model for exchangeable variances, as we use in previous sections. Simplifying, we can write

$$y_{gr} \sim N\left(x_g, \sigma_g^2\right)$$
$$\sigma_g^2 \sim \text{logNorm}(\mu, \eta^2)$$
$$(\mu, \eta^2) \sim N(0, 10^5)\text{Gamma}(10^{-3}, 10^{-3}) \tag{3.10}$$

Suppose we are interested in the gene variances. We choose the test statistic T_g to be the sample variance S_g^2 for gene g. In posterior predictive checks these are simply calculated from the posterior predictive distribution: $y_{gr}^{(\text{pred})} \sim N(x_g, \sigma_g^2)$. For mixed predictive checks new intermediate parameters are predicted within the model, $\sigma_g^{2\,(\text{mixpred})} \sim \text{logNorm}(\mu, \eta^2)$, and the predicted "data" is conditioned on these predicted parameters: $y_{gr}^{(\text{mixpred})} \sim N(x_g, \sigma_g^{2\,(\text{mixpred})})$. To highlight the conditioning used, Figure 3.9 shows the directed acyclic graph for the above model, along with the extra parameters needed to calculate mixed predictive p values.

Mixed predictive checks have been shown to be much less conservative than posterior predictive checks (Marshall and Spiegelhalter 2003). This is because in the latter the information in the posterior predictive distribution for any given gene comes mainly from the data from that gene (from the posterior on σ_g^2 in

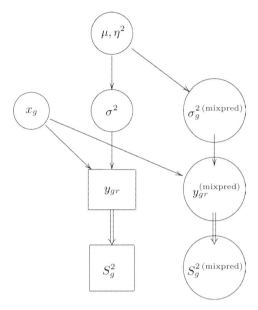

Fig. 3.9. Directed acyclic graph for the model in equation (3.10), with additional parameters used in the calculation of mixed predictive *p*-values. Rectangles represent data; circles represent stochastic parameters. Double arrows indicate that one quantity is a deterministic function of another.

our example), whereas in the former the information about a given gene only contributes through the estimation of the hyperparameters (μ, η^2), which have been informed by all the genes.

As an example, we calculate mixed predictive *p* values for the model in Section 3.3. We have done this for two data sets. The first consists of MAS 5.0 expression values for three Affymetrix arrays of wild-type mouse data, discussed in Lewin et al. (2005). The *p* values for this data set are shown in Figure 3.10. They are almost uniform, suggesting that the exchangeable variance model is appropriate for this data set. The second data set is the C group of the Choe data set (Choe et al. 2005) described in Section 3.2.2. For this data set the *p* values are not uniform, suggesting that the exchangeable model on the variances could be improved.

Software

Software for the hierarchical models described is available at http://www. bgx.org.uk/. The code for the BGX model is written in C++, with an R interface. The model in Section 3.3 is implemented in WinBUGS.

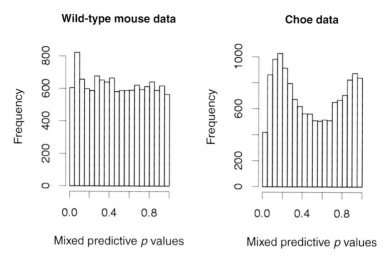

Fig. 3.10. Mixed and posterior predictive *p* values for a set of wild-type mouse data and for the Choe data.

Acknowledgment

This work was supported by BBSRC "Exploiting Genomics" grant 28EGM16093.

Bibliography

Bayarri, M. J. and Berger, J. (2000). P-values for composite null models. *Journal of the American Statistical Association* **95**, 1127–1142.

Benjamini, Y. and Hochberg, Y. (1995). Controlling the false discovery rate: A practical and powerful approach to multiple testing. *Journal of the Royal Statistical Society, Series B* **57**, 289–300.

Carroll, R. J., Ruppert, D., and Stefanski, L. A. (1995). *Measurement Error in Nonlinear Models.* London: Chapman and Hall/CRC.

Choe, S. E., Boutros, M., Michelson, A. M., Church, G. M., and Halfon, M. S. (2005). Preferred analysis methods for Affymetrix GeneChips revealed by a wholly defined control dataset. *Genome Biology* **6**, R16.

Durbin, B. P., Hardin, J. S., Hawkins, D. M., and Rocke, D. M. (2002). A variance-stabilizing transformation for gene-expression microarray data. *Bioinformatics* **18**, S105–S110.

Gelman, A., Meng, X.-L., and Stern, H. (1996). Posterior predictive assessment of model fitness via realized discrepancies. *Statistica Sinica* **6**, 733–807.

Gilks, W. R., Richardson, S., and Spiegelhalter, D. J. (1996). *Markov Chain Monte Carlo in Practice.* London: Chapman and Hall.

Green, P. J., Hjort, N. L., and Richardson, S. (2003). *Highly Structured Stochastic Systems.* Oxford: Oxford University Press.

Hein, A. K., Richardson, S., Causton, H. C., Ambler, G. K., and Green, P. J. (2005). BGX: A fully Bayesian integrated approach to the analysis of Affymetrix GeneChip data. *Biostatistics* **6**, 349–373.

Hubbell, E., Liu, W., and Mei, R. (2002). Robust estimators for expression analysis. *Bioinformatics* **18**, 1585–1592.

Huber, W., von Heydebreck, A., Sültmann, H., Poustka, A., and Vingron, M. (2002). Variance stabilization applied to microarray data calibration and to the quantification of differential expression. *Bioinformatics* **18**, S96–S104.

Irizarry, R., Hobbs, B., Collin, F., Beazer-Barclay, Y., Antonellis, K., Scherf, U., and Speed, T. (2003). Exploration, normalization, and summaries of high density oligonucleotide array probe level data. *Biostatistics* **4**, 249–264.

Kerr, M. K., Martin, M., and Churchill, G. A. (2000). Analysis of variance for gene expression microarray data. *Journal of Computational Biology* **8**, 819–837.

Lewin, A., Richardson, S., Marshall C., Glazier A., and Aitman T. (2006). Bayesian modelling of differential gene expression. *Biometrics* **62**, 1–9.

Li, C. and Wong, W. (2001). Model-based analysis of oligonucleotide arrays: Expression index computation and outlier detection. *Proceedings of the National Academy of Sciences USA* **98**, 31–36.

Lockhart, D. J., Dong, H., Byrne, M. C., Follettie, M. T., Gallo, M. V., Chee, M. S., Mittmann, M., Wang, C., Kobayashi, M., Horton, H., and Brown, E. L. (1996). Expression monitoring by hybridization to high-density oligonucleotide arrays. *Nature Biotechnology* **14**, 1675–1680.

Marshall, E. C. and Spiegelhalter, D. J. (2003). Approximate cross-validatory predictive checks in disease mapping models. *Statistics in Medicine* **22**, 1649–1660.

O'Hagan, A. (2003). Highly structured stochastic systems model criticism. In *Highly Structured Stochastic Systems*, Green, P. J., Hjort, N. L., and Richardson, S. eds. Oxford: Oxford University Press.

Smyth, G. K. (2004). Linear models and empirical Bayes methods for assessing differential expression in microarray experiments *Statistical Applications in Genetics and Molecular Biology*, **3**(1), 3.

Storey, J. D. (2002). A direct approach to false discovery rates. *Journal of the Royal Statistical Society, Series B* **64**, 479–498.

Tusher, V. G., Tibshirani, R., and Chu, G. (2001). Significance analysis of microarrays applied to the ionizing radiation response. *PNAS* **98**, 5116–5121.

4

Bayesian Process-Based Modeling of Two-Channel Microarray Experiments: Estimating Absolute mRNA Concentrations

MARK A. VAN DE WIEL

Vrije Universiteit, Amsterdam

MARIT HOLDEN

Norwegian Computing Center

INGRID K. GLAD

University of Oslo

HEIDI LYNG

Norwegian Radium Hospital

ARNOLDO FRIGESSI

University of Oslo

Abstract

We present a Bayesian process-based model for spotted microarray data incorporating available information about the experiment from target gene preparation to image analysis. We demonstrate that, using limited calibration data, our method can estimate absolute gene concentrations from spotted microarray intensity data. Number of transcripts (copies of the gene sequence) per microgram total RNA are obtained for each gene, enabling comparisons of transcript levels within and between samples. All parameters are estimated in one Markov chain Monte Carlo run thereby propagating uncertainties throughout the model. We reparameterize the core of the model, binomial selection, and show identifiability of the parameters. Using a small data set, we illustrate potentials of our method discriminating it from conventional, ratio-based methods. This chapter gives a thorough description of the statistical methodologies that form the foundation of the biology-focused companion paper [11].

4.1 Introduction

Analysis of microarray data is challenging due to the huge number of measurements made in each experiment and the large uncertainty associated with it.

When spotted cDNA microarrays are used, gene expression levels are generally measured as a log-ratio of the fluorescence intensity of two cDNA samples to reduce systematic effects in the data, though biological information that lies in the absolute concentrations may be lost [7, 21]. Samples are derived from mRNA by reverse transcription and dye labeling and cohybridized to an array of DNA probes on a microscope slide. The intensities are measured by imaging the array in an optical scanner. There are several sources of variation associated with each step in the experimental procedure that influence the measured intensities, and hence the expression. Experimental variation is present, and includes measurement error and unstable experimental settings, such as the RNA purity and amount, the cDNA length and extent of dye incorporation, the quality and quantity of probe material, and the optical characteristics of the dyes. The large and unknown uncertainty in the data has important implications on the strategy used to identify differentially expressed genes and to group genes or samples with similar characteristics.

The process-based Bayesian approach we present here is based on a completely novel strategy. We follow the various steps of the microarray experiment and build a hierarchical model, incorporating technical and scientific knowledge in terms of explanatory covariates and known qualitative effects. The effects of all factors and all gene expressions are estimated in one single Bayesian procedure. Moreover, our method is able to estimate absolute concentrations of mRNA for each gene rather than ratios. The need for developing tools to obtain these absolute concentrations instead of or next to ratios has been expressed by the genomics community [6, 17]. Not only are these interesting quantities per se, but also can they be directly compared between experiments and between genes (as opposed to ratios), and are very useful for meta-analysis.

Commonly used methods to identify differentially expressed genes rely on a normalization of the data, which has the aim to filter out the biological content in the data from the experimental variability, by adjusting for dye-bias, for scanner properties, and for variation not due to mRNA differences [22]. Normalization methods are based on strong prior assumptions about relations in the data, which are then transformed in order to recreate such expected behaviors [22]. Typically, several noncommutative adjustments are performed sequentially, with no propagation of uncertainty. Such normalized data are then plugged into expression analyzers as if they were the original data, mostly ignoring the distributional consequences of the specific assumptions they were based upon and the transformations undergone. This can lead to diminished ability to detect genes that are differentially expressed [24]. Furthermore, all these methods are based on log-ratios and do not utilize the information that lies in the intensities per se.

Improving methods for extracting the significant information from microarray data is crucial to realize the full potential of the technology. Model-based approaches, such as two-step ANOVA [18], incorporate knowledge of inherent characteristics of variations. Our method is a further step in this direction. Our model follows the experimental setting more closely, including the imaging technology, and takes advantage of available experimental covariates (for example, specific probe-related measurements) to explain experimental variation.

In this study we present and discuss in depth the mathematical model and related Markov chain Monte Carlo (MCMC)-based Bayesian inference. Bayesian statistics is widely recognized as a fundamental tool for discovery in genetics [3] and the present study is a further demonstration of its use. Other Bayesian approaches to microarray data can be found in [2, 5, 20].

Estimates of absolute concentrations for spotted cDNA microarrays have been obtained before (see, e.g., [10] and [16]). However, in these approaches, each gene needs individual calibration, leading to very unusual and expensive chip requirements. Our process-based model enables estimation of absolute concentrations of mRNA targets using only chipwise calibration. We validated this claim extensively in a large study elsewhere [11].

The basic idea of our model is to follow the mRNA molecules from transcription to hybridization and imaging. Hence, we have adopted a Bayesian process-based approach. Such an approach is somewhat similar to the integrated hierarchical model approach in [14] for Affymetrix data, because these approaches share the philosophy of propagating uncertainties. Our model, however, follows the process more closely. We interpret the microarray experiment as a selection procedure, where the mRNA molecules initially present in a tissue solution are stepwise selected, until eventually the intensities are measured. Starting from the unknown number of mRNAs for each gene, each step of a typical microarray protocol is represented as a selection, where each molecule has a certain probability of being kept in the experiment. This probability is different for each step, gene, and sample, and is modulated by probe-related covariates and experimental settings. For example, on some microarrays more than one probe sequence is used to hybridize with the same target, but it is unlikely that all these sequences are equally efficient. Also, the amount of probe is varying and likely to be important. We show that by using quality- and quantity-related probe information, we are able to explain much of the spot-to-spot variation of measured intensities in our data. We treat the imaging after hybridization and washing as an integral part of the model. This means that we propagate uncertainty due to the imaging in the rest of the model, taking special care of the crucial relationship between the value of the photomultiplier tube (PMT value: an adjustable setting of the scanner) and the measured intensities.

Given the measured intensities of the finally remaining molecules per spot, we estimate backwards all parameters related to the various covariates and the concentration ratios (or absolute concentrations) per gene. These estimates can be considered as normalized data, since most variation due to the technology rather than to biological differences has been subtracted. Since all concentration ratios (or absolute concentrations) are jointly estimated and since we use each data channel separately, our method easily deals with complex multisample experiments as well as single channel arrays.

Our method, which we named TransCount, is illustrated here with data from a simple experiment with four arrays only. The data are from a standard tissue (reference) and three tumor biopsies. We concentrate on questions that are difficult to solve with conventional methods, since these problems require explicit knowledge of the joint expression distribution and knowledge of absolute concentrations.

4.2 The Hierarchical Model

The model we construct is able to estimate actual target concentrations, which is the number of target molecules per microgram total RNA. When selecting genes, one may choose to use such estimated concentrations, the estimated ratios, or both. The model contains three levels: first, a selection process modeling the proportion of target molecules that have survived the several steps of the microarray experiment; second, the translation of the number of imaged target molecules into pixel-wise intensities; and third, the final measurement process. We go through the several steps of the experiment and discuss which covariates correlate with molecule survival. Furthermore, we introduce scaling factors that scale the number of molecules that have hybridized to a total number of molecules in the solution. The resulting hierarchical model then propagates uncertainties properly. We describe here the experimental protocol in use at the Norwegian Cancer Hospital, which is standard, but other protocols could be modeled similarly.

The several selections of molecules in the microarray experiment are modeled as Bernoulli trials. That is, we assume that in each step the target molecules act independently with a success probability modulated by covariates, target, experiment, and probe dependence. We use $p_s^{t,a}$ to denote the multiplicative effect on spot s, array a, and sample t of the experimental steps described below. The following discussion introduces the relevant covariates that we will later use to model $p_s^{t,a}$.

Preparation of the mRNA solution. The known quantity of material for sample t ($t = 1, 2, \ldots, T$) on array a is denoted $q^{t,a}$, for example the weight of mRNA after amplification. For each gene $i = 1, 2, \ldots, G$ in the study, let K_i^t denote the unknown number of transcripts per weight unit in sample t.

Reverse transcription and dye labeling. Dye-labeled cDNAs are achieved by incorporation of Cy3-dUTP and Cy5-dUTP during or after cDNA synthesis of the mRNAs. The amount of dye and nucleotides are assumed to be in excess, so that all mRNA molecules can in principle be reverse-transcribed and labeled. First assume that purity is high and homogeneous, and that the expected number of actually bound Cy3- or Cy5-dUTPs is the same for all transcripts of all genes, since the number of binding sites, though different, is always large enough to allow for such a geometric approximation. The expected number of actually bound CyX-dUTPs often depends on dye, that is, there is a chemical dye effect. This effect will be important in the imaging step described below. We assume the $q^{t,a} \cdot K_i^t$ molecules in the solution to be reverse-transcribed and labeled independently of each other. The probability to do so may depend on gene-, array-, and sample-specific properties, such as the sample purity.

Purification. The two solutions are mixed. Excessive CyX-dUTP molecules are washed away. During this process some of the cDNA target molecules will also be lost. We expect that the success probability depends on the target molecule length of gene i. Target length possibly influences purification since longer molecules are less likely to be mistakenly washed off. Currently, target length has not been included directly in the model because it is not available. Differences in the success probability specifically caused by target length will instead be absorbed in a gene-specific parameter.

Microarray production. The variability of probe material and microarray production modulates the probability of successful hybridization. For a certain spot the microarray, the pen, and the probe used influence this probability. Consequently, both microarray and pen are included as covariates in the model, in addition to probe quantity- and quality-dependent covariates. Because each of the pens is used on a specific sub-grid of the microarray, the pen effect may confound with spatial effects. Quantity of the probe material also varies. A test slide of the printing batch is stained with SYBR green, a fluorophore with specific affinity for the DNA probes. The fluorescence intensity is used as a measure of probe quantity of each spot and is included as a covariate in the model. Quality of the probe material may also vary. We distinguish two probe-related covariates. First, the probe identification number (PID), which is unique for a specific sequence of cDNA. Second, the replication identification number (RID), distinguishing between replications with the same PID. We do not distinguish here between spot center and periphery, assuming for simplicity that each part of a spot is equally covered by probe.

Hybridization. We assume that the spatial distribution of each target molecule is uniform over the slide and target molecules do not cluster nor repulse, except for interaction with the corresponding probe. Let n_s^a be the total number of pixels in spot s on array a. After successful cDNA synthesis, labeling, and purification, a proportion $c \cdot n_s^a$ of the target molecules present in the purified solution may reach spot s for hybridization. Here c is a hybridization scaling factor, determination of which we discuss later. The success probability depends on probe molecule properties and technical experimental conditions as well as on target molecule properties, including probe quantity, probe length, PID, RID, pen, and microarray. Target molecule length possibly describes the diffusion coefficient of target molecules and could have been included here also. Hybridization is assumed to be dye-independent [23] and the hybridization probability is assumed to be constant in time. The model does not include cross-hybridization.

Washing. We assume that all nonhybridized material, including nontarget CyX-dUTPs, is removed during microarray washing. Some hybridized molecules might however also drop out. The success probability may depend on probe length reflecting the binding strength and on microarray effects. We denote the number of molecules from sample t which have survived all the aforementioned selection processes and are ready for imaging on spot s on array a by $J_s^{t,a}$.

Imaging. The microarray is gridded and segmented into spots. The PMT scanning voltage, possibly varying between both channels and arrays, and the scanner-dependent amplification factor [19] are included in the model. Assume that the background captures local luminescence features. Let $\mathcal{S}_s^a$ be the set of n_s^a pixels in the spot and $\mathcal{B}_s^a$ the set of background pixels for the same spot. Assume for simplicity that segmentation is perfect, that is, $\mathcal{S}_s^a$ covers exactly the spot on the slide. Let $L_{j,s}^{t,a}$ be the intensity measured for sample t in array a in pixel j of spot s. Assume that the hybridized molecules $J_s^{t,a}$ are on average homogeneously spread over the pixels j in $\mathcal{S}_s^a$, so that the expected intensity is the same for each pixel in a spot; hence we do not model any variability between the center of the spot and its periphery. We then model the measured intensity as

$$L_{j,s}^{t,a} = \frac{\mu_s^{t,a}}{n_s^a} + \epsilon_{j,s}^{t,a} \tag{4.1}$$

if pixel j is in $\mathcal{S}_s^a$ and n_s^a is the number of pixels in spot s on array a. Here $\mu_s^{t,a}$ is the expected intensity from hybridized material in a pixel of spot s, and $\epsilon_{j,s}^{t,a}$, representing an additive measurement error in the imaging process, is a zero-mean normal variable with variance $(\tau_s^{t,a})^2$. We currently plug in estimated spot variances. Standard calculations for normal densities show that the sample mean and sample variance of pixel-wise values are sufficient statistics to estimate both $\mu_s^{t,a}$ and $\tau_s^{t,a}$.

It is sometimes advisable to assume that the background intensity adds to the intensity from the hybridized material to form the total spot intensity. In this case, $L_{j,s}^{t,a} = \mu_s^{t,a}/n_s^a + \xi_s^{t,a}/n_s^a + \epsilon_{j,s}^{t,a}$ if pixel j is in S_s^a, while $L_{j,s}^{t,a} = \xi_s^{t,a}/n_s^a + \nu_{j,s}^{t,a}$, if j is in B_s^a. Here $\xi_s^{t,a}$ is the expected background intensity in a pixel belonging to the background of spot s, while $\epsilon_{j,s}^{t,a}$ and $\nu_{j,s}^{t,a}$ are error terms. In this paper we do not use background correction. Intermediate solutions are also possible.

The expected scanned intensity on spot s, array a, is modeled as

$$\mu_s^{t,a} = 2^{f_{\text{dye}(t,a)}\text{PMT}^{t,a}} J_s^{t,a} \alpha_{\text{dye}(t,a)}, \qquad (4.2)$$

where $\text{dye}(t,a)$ and $\text{PMT}^{t,a}$ are the dye and PMT voltage used during scanning of sample t on array a, f_{Cy3} and f_{Cy5} are the known scanner amplification factors, and α_{Cy3} and α_{Cy5} are unknown chemical and optical dye effects. Scanning has to be performed so that all spot and background intensities are within the $\log_2$-linear range of the scanner [19]. In that case (4.2) holds. Extension to sample-dependent dye effects (i.e., $\alpha_{\text{dye}(t,a)}^t$) is possible.

4.2.1 Collapsed Model and Link Function

Each step (labeling-transcription, purification, hybridization, washing, and imaging) is modeled conditionally on the preceding one and depends on co-variates, the effects of which are estimated together with the unknown mRNA concentrations K_i^t. We shall perform Bayesian inference on all parameters of interest based on the joint posterior density. Since for binomials it holds that if $X \sim \text{Bin}(Y, p)$ and $Y \sim \text{Bin}(Z, q)$ then $X \sim \text{Bin}(Z, pq)$, the nested selection process from K_i^t to $J_s^{t,a}$ can simply be modeled as one binomial process. We get

$$J_s^{t,a} \sim \text{Binomial}\left(c \cdot n_s^a \cdot q^{t,a} \cdot K_{g(s,a)}^t, p_s^{t,a}\right), \qquad (4.3)$$

where c is a scaling constant related to the hybridization process and $g(s,a)$ is the index of the gene on spot s on array a. Knowledge of the scaling constant c is needed for the interpretation of $K_{g(s,a)}^t$ as an absolute concentration.

A calibration experiment with known quantities (spikes) is the best way to estimate c. Note that this can be a relatively modest experiment, since c does not depend on genes (see [11] for discussion of this off-line experiment). Alternatively, we can assume $c = A'/A$, where A is the area of the array and A' is the attraction area of a spot. It is difficult to define A' exactly, but in case of manual hybridization (where there is limited movement of the hybridization solution) a rough estimate of A' is simply the spot area. We will use this in our illustration example in Section 4.6.

We regress the overall success probability parameter $p_s^{t,a}$ on the several covariates. We use the following covariates in the selection process: purity (P'), microarray, probe length (pl_s^a), SYBR green (SG_s^a), probe identification number, replication identification number, and pen, which correspond to parameters γ, $\beta_{1,a}$, β_2, β_3, $\beta_{4,i}$, $\beta_{5,j}$, and $\beta_{6,p}$, respectively. Moreover, we introduce γ_0 as a common baseline parameter and γ_i, $i = 1, \ldots, G$ as a gene-specific parameter, which represents gene-specific properties that may alter success probability $p_s^{t,a}$. Let $PID(s, a)$, $RID(s, a)$, and $p(s, a)$ denote probe identification number, replication identification number, and pen, respectively, applied to spot s and array a. We use the following regression:

$$
\begin{aligned}
p_s^{t,a} &= L^{-1}\left(\gamma_0 + \gamma_{g(s,a)} + \gamma P' + \beta_{1,a} + \beta_2\, pl_s^a + \beta_3\, SG_s^a \right.\\
&\qquad \left. + \beta_{4,PID(s,a)} + \beta_{5,RID(s,a)} + \beta_{6,p(s,a)}\right) \\
&= L^{-1}\left(\gamma_0 + \gamma_{g(s,a)} + \gamma\, P' + \bar{\beta} X_s^a\right),
\end{aligned}
\tag{4.4}
$$

where L is a link function that maps the sum to a number between 0 and 1. The matrix X_s^a contains all covariates that can differ *within* repeated measurements on the same gene. We used the censored log link $L^{-1}(x) = \min(1, \exp(x))$. An alternative is the logit link $L^{-1}(x) = \text{logit}^{-1}(x) = 1/(1 + \exp(-x))$, which did not give very different results.

4.3 Reparameterization and Identifiability

The hierarchical model consists of four levels:

$$
\begin{aligned}
L_{j,s}^{t,a} &= \mu_s^{t,a}/n_s^a + \epsilon_{j,s}^{t,a} \\
\mu_s^{t,a} &= 2^{f_{dye(t,a)} \cdot PMT^{t,a}} J_s^{t,a} \alpha_{dye(t,a)} \\
J_s^{t,a} &\sim \text{Binomial}\left(c \cdot n_s^a \cdot q^{t,a} \cdot K_{g(s,a)}^t, p_s^{t,a}\right) \\
p_s^{t,a} &= \min\left[1, \exp\left(\gamma_0 + \gamma_{g(s,a)} + \gamma P' + \bar{\beta} X_s^a\right)\right].
\end{aligned}
$$

We use the normal approximation to the binomial:

$$
J_s^{t,a} \sim N\left(C_s^{t,a} \cdot K_{g(s,a)}^t \cdot p_s^{t,a}, \; C_s^{t,a} \cdot K_{g(s,a)}^t \cdot p_s^{t,a}\left(1 - p_s^{t,a}\right)\right),
\tag{4.5}
$$

where $C_s^{t,a} = c \cdot n_s^a \cdot q^{t,a}$. For obtaining easier convergence of the MCMC, we reparameterize (4.5) in such a way that only parameters directly identifiable based on the expectation occur in the expectation, while all the others appear only in the variances. To perform this reparameterization, it is easier to use the link function $\exp(x)$ instead of $\min(1, \exp(x))$. Note that identifiability under the relaxed link function implies identifiability under the $\min(1, \exp(x))$ link function, because for the latter the parameter space is smaller due to the constraint. Then, let

$$\alpha_{\text{dye}(t,a)} = \alpha'_{\text{dye}(t,a)}\alpha,$$

where $\alpha'_{Cy5} = 1$, and α'_{Cy3} and α are the new parameters to be estimated, replacing α_{Cy3} and α_{Cy5}. In addition $\tilde{J}$'s and $\tilde{K}$'s replacing the J's and K's are defined as

$$\tilde{J}_s^{t,a} = J_s^{t,a}\alpha$$
$$\tilde{K}_i^t = K_i^t \alpha\, e^{\gamma_0+\gamma_i+\gamma\, P^t}. \tag{4.6}$$

Then, we observe that

$$\tilde{J}_s^{t,a} \sim N\big(C_s^{t,a} \cdot \tilde{K}_{g(s,a)}^t \cdot \exp\big(\bar{\beta}X_s^a\big),\ C_s^{t,a} \cdot \tilde{K}_{g(s,a)}^t \exp\big(\bar{\beta}X_s^a\big)$$
$$\times \big(1 - \exp\big(\gamma_0 + \gamma_{g(s,a)} + \gamma P^t + \bar{\beta}X_s^a\big)\big) \cdot \alpha\big). \tag{4.7}$$

Since $E[n_s^a L_{j,s}^{t,a}] = C_s^{t,a} \cdot \tilde{K}_{g(s,a)}^t \alpha'_{\text{dye}} \exp(\bar{\beta}X_s^a)$, all parameters except γ_0, the γ_i's, γ, and α are estimable based on the mean pixel-wise values with the described reparameterization, provided that the regression of this mean on the covariates X_s^a is identifiable, which can easily be checked by studying the design-matrix of the study. This identifiability based on the mean values only is equivalent to identifiability under a Poisson selection model. The parameters γ_0, γ_i's, γ, and α are estimable based on the variances and none of them occur in the expressions for the means. When there are pieces of data without repeats (e.g., samples hybridized only once and genes spotted only once), such single data points must be excluded when variance-related parameters are estimated, otherwise these estimates are shrunken. For estimating all parameters we use a two-step procedure. First, all parameters are estimated using all data except such special single data points. Then, the remaining unestimated concentrations are estimated using only single data points and the posterior distributions of all parameters as priors. In practice, both steps are done within a single MCMC run.

We further constrained the categorical parameters for identifiability. In order to assure identifiability of the pen parameters, we use the constraint $\sum_p \beta_{6,p} = 0$. A similar constraint is used for the array parameter $\beta_{1,a}$ and the gene-related parameters γ_i. Moreover, the mean effect of all probes per gene sums to zero ($\sum_j \beta_{4,j} = 0$) where summation runs over all probes in the probe set of each gene. Similarly, $\sum_j \beta_{5,j} = 0$, for all probes, where summation runs over all replicates for the particular probe. In addition, microarray ($\beta_{1,a}$), pen

$(\beta_{6,p})$, gene-dependent selection efficiency (γ_i), probe identification number $(\beta_{4,j})$, and replication identification number $(\beta_{5,j})$ are modeled as random effects, that is, we have $\beta_{1,a} \sim \text{Normal}(0, (\sigma_A)^2)$, $\beta_{6,p} \sim \text{Normal}(0, (\sigma_P)^2)$ and $\gamma_i \sim \text{Normal}(0, (\sigma_G)^2)$. Since the number of probe products per gene is usually small, we do not use separate variance parameters for each gene, but instead we have $\beta_{4,j} \sim \text{Normal}(0, (\sigma_{\text{PID}})^2)$ for all probe sequences. Similarly, we have $\beta_{5,j} \sim \text{Normal}(0, (\sigma_{\text{RID}})^2)$ for all replications. Otherwise, all hyperparameters are equipped with flat improper noninformative priors.

We have discussed reparameterization and identifiability under the log-link. However, use of a logit or censored log-link is important since it conserves the complicated nonproportional effects of factors.

4.4 MCMC-Based Inference

Markov chain Monte Carlo is needed to sample from the posterior model. We implement a single-update random-walk Metropolis-Hastings sampler. For all the parameters we use a simple uniform proposal: let v be the current value of the parameter p for which a new value will be proposed, and let $c_{p,0}$ and $c_{p,1}$ be two constants. If the parameter is not restricted to be positive, and its prior is $\text{Normal}(0, \sigma_p^2)$, we draw from the uniform density $U[v - c_{p,1}\sigma_p, v + c_{p,1}\sigma_p]$, otherwise we draw from $U[v - (c_{p,1}|v| + c_{p,0}), v + (c_{p,1}|v| + c_{p,0})]$. If the parameter is restricted to be positive, we draw the logarithm of the parameter from

$$U[\log(v) - (c_{p,1}|\log(v)| + c_{p,0}), \log(v) + (c_{p,1}|\log(v)| + c_{p,0})].$$

The two constants $c_{p,0}$ and $c_{p,1}$ for each parameter p were tuned such that acceptance rates between 0.2 and 0.6 were observed. Initial values for the parameter α'_{Cy3} and the β's are found from the data using linear regression. Initial values for the variances of the random effects, for the $\ddot{J}$'s and the $\breve{K}$'s, are then computed from these estimates. In all these computations we substitute all random variables with their expectations. The parameters γ_0, γ, and the γ_i's are initialized such that for each gene i, the geometric mean of the success probabilities $p_s^{t,a}$ becomes 0.5. This is necessary to keep the model away from its Poisson approximation, which would not allow estimation of parameters only present in the variance. Finally, α is set equal to the geometric mean of

$$\left(J_s^{t,a} - c \cdot K_g^t \cdot p_s^{t,a}\right)^2 / \left(c \cdot K_g^t \cdot p_s^{t,a} \cdot (1 - p_s^{t,a})\right).$$

Convergence and mixing of the MCMC chain were assessed by comparing the results of three to six different runs and observing similar results. Details on the MCMC, such as the number of iterations, are reported on the TransCount Web site.

4.5 Validation

Validation of our model is described in detail in [11] on the basis of a spike experiment, where spikes are gene-like molecules of which the concentrations are known exactly. The validation experiment consists of 12 dye-swaps (24 arrays in total), where all dye-swaps contained the same reference material, but 12 different cervix tumor samples. The experiment was split in two parts on two different days; next, the hybridization scaling constant c (4.3) was determined for the first part and the model was fitted from data of the second part, using the estimate of the hybridization constant c. Indeed, we found a good agreement between the estimates and the true values. Moreover, an independent qRT-PCR validation was performed for eight genes covering the whole concentration range. It was shown that the absolute concentration estimates correlate very well with the qRT-PCR results, even better so than the ratios do.

4.6 Illustration

We illustrate the use of the full Bayesian approach to estimate posterior uncertainty of complex quantities. Our cDNA microarray slides were produced at the cDNA Microarray Facility at The Norwegian Radium Hospital. The probes were cDNA clones, representing named human genes or expressed sequence tags (ESTs). The example we describe here includes four microarrays. Spots at the same location on each of the four microarrays contain identical probe material and they are printed under the same conditions. Hence, these spots have equal values for the spot-related covariates in our model. Some probes were printed in duplicate with different pens, enabling estimation of a pen effect on the intensities. Moreover, some probes with different cDNA sequence represented the same genes, enabling the estimation of a probe length and probeID effect on the intensities. Finally, some probes with the same cDNA sequence, but with a slightly different amplification treatment, were duplicated at different positions on the microarray. These correspond to different values of $RID(s, a)$. A test slide of each printing series was stained with SYBR green to assess probe quantity. A small percentage of the spots corresponded to very low SYBR green intensities. SYBR green served as a covariate to predict success of hybridization.

Sample preparation, hybridization, and imaging. Total RNA was isolated from tumor tissues. Labeled cDNA was produced from 50 to 60 µg total RNA.

Table 4.1. *Design of Tumor Heterogeneity Study*

Microarray	Sample, dye Cy3	Sample, dye Cy5
1	Ref	A
2	A	B1
3	B1	B2
4	B2	Ref

The labeled samples were suspended in hybridization buffer and applied to the array slides. Three biopsies (A, B1, B2) and a reference (Ref) were considered. The study design is displayed in Table 4.1.

We have a loop design and a dye-swap for each sample. In this example we focus on 100 genes corresponding to 158 spots of each microarray. Of these 100 genes 27 genes are in duplicate with different probe sequences (PID), 31 genes are in duplicate with different replications of probe material (RID), and 42 genes are singles. The 100 genes were printed with five different pens. The probe lengths of these 100 genes were available. The four arrays were produced in batch and a SYBR green measurement was carried out for one of them. Since purity of the three samples was high and very similar among the three, it is not included in the model. This design is unbalanced. Our method can be equally used for larger data sets of thousands of genes and many samples, as shown in [11]. To provide concentrations, the estimated numbers of transcripts were related to the known weight of the total RNA. In this illustration experiment we did not calibrate estimates to represent actual absolute concentrations (see [11] for a discussion on this). Results presented here are hence correct up to a common constant factor.

In the imaging process a laser power of 100% was used. The PMT voltage was adjusted for the red and green channel individually to ensure that the intensity of the weakest spots and background segments was within the linear range of the scanner. Saturated spot intensities were corrected using the algorithm in [19]. The GenePix 3.0 image analysis software was used for spot segmentation and intensity calculation. Bad spots and regions with high unspecific binding of dye were manually flagged and excluded from the analysis. No normalization of the data was performed.

Results. Table 4.2 displays the concentration estimates for genes with rank 1, 10, 50, 90, and 100 when ranked according to the median posterior mode computed over the biopsies. We summarize the results of the parameter estimates in Table 4.3. For the random effect parameters, we only show the variance hyperparameters here. Complete tables containing all parameter estimates and their 95% credibility intervals may be found on the TransCount Web site.

Table 4.2. *Transcript Concentration Estimates* ($*10^6$)

Gene number and rank	Reference mode and credibility interval		Biopsy B1 mode and credibility interval		Biopsy B2 mode and credibility interval		Biopsy A mode and credibility interval	
16, 1	0.06	(0.03, 0.14)	0.04	(0.02, 0.13)	0.05	(0.02, 0.13)	0.05	(0.02, 0.13)
36, 5	0.06	(0.03, 0.16)	0.07	(0.03, 0.19)	0.02	(0.04, 0.22)	0.09	(0.043, 0.21)
95, 50	0.42	(0.25, 0.92)	0.27	(0.13, 0.52)	0.24	(0.16, 0.59)	0.35	(0.19, 0.66)
42, 90	2.25	(1.30, 5.40)	1.31	(0.62, 2.75)	1.60	(0.81, 3.25)	1.89	(1.05, 4.55)
49, 100	0.53	(0.27, 1.51)	9.24	(3.80, 20.5)	8.57	(4.23, 20.9)	6.46	(2.64, 14.8)

Table 4.3. *Parameter Estimates*

Parameter	Mode	95% credibility interval	Parameter	Mode	95% credibility interval
γ_0	−2.343	(2.614, −2.074)	σ_{PID}	0.599	(0.53, 0.702)
α	1.589	(1.195, 2.102)	σ_{RID}	0.556	(0.485, 0.61)
α'_{Cy3}	0.365	(0.355, 0.383)	σ_P	0.041	(0.011, 0.346)
β_2	−0.17	(−0.335, 0.036)	σ_A	0.34	(0.2, 1.031)
β_3	0.254	(0.106, 0.431)	σ_G	0.034	(0.011, 0.365)
σ	0.294	(0.269, 0.321)			

From Table 4.2 it is obvious that the information from absolute concentrations may be quite different from that of the ratios computed with respect to the reference. Besides the absolute concentrations, the estimated experimental parameters may also be of use, for example to understand critical parameters in the hybridization process and to improve protocols. Here, we observe that the probe length effect β_2 was negative meaning that probes with short length have a higher probability to retain molecules for imaging, after hybridization and washing. The positive sign and magnitude of β_3 imply that the SYBR green measurement is quite useful to incorporate and indeed large SYBR green values indicate a positive effect on hybridization.

We verified whether the results for the estimates per sample confirmed our prior expectation: expression profiles from biopsies B1 and B2 are expected to be more similar to each other than to expression profiles from biopsy A, since B1 and B2 were closer to each other in the tumor. The scale of the concentration estimates was very similar for all three biopsies. However, the correlation of estimated concentrations for B1 and B2 was as high as $\rho(B1, B2) = 0.993$, while

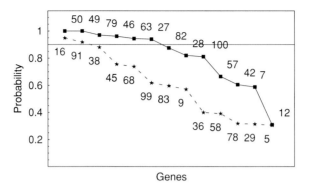

Fig. 4.1. Probabilities of genes to be among the 10 genes with the highest (solid) and lowest (dashed) mRNA concentrations.

the others were lower: $\rho(A, B1) = 0.912$ and $\rho(A, B2) = 0.928$. Moreover, all correlations with the estimates for the reference were much lower, for example, $\rho(B1, Ref) = 0.258$. Hence, the results were consistent with our prior expectations.

Potentials. We illustrate the potentials of our approach by considering specific issues. These problems are particularly hard to solve with standard methods, since their solution either requires knowledge of the joint distribution of gene expression values or the ability to estimate absolute concentrations (possibly up to a constant factor). They are solved using this approach. The gene numbers correspond to those in the complete tables on the Web site.

(1) We evaluated the probability that any single gene in turn had a mean concentration among the highest (or lowest) 10. We then ranked all genes according to this probability (Figure 4.1). There are six genes with probability larger than 0.90 to have mRNA concentration among the 10 highest, and two genes to have concentrations among the 10 lowest ones. The value of the success probability (here chosen as 0.90) should be as high as possible, but still such that enough genes are selected for the purpose of the study. Low concentrations are associated with more uncertainty than high ones, resulting in less candidate genes with low concentration. This ranking is independent of any reference sample.

Alternatively, we can summarize the same inference by plotting against n the probability of a gene being among the n highest (Figure 4.2). This involves a 100-dimensional integration of the posterior joint distribution performed with MCMC. The plots clearly indicate if a gene is among those with high (gene 46), intermediate (genes 13 and 33), or low (gene 91) concentration. The

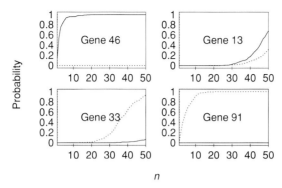

Fig. 4.2. Probability of four genes to be among the n genes with the highest (solid) or lowest (dashed) mRNA concentration.

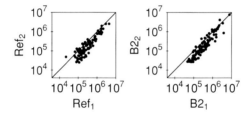

Fig. 4.3. Comparison of the absolute transcript levels in a reference and a human cervical tumor sample, estimated from two different experiments.

steepness of the curve describes the level of concentration of a gene compared to others.

(2) We investigated the potential for analysis of nontransitive designs and check reproducibility of our results by splitting the data into two sets of two arrays each: (Ref-B1, B1-B2) and (B2-A, A-Ref). We analyzed these separately, pretending samples were not shared. Figure 4.3 demonstrates the high reproducibility in our results. Estimated mRNA concentrations (number of mRNA molecules per microgram of total RNA; posterior modes) are plotted for each gene and sample. The two independently estimated concentrations Ref_1 and Ref_2 for the reference and $B2_1$ and $B2_2$ for sample B2 were similar and highly correlated. A small difference was observed for both samples, 0.188 in $\log_{10}$-scale for Ref and 0.231 for B2. This difference originated from the uncertainty in the estimation of γ_0, a difficult task with just two arrays. This similarity supports our claim that estimated numbers

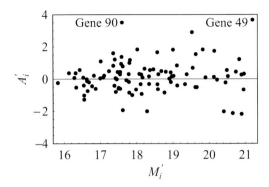

Fig. 4.4. Estimate-based MA plot.

of transcripts of different samples can be compared and combined, also when originating from separate experimental schemes, with a nontransitive design.

(3) We graphically combined fold with absolute concentration estimates (Figure 4.4). Gene selection methods based on either folds or absolute concentrations alone are simplistic: a ratio of 2 "means" something different when it is, say, 20,000/10,000 (both signals high) than when it is 20/10 (both signals low). The same holds for absolute concentrations: two absolute concentrations of 20,000 in tumor tissue have a different interpretation when their reference concentrations are, say, 5,000 and 15,000. We believe it is important to visualize both ratios and absolute concentrations simultaneously. In analogy to data-based $\log_2$-intensity and $\log_2$-ratio, define the estimate-based mean $\log_2$-intensity and mean $\log_2$-ratio as

$$M_i' = \left[\sum_{t=2}^{4} \log_2\left(\hat{K}_i^t * \hat{K}_i^1 \right)/2 \right] \bigg/ 3 \quad \text{and} \quad A_i' = \left[\sum_{t=2}^{4} \log_2\left(\frac{\hat{K}_i^t}{\hat{K}_i^1} \right) \right] \bigg/ 3,$$

where $\hat{K}_i^1$ refers to the estimated reference concentration, based on the mode of the MCMC trace, for gene i. Figure 4.4 displays M_i' versus A_i' for all 100 genes. This plot is an analogue to the well-known MA plot (which shows average $\log_2$-intensity versus $\log_2$-ratio for each array). We observe that gene 49 expresses roughly 12 times more than gene 90 in absolute sense. Therefore, one might, for example, conclude that gene 49 is more important than gene 90, although both correspond to an approximate mean $\log_2$ ratio equal to 3.5. Of course, for final gene selection one would need to take the uncertainties of the estimates into account as well.

4.7 TransCount Web Site and Computing Times

A C++ implementation of our model applied to the data in this chapter is available on `www.nr.no/pages/samba/area_emr_smbi_transcount2`.

The Web site also contains further information on how to run TransCount. The software and a demo data set is also available as a plug-in in BASE and may be downloaded together with a demo data set from the aforementioned Web site. We illustrated our approach on a small data set in terms of the number of spots and parameters. For this illustration data set, convergence was reached after a few hours. We are currently working on several solutions for speeding up the algorithm such as making the program suitable for parallel computing.

4.8 A Statistical Discussion of the Model

In this section, we concentrate on some statistical issues that may be of more general use than the context of this model. Our model is a complex variant of a simple Binomial(K, p) model with both K and p unknown. General methods to identify K and p together have been discussed in [9]. Moreover, the simple Binomial(K, p) model is studied in [4] in which K is the parameter of interest and p a nuisance parameter, using an integrated likelihood approach. In our case, γ_0, γ_i's, γ, and α are nuisance parameters and MCMC effectively integrates these out, to find the posterior distribution of K_i^t. Still, acknowledging that estimation of both binomial parameters is problematic, one may wonder why it works in our setting.

First of all, the scaling parameter c is important. It is crucial to use this typically small value in (4.3) to discriminate the binomial from the Poisson distribution. If c would not be introduced, it would be absorbed by p, which would become very small and the two distributions would become indistinguishable. In the validation study, c was determined by use of spikes, which are gene-like molecules of *known* concentration that undergo the same experiment as the genes.

Secondly, some of the covariates in the regression of p [in (4.4)] are shared by many genes, which allows for better estimation of their effect and hence also of p.

Thirdly, we assumed a $N(0, (\sigma_G)^2)$ prior for the gene-wise hybridization efficiency parameter γ_i (4.4), using one common variance parameter. Note that γ_i is difficult to estimate. However, use of this prior shrinks the γ_i estimates to the mean. The parameter γ_i describes the efficiency of hybridization for gene i independently of any other factor, including probe quantity. We can safely assume that hybridization efficiency is not very low for the majority of genes, so that we will obtain reasonably precise estimates of K_i^t for most genes; for those few genes that do correspond to low efficiencies, K_i^t is estimable due to this prior, but the estimates are (and should be) unprecise.

Finally, while the reference design is currently seen with scepticism, it is in fact very useful in the context of our full mechanistic parameterization. The large amount of data on the reference material in the validation study (at least 24 intensities per gene) is very useful for this model. The reason for this is that the reference material and the tumor tissues share most regression parameters, including the "difficult" γ_i, in equation (4.4). Since the reference intensities share the same K_i^1 for all genes, these parameters will adapt to the mean and variance of these 24 data points. This makes it easier to estimate K_i^t for $t \geq 2$.

We note that estimating parameters appearing only in the variance of a model requires the exclusion of nonrepeated single data pieces, which otherwise would reduce posterior uncertainty. It is easy to cope with such a situation in a two-step scheme, where the posterior of the first step becomes the prior in the second one.

The reparameterization as introduced in Section 4.3 may be of general use as a way to speed up convergence in a model where mean-related parameters are also present in the variance. It effectively separates the contribution to the variance of those parameters contributing also to the mean from those not contributing to the mean. It improves orthogonality of the joint posterior of the mean and variance parameters of $\tilde{J}_s^{t,a}$ in (4.7) with respect to those of $J_s^{t,a}$ in (4.5). In an MCMC setting, where parameters would be updated sequentially, this helps: suppose one temporarily fixes the means of the normals, then, when using parameterization (4.7) instead of (4.5), many parameters may be varied independently to fit the variance of the normal to the "data".

Our process-based model should be considered in the context of model validation. Each of the levels is motivated by interpretation of physical processes, which is a large advantage over conventional hierarchical Bayes modeling, where the levels are only vaguely connected with the system. Several levels of our model are validated by independent studies. First of all, the relationship between the observed intensity and the scanner settings (4.2) was extensively checked in [19]. The normality assumption for the within-spot variability described in (4.1) is easily checked and tested for and seemed reasonable in our data. The core of the process-based model, the binomial selection (4.3), is mainly based on the assumption that for the majority of genes the hybridization experiment is reasonably efficient (meaning $p \gg 0$). We indeed found that this was true for most genes. However, it may be useful to test it more extensively using spike data (known K_i^t), preferably under constant conditions to obtain true replicates. Note that binomial selection was used before for modeling gene expression data in [1]. We did not find large differences in the estimates for K_i^t between the use of censored log-link or logit-link (4.4), but a broader class of link functions could be tried and tested for, like in [8]. When a reasonable amount of replicates of K_i^t is available (at least for some genes), cross-validation techniques may be useful to validate results of the model as a whole. For example, one could test whether the credibility intervals for K_i^t are of correct size. Model validation techniques are extensively discussed in [13].

4.9 Discussion

We developed a process-based Bayesian model for a typical cDNA microarray experiment, which allows to estimate with sufficient precision absolute and relative mRNA concentrations. This allows a more precise assessment of differential gene expressions than usual normalization. Furthermore, as described in [11], the method does not require transitivity in the experimental design, and hence opens for the possible merging of data obtained without common reference. In addition, there is no need to impute missing values, since our method naturally copes with unbalanced designs. The hierarchical setting is very flexible and allows to introduce in the future deeper knowledge about the technology and biology. The process-based model allows to include a plausible mechanistic description of the experimental phenomena, making the global model more realistic and reliable. We make explicit use of available covariates and treat the unequal number of replicates per gene. This in turn allows to attribute backwards dependencies observed in the data to various experimental factors (experienced by molecules), while the rest is interpretable as biological dependency between the levels of transcripts for each gene. The model we have constructed is also useful as a cDNA microarray data simulator.

Extensions. The model can be improved by inclusion of more covariates. When available, hybridization settings like temperature, humidity, and ozone concentration could be included. Also, spatial related covariates (grids of the array) may improve the fit of the model. It is possible to include competition between target molecules in our model in terms of density dependence, for example by adding the term $\beta_7 K_{g(s,a)}^t$ to $p_s^{t,a}$ in (4.4). Then, we expect β_7 to be negative: the larger $K_{g(s,a)}^t$, the more competition and hence the smaller the probability to hybridize. However, inclusion of such a term seriously increases computing times of the MCMC. For the same reason, we did not implement a more advanced hybridization model, such as the Langmuir model in [15], describing the kinetics of the mRNA molecules in greater detail. Nevertheless, it is very interesting to find the value of β_7 (or the parameters in the Langmuir model) to infer what the impact of competition is, possibly using an experiment with few genes only to keep computing times manageable. The imaging and segmentation part of the model could also be extended, like in [12], possibly again with some efficiency loss. If non-(log)-linear dye-effects occur, for example in the low expression regions, this is probably due to the scanner. Therefore, such effects should be included in the calibration formula (4.2) if one wishes to include those genes.

Currently, we do not explicitly use the pixel-wise values, which are available for each spot. In fact, we only model the spot mean as a function of the absolute concentrations. The (spread of) pixel-wise values may give additional information on the binomial selection process. Note that under normality, modeling the spot mean and variance simultaneously would be sufficient.

It is also possible to make more explicit use of the spike information. Currently, we use it only to determine the scaling constant c in an off-line experiment. However, for example, a more informative prior on γ_i may be based on the estimated γ_i's for the spike experiment.

Addition of clinical levels. After obtaining the absolute concentrations, K_i^t, for all samples including the reference, an obvious task is to relate these to clinical data (testing, survival, group membership, effect of treatment over time, etc.). In principle, all types of analyses for ratio data may be applied to absolute concentrations. Which type of data is more useful may depend on the clinical issue at hand.

For example, clustering of genes may be more natural on absolute concentrations, because this is not biased by what happens for those genes in the reference material. We may now directly compare genes with another, which is potentially very useful for drug targeting. Note that statistical comparison of genes is conceptually not different from comparing samples for the same gene. As noted before (Figure 4.4) it may be interesting to combine the two measures of gene expression. One would then hope that there is more biologically relevant information in the pair (K_i^t, f_i^t) than there is in either of the two. For example, one can speculate that a classifier based on both ratios and absolute concentrations is more powerful and robust than one that is based on either of these gene expression measures, simply because ratios and absolute concentrations are different pieces of biological information. However, several hurdles need to be taken here, since the two quantities are obviously dependent and with twice as many variables the dimension problem becomes larger.

Acknowledgments

We thank Lars Holden and the editors for useful discussions and comments on the manuscript. Financial support was provided by The Norwegian Research Council, FUGE, the TMR-EU program "Computational and Spatial Statistics,"

The Norwegian Microarray Consortium, The Norwegian Radium Hospital, The Norwegian Cancer Society, and the Dutch BSIK/BRICKS consortium.

Bibliography

[1] Baggerly, K.A., K.R. Coombes, K.R. Hess, D.N. Stivers, L.V. Abruzzo, and W. Zhang (2001). Identifying differentially expressed genes in cDNA microarray experiments. *J. Comput. Biol.*, **8**, 639–659.

[2] Baldi, P., and A.D. Long (2001). A Bayesion framework for the analysis of microarray expression data: Regularized t-test and statistical inferences of gene changes. *Bioinformatics*, **17**, 509–519.

[3] Beaumont, M.A., and B. Rannala (2004). The Bayesian revolution in genetics. *Nat. Rev. Genet.*, **5**, 251–261.

[4] Berger, J.O., B. Liseo, and R.L. Wolpert (1999). Integrated likelihood methods for eliminating nuisance parameters. *Stat. Sci.*, **14**, 1–28.

[5] Broët, P., A. Lewin, S. Richardson, C. Dalmasso, and H. Magdelenat (2004). A mixture model-based strategy for selecting sets of genes in multiclass response microarray experiments. *Bioinformatics*, **20**, 2562–2571.

[6] Butte, A. (2002). The use and analysis of microarray data. *Nat. Rev. Drug Discov.*, **1**, 951–960.

[7] Churchill, G.A. (2002). Fundamentals of experimental design for cDNA microarrays. *Nat. Genet.*, **32**, 490–495.

[8] Czado, C., and A. Munk (2000). Noncanonical links in generalized linear models – When is the effort justified? *J. Statist. Plann. Inference*, **87**, 317–345.

[9] DasGupta, A., and H. Rubin (2005). Estimation of binomial parameters when both n, p are unknown. *J. Statist. Plann. Inference*, **130**(1–2), 391–404.

[10] Dudley, A.M., J. Aach, M.A. Steffen, and G.M. Church (2002). Measuring absolute expression with microarrays with calibrated reference sample and an extended signal intensity range. *Proc. Natl. Acad. Sci. U.S.A.*, **99**, 7554–7559.

[11] Frigessi, A., M.A. van de Wiel, M. Holden, I.K. Glad, D.H. Svendsrud, and H. Lyng (2005). Genome-wide estimation of transcript concentrations from spotted cDNA microarray data. *Nucleic Acids Res. – Methods Online*, **33**, e143.

[12] Gottardo, R., J.A. Pannucci, C.R. Kuske, and T. Brettin (2004). Statistical analysis of microarray data: A Bayesian approach. *Biostatistics*, **4**, 597–620.

[13] Hamilton, M.A. (1991). Model validation: An annotated bibliography. *Comm. Statist. Theory Methods*, **20**(7), 2207–2266.

[14] Hein, A.M.K., S. Richardson, H.C. Causton, G.K. Ambler, and P.J. Green (2005). BGX: A fully Bayesian integrated approach to the analysis of Affymetrix GeneChip data. *Biostatistics*, **6**, 349–373.

[15] Hekstra, D., A.R. Taussig, M. Magnasco, and F. Naef (2003). Absolute mRNA concentrations from sequence-specific calibration of oligonucleotide arrays. *Nucleic Acids Res.*, **31**, 1962–1968.

[16] Held, G.A., G. Grinstein, and Y. Tu (2003). Modeling of DNA microarray data by using physical properties of hybridization. *Proc. Natl. Acad. Sci.*, **100**, 7575–7580.

[17] Holloway, A.J., R.K. van Laar, R.W. Tothill, and D.D.L. Bowtell (2002). Options available – from start to finish – for obtaining data from DNA microarrays II. *Nat. Genet. Suppl.*, **32**, 481–489.

[18] Kerr, M.K., M. Martin, and G.A. Churchill (2000). Analysis of variance for gene expression microarray data. *J. Comput. Biol.*, **7**, 819–837.

[19] Lyng, H., A. Badiee, D.H. Svendsrud, E. Hovig, O. Myklebost, and T. Stokke (2004). Profound influence of non-linearity in microarray scanners on gene expression ratios: Analysis and procedure for correction. *BMC Genomics*, **5**, 10.

[20] Newton, M.A., C.M. Kendziorski, C.S. Richmond, F.R. Blattner, and K.W. Tsui (2001). On differential variability of expression ratios: Improving statistical inference about gene expression changes from microarray data. *J. Comput. Biol.*, **8**, 37–52.

[21] Quackenbush, J. (2002). Microarray data normalization and transformation. *Nat. Genet.*, **32**, 496–501.

[22] Smyth, G.K., Y.H. Yang, and T. Speed (2003). Statistical issues in cDNA Microarray data analysis. *Methods Mol. Biol.*, **224**, 111–136.

[23] Wang, Y., X. Wang, S.-W. Guo, and S. Ghosh (2002). Conditions to ensure competitive hybridization in two-color microarray: A theoretical and experimental analysis. *Biotechniques*, **32**, 1342–1346.

[24] Yang, Y.H., S. Dudoit, P. Luu, D. M. Lin, V. Peng, J. Ngai, and T.P. Speed (2002). Normalisation for cDNA microarray data: A robust composite method addressing single and multiple slide systematic variation. *Nucleic Acids Res.*, **30**(4), e15.

5

Identification of Biomarkers in Classification and Clustering of High-Throughput Data

MAHLET G. TADESSE
University of Pennsylvania

NAIJUN SHA
University of Texas at El Paso

SINAE KIM
University of Michigan

MARINA VANNUCCI
Texas A&M University

Abstract

Variable selection has been the focus of much research in recent years. In this chapter we review our contributions to the development of Bayesian methods for variable selection in problems that aim at either classifying or clustering samples. These methods are particularly relevant for the analysis of genomic studies, where high-throughput technologies allow thousands of variables to be measured on individual samples. We illustrate the methodologies using a DNA microarray data example.

5.1 Introduction

One of the major challenges in analyzing genomic data is their high-dimensionality. Such data comes with an enormous amount of variables, which is often substantially larger than the sample size. A typical example with this characteristic, and one that we use to illustrate our methodologies, is DNA microarray data. Commonly used approaches for analyzing gene expression data proceed in two steps. First, the dimension of the data is reduced either by assessing each gene one at a time and removing those that do not pass a certain threshold, or by using a dimension reduction technique such as principal component analysis. Then, in a second stage of the analysis, a statistical model is applied to the reduced data. A limitation of the univariate screening approach is that it does not assess the joint effect of multiple variables and could throw away potentially valuable markers, which are not significant individually but may be important in conjunction with other variables. With the dimension reduction techniques, one drawback is that the actual markers are not assessed, since principal components, for example, are linear combinations of all the original variables. The Bayesian methods reviewed here overcome these limitations and address the selection and prediction problems in a unified manner.

In high-throughput genomic and proteomic studies, there is often interest in identifying markers that discriminate between different groups of tissues. The distinct classes may correspond to different subtypes of a disease or to groups of patients who respond differently to treatment. The problem of locating relevant variables could arise in the context of a supervised or an unsupervised analysis. In the supervised setting, a training data is available in which the group membership of all samples is known. The goal of variable selection in this case is to locate sets of variables that relate to the prespecified groups, so that the class membership of future samples can be predicted accurately. In the unsupervised setting, instead, the samples' outcomes are not observed and the goal of the analysis is to identify variables with distinctive expression patterns while uncovering the latent classes. In statistics the supervised and unsupervised frameworks are respectively referred to as classification and clustering. The problem of variable selection is inherently different in the two settings and requires different modeling strategies.

The practical utility of variable selection is well recognized and this topic has been the focus of much research. Variable selection can help assess the importance of explanatory variables, improve prediction accuracy, provide a better understanding of the underlying mechanisms generating the data, and reduce the cost of measurement and storage for future data. A comprehensive account of widely used classical methods, such as stepwise regression with forward and backward selection, can be found in [18]. In recent years, procedures that specifically deal with very large number of variables have been proposed. One such approach is the least absolute shrinkage and selection operator (lasso) method of Tibshirani [29], which uses a penalized likelihood approach to shrink to zero coefficient estimates associated with unimportant covariates. For Bayesian variable selection methods, pioneering work in the univariate linear model setting was done by Leamer [16], Mitchell and Beauchamp [19], and George and McCulloch [12], and in the multivariate setting by Brown et al. [3]. The key idea of the Bayesian approach is to introduce a latent binary vector to index possible subsets of variables. This indicator is used to induce a mixture prior on the regression coefficients, and the variable selection is performed based on the posterior model probabilities.

Standard methods for classification include linear and quadratic discriminant analyses. When dealing with high-dimensional data, where the sample size n is smaller than the number p of variables, a dimension reduction step, such as partial least squares [21] or singular value decompositions [33], is often used. Methods that directly perform variable selection in classification, such as support vector machines [32] and the shrunken centroid approach [30], have also been developed in recent years. For cluster analysis, the most popular algorithms include k-means and hierarchical clustering, which group observations based on similarity or distance measures [13]. Model-based clustering methods, which view the data as coming from a mixture of probability distributions, offer an attractive alternative [17]. In this approach, a latent vector is introduced to identify the sample allocations and is estimated using the expectation–maximization algorithm [5] or Markov chain Monte Carlo (MCMC) techniques. Diebolt and Robert [6] present MCMC strategies when the number of mixture components is known. Richardson and Green [22] and Stephens [26] propose methods for handling finite mixture models with an unknown number of components. This general case can also be addressed via infinite mixture models that use Dirichlet process priors [2, 8]. A few procedures that combine the variable selection and clustering tasks have been proposed. For instance, Fowlkes et al. [9] use a forward selection approach in the context of hierarchical clustering. Recently, Friedman and Meulman [10] have proposed a hierarchical clustering procedure that uncovers cluster structure on separate subsets of variables.

In this chapter we review our work on Bayesian variable selection techniques for classification and clustering. In the classification setting, we build the variable selection procedure in a multinomial probit model and use the latent variable selection indicator to induce mixture priors on the regression coefficients. In the clustering setting, the group structure in the data is uncovered by specifying mixture models. We discuss both finite mixtures with an unknown number of components and infinite mixture models with Dirichlet process priors. The discriminating covariates are selected via a latent binary vector, which in this case indicates variables that define a mixture distribution for the data, versus those that favor a single multivariate distribution across all samples. In both classification and clustering settings, we specify conjugate priors and integrate out some of the parameters to accelerate the model fitting. We use MCMC techniques to identify the high probability models.

This chapter is organized as follows. In Section 5.2, we briefly review the Bayesian stochastic search variable selection method in the linear models setting. In Section 5.3, we describe extensions of this method to handle classification problems. We discuss variable selection in the context of clustering in Sections 5.4 and 5.5 by formulating the clustering problem respectively in terms of finite mixture models with an unknown number of components and infinite mixture models using Dirichlet process priors. We conclude the chapter in Section 5.6 with an application of the methods to a DNA microarray data set.

5.2 Bayesian Variable Selection in Linear Models

In the multivariate linear model setting an $n \times q$ continuous response $\boldsymbol{Y}$ is related to the $n \times p$ covariate matrix $\boldsymbol{X}$ via a model of the form

$$\boldsymbol{Y}_i = \boldsymbol{1}\alpha' + \boldsymbol{X}_i'\boldsymbol{B} + \boldsymbol{\varepsilon}, \quad \boldsymbol{\varepsilon} \sim \mathcal{N}(\boldsymbol{0}, \Sigma), \qquad i = 1, \ldots, n, \qquad (5.1)$$

where $\boldsymbol{B}$ is the $p \times q$ matrix of regression coefficients. Often, not all the covariates in $\boldsymbol{X}$ explain changes in $\boldsymbol{Y}$ and the goal is to identify the promising subset of predictors. For instance, in DNA microarray studies where thousands of variables (genes) are measured, a large number of them provide very little, if any, information about the outcome. This is a problem of variable selection. In the Bayesian framework, variable selection is accomplished by introducing a latent binary vector, $\boldsymbol{\gamma}$, which is used to induce mixture priors on the regression coefficients [3, 12]

$$\boldsymbol{B}_j \sim \gamma_j \mathcal{N}\left(0, \tau_j^2 \Sigma\right) + (1 - \gamma_j)\mathcal{I}_0, \qquad (5.2)$$

where $\boldsymbol{B}_j$ indicates the jth row of $\boldsymbol{B}$ and $\mathcal{I}_0$ is a vector of point masses at 0. If $\gamma_j = 1$, variable X_j is considered meaningful in explaining the outcome; if $\gamma_j = 0$, the corresponding vector of regression coefficients has a prior with point mass at 0 and variable X_j is therefore excluded from the model and deemed unimportant.

Suitable priors can be specified for $\boldsymbol{\gamma}$, the simplest choice being independent Bernoulli priors

$$p(\boldsymbol{\gamma}) = \prod_{j=1}^{p} \theta^{\gamma_j}(1 - \theta)^{1 - \gamma_j}, \qquad (5.3)$$

where $\theta = p_{\text{prior}}/p$ and p_{prior} is the number of variables expected a priori to be included in the model. This prior can be relaxed, for example, by putting a beta distribution on θ. Conjugate normal- and inverse-Wishart priors can be specified for the parameters $\boldsymbol{B}$ and Σ, respectively.

For posterior inference, fast and efficient MCMC can be implemented by integrating out $\boldsymbol{B}$ and Σ, so that $\boldsymbol{\gamma}$ becomes the only parameter that needs to be updated. Posterior samples for $\boldsymbol{\gamma}$ can be obtained via Gibbs sampling or a Metropolis algorithm. For instance, the latent vector can be updated using a

Metropolis algorithm that generates at each iteration a new candidate γ^{new} by randomly choosing one of these transition moves:

(i) Add/Delete: Randomly pick one of the indices in γ^{old} and change its value.
(ii) Swap: Draw independently and at random a 0 and a 1 in γ^{old} and switch their values.

The new candidate is accepted with probability

$$\min\left\{1, \frac{f(\gamma^{\text{new}}|\boldsymbol{Y}, \boldsymbol{X})}{f(\gamma^{\text{old}}|\boldsymbol{Y}, \boldsymbol{X})}\right\}. \tag{5.4}$$

The MCMC procedure results in a list of visited models, $\gamma^{(0)}, \ldots, \gamma^{(T)}$ and their corresponding posterior probabilities. Posterior inference for selecting variables can then be based on the γ vectors with largest posterior probabilities among the visited models, that is,

$$\hat{\gamma} = \underset{1 \leq t \leq T}{\operatorname{argmax}} \, p(\gamma^{(t)}|\boldsymbol{Y}, \boldsymbol{X}). \tag{5.5}$$

Alternatively, one can estimate marginal posterior probabilities for inclusion of each γ_j by

$$p(\gamma_j = 1|\boldsymbol{X}, \boldsymbol{Y}) \approx \sum_{t:\gamma_j=1} p(\boldsymbol{Y}|\boldsymbol{X}, \gamma^{(t)}) p(\gamma^{(t)}) \tag{5.6}$$

and choose those γ_j's with marginals exceeding an arbitrary cutoff. As for prediction of future observations, this can be achieved via least squares prediction based on a single "best" model or using Bayesian model averaging, which accounts for the uncertainty in the selection process by averaging over a set of a posteriori likely models to estimate $\boldsymbol{Y}_f$ as

$$\widehat{\boldsymbol{Y}}_f = \sum_{\gamma} \left(\boldsymbol{1}\tilde{\alpha}' + \boldsymbol{X}_{f(\gamma)}\tilde{\boldsymbol{B}}_{(\gamma)}\right) p(\gamma|\boldsymbol{Y}, \boldsymbol{X}), \tag{5.7}$$

where $\boldsymbol{X}_{f(\gamma)}$ consists of the covariates selected by γ, $\tilde{\alpha} = \bar{\boldsymbol{Y}}$, $\tilde{\boldsymbol{B}}_\gamma = (\boldsymbol{X}_{\gamma'}\boldsymbol{X}_\gamma + \boldsymbol{H}_\gamma^{-1})^{-1}\boldsymbol{X}_{\gamma'}\boldsymbol{Y}$ and $\boldsymbol{H}$ is the prior row covariance matrix of $\boldsymbol{B}$.

5.3 Bayesian Variable Selection in Classification

In classification, the observed outcome is a categorical variable that takes one of K values identifying the group from which each sample arises. A multinomial probit model can be used to link the categorical outcome $\boldsymbol{Z}$ to the linear predictors $\boldsymbol{X}$ by using a data augmentation approach, as in [1]. This approach introduces a latent matrix $\boldsymbol{Y}_{n\times(K-1)}$ where the row vector $\boldsymbol{Y}_i = (y_{i,1}, \ldots, y_{i,K-1})$ indicates the propensities of sample i to belong to one of the

K classes. A correspondence between the categorical outcome Z_i and the latent continuous outcome $\boldsymbol{Y}_i$ is defined by

$$
z_i = \begin{cases} 0 & \text{if } \max_{1 \le k \le K-1} \{y_{i,k}\} \le 0 \\ j & \text{if } \max_{1 \le k \le K-1} \{y_{i,k}\} > 0 \text{ and } y_{i,j} = \max_{1 \le k \le K-1} \{y_{i,k}\}. \end{cases} \tag{5.8}
$$

Here we view the first category as a "baseline." The data augmentation allows us to express the classification problem as a multivariate regression model of the form (5.1), in terms of the latent continuous outcome $\boldsymbol{Y}$.

If Z is an ordered categorical outcome, such as the stage of a tumor, we account for the ordering by introducing a latent continuous vector Y and modifying the correspondence between y_i and z_i to

$$
z_i = j \quad \text{if } \delta_j < y_i \le \delta_{j+1}, \quad j = 0, \ldots, K-1, \tag{5.9}
$$

where the boundaries δ_j are unknown and $-\infty = \delta_0 < \delta_1 < \cdots < \delta_{K-1} < \delta_K = \infty$. In this case the classification problem reduces to a linear regression model that is univariate in the response.

Bayesian variable selection can then be implemented for these models as described in Section 5.2 by introducing a latent binary vector $\boldsymbol{\gamma}$ that induces mixture priors on the regression coefficients and using MCMC techniques to explore the posterior space of variable subsets. The model fitting in the classification setting, however, is a bit more intricate because the regression model is defined in terms of latent outcomes. The MCMC procedure needs to account for this and includes a step that updates the latent values $\boldsymbol{Y}$ from their full conditionals. For classification into nominal categories, $\boldsymbol{Y}|(\boldsymbol{\gamma}, \boldsymbol{X}, \boldsymbol{Z})$ follows a truncated matrix-variate t-distribution. For ordered classes, $\boldsymbol{Y}|(\boldsymbol{\gamma}, \boldsymbol{X}, \boldsymbol{Z})$ follows a multivariate truncated normal distribution and we also need to update the boundary parameters δ_j from their posterior densities, which are uniform on the interval

$$
\left[\max\{\max\{Y_i : Z_i = j - 1\}, \delta_{j-1}\}, \min\{\min\{Y_i : Z_i = j\}, \delta_{j+1}\} \right]
$$

with $j = 1, \ldots, K - 1$. The variable selection indicator $\boldsymbol{\gamma}$ is updated using a Metropolis algorithm as discussed in the previous section.

Posterior inference for the discriminating variables can be based on the joint posterior probability of the vector $\boldsymbol{\gamma}$ or the marginal posterior probabilities of the γ_j's, as described in Section 5.2. The class membership for future samples can be predicted by estimating their latent outcomes, $\boldsymbol{Y}_f$, then using the correspondence defined between $\boldsymbol{Y}$ and $\boldsymbol{Z}$. The details of the method and its implementation along with applications to DNA microarray data from arthritis studies can be found in Sha et al. [24, 25]. In Sha et al. [24], markers were identified for the classification of two forms of arthritis, rheumatoid arthritis (RA) and osteoarthritis (OA), which have a similar clinical endpoint but different underlying molecular mechanisms. Because of the inflammatory component that characterizes RA, the discrimination between established RA and OA represents an ideal scenario to assess the significance of classification methods. The study aimed at selecting the genes that best characterize the different classes. In Sha et al. [25], the methodology was applied to the identification of molecular signatures predictive of different stages of RA. The goal was to understand how the immune cells in the peripheral blood modify their molecular profiles with the progression of the disease. The small subset of genes identified led to good classification results. In addition, some of the selected genes were clearly correlated with known aspects of the biology of arthritis.

5.4 Bayesian Variable Selection in Clustering via Finite Mixture Models

In recent years, there has been an increased interest in using DNA microarray technologies to uncover disease subtypes and identify discriminating genes. There is a consensus that the existing disease classes for various malignancies are too broad and need to be refined. Indeed, patients receiving the same diagnosis often follow significantly different clinical courses and respond differently to therapy. It is believed that gene expression profiles can capture disease heterogeneities better than currently used clinical and morphological diagnostics. The goal is to identify a subset of genes whose expression profiles can help stratify samples into more homogeneous groups. This is a problem of variable selection in the context of clustering samples.

From a statistical point of view, this is a more complicated problem than variable selection for linear models or classification, where the outcomes are observed. In clustering, the discriminating genes need to be selected and the different classes need to be uncovered simultaneously. The appropriate statistical approach therefore must identify genes with distinctive expression patterns, estimate the number of clusters and allocate samples to the different uncovered classes. We have proposed model-based methodologies that provide a unified approach to this problem. In Tadesse et al. [28] we formulate the clustering problem in terms of finite mixture models with an unknown number of components and use a reversible jump MCMC technique to allow creation and deletion of clusters. In Kim et al. [15] we propose an alternative approach that uses infinite mixture models with Dirichlet process priors. In both models, for the variable selection we introduce a latent binary vector γ and use stochastic search MCMC techniques to explore the space of variable subsets. The definition of this latent indicator and its inclusion into the models, however, are inherently different from the regression settings. In this section we present the method under the finite mixture models formulation, and describe the approach using infinite mixture models in the subsequent section.

5.4.1 Model

In model-based clustering, the data are viewed as coming from a mixture of distributions:

$$f(\boldsymbol{x}_i|\boldsymbol{w}, \boldsymbol{\phi}) = \sum_{k=1}^{K} w_k f(\boldsymbol{x}_i|\boldsymbol{\phi}_k), \tag{5.10}$$

where $f(\boldsymbol{x}_i|\boldsymbol{\phi}_k)$ is the density of sample $\boldsymbol{x}_i$ from group k and $\boldsymbol{w} = (w_1, \ldots, w_K)^T$ are the cluster weights ($\sum_k w_k = 1$, $w_k \geq 0$) [17]. We assume that K is finite but unknown. In order to identify the cluster from which each observation is drawn, we introduce latent variables $\boldsymbol{c} = (c_1, \ldots, c_n)^T$, where $c_i = k$ if the ith sample comes from group k. The sample allocations c_i are assumed to be independently and identically distributed with probability mass function $p(c_i = k) = w_k$. We assume that the mixture distributions are multivariate normal with component parameters $\boldsymbol{\phi}_k = (\boldsymbol{\mu}_k, \boldsymbol{\Sigma}_k)$. Thus, for sample i, we have

$$\boldsymbol{x}_i|c_i = k, \boldsymbol{w}, \boldsymbol{\phi} \sim \mathcal{N}(\boldsymbol{\mu}_k, \boldsymbol{\Sigma}_k). \tag{5.11}$$

When dealing with high-dimensional data, it is often the case that a large number of collected variables provide no information about the group structure of the observations. The inclusion of too many unnecessary variables in the model could mask the true grouping of the samples. The discriminating variables therefore need to be identified in order to successfully uncover the clusters. For this, we introduce a latent binary vector $\boldsymbol{\gamma}$ to identify relevant variables

$$\begin{cases} \gamma_j = 1 & \text{if variable } j \text{ defines a mixture distribution,} \\ \gamma_j = 0 & \text{otherwise.} \end{cases} \tag{5.12}$$

In particular, $\boldsymbol{\gamma}$ is used to index the contribution of the variables to the likelihood. The set of variables indexed by a $\gamma_j = 1$, denoted $\mathbf{X}_{(\gamma)}$, define the mixture distribution, while the variables indexed by $\gamma_j = 0$, $\mathbf{X}_{(\gamma^c)}$, favor one multivariate normal distribution across all samples. The distribution of sample i is then given by

$$\boldsymbol{x}_{i(\gamma)}|c_i = k, \boldsymbol{w}, \boldsymbol{\phi}, \boldsymbol{\gamma} \sim \mathcal{N}(\boldsymbol{\mu}_{k(\gamma)}, \boldsymbol{\Sigma}_{k(\gamma)})$$
$$\boldsymbol{x}_{i(\gamma^c)}|\boldsymbol{\psi}, \boldsymbol{\gamma} \sim \mathcal{N}(\boldsymbol{\eta}_{(\gamma^c)}, \boldsymbol{\Omega}_{(\gamma^c)}), \tag{5.13}$$

where $\boldsymbol{\psi} = (\boldsymbol{\eta}, \boldsymbol{\Omega})$. Notice that the use of the variable selection indicator here is different from the linear model context, where $\boldsymbol{\gamma}$ was used to induce mixture priors on the regression coefficients. In clustering, the outcome is not observed and the elements of the matrix $\mathbf{X}$ are viewed as random variables.

5.4.2 Prior Setting

The elements of $\boldsymbol{\gamma}$ can be taken to be independent Bernoulli random variables. For the vector of component weights, we specify a symmetric Dirichlet prior. We assume that the number of components, K, is unknown and choose a truncated Poisson or a discrete Uniform prior on $[1, \ldots, K_{\max}]$, where $K_{\max}$ is chosen arbitrarily large. As $\boldsymbol{\gamma}$ gets updated, the dimensions of the model parameters $\boldsymbol{\phi}_{k(\gamma)} = (\boldsymbol{\mu}_{k(\gamma)}, \boldsymbol{\Sigma}_{k(\gamma)})$ and $\boldsymbol{\psi}_{(\gamma^c)} = (\boldsymbol{\eta}_{(\gamma^c)}, \boldsymbol{\Omega}_{(\gamma^c)})$ change. Posterior inference on these parameters therefore requires a sampler that moves between different dimensional spaces. An efficient sampler can be implemented by working with a marginalized likelihood where these model parameters are integrated out. The integration is facilitated by taking conjugate normal-Wishart priors on both $\boldsymbol{\phi}$ and $\boldsymbol{\psi}$. Some care is needed in the choice of the hyperparameters. In particular, the variance parameters need to be specified within the range of variability of the data. An extensive discussion on the prior specification and the MCMC procedure can be found in [28].

5.4.3 MCMC Implementation

The MCMC procedure iterates the following steps:

(i) Update $\boldsymbol{\gamma}$ using a Metropolis algorithm. The transition moves described in Section 5.2 for the linear setting can be used.
(ii) Update the component weights, $\boldsymbol{w}$, from their full conditionals.
(iii) Update the sample allocation vector, $\boldsymbol{c}$, from its full conditional.
(iv) Split/merge moves to create/delete clusters. We make a random choice between attempting to divide or combine clusters. The number of components may therefore increase or decrease by 1, and the necessary corresponding changes need to be made for the sample allocations and the component parameters. These moves require a sampler that jumps between different dimensional spaces, which is not a trivial task in the multivariate setting.
(v) Birth/death of empty components.

The MCMC output can then be used to draw posterior inference for the sample allocations and the variable selection. Posterior inference for the cluster structure is complicated by the varying number of components. A simple approach for estimating the most probable cluster structure $\boldsymbol{c}$ is to use the maximum a posteriori (MAP) configuration, which corresponds to the vector with highest conditional posterior probability among those visited by the MCMC sampler. An alternative is to estimate the number of clusters, K, by the value most frequently visited by the MCMC sampler and then draw inference conditional on $\widehat{K}$. With this approach, we first need to address the label switching problem using for instance Stephens' relabeling algorithm [27]. The sample allocation vector, c, can then be estimated by the mode of the marginal posterior probabilities given by

$$\hat{c}_i = \underset{1 \leq k \leq K}{\operatorname{argmax}}\{p(c_i = k|\boldsymbol{X}, \widehat{K})\}. \tag{5.14}$$

Several other inferential approaches are possible. An alternative estimator, for example, is the one proposed by Dahl [4], which relies on the posterior pairwise probabilities of allocating samples to the same cluster.

For the variable selection, inference can be based on the $\boldsymbol{\gamma}$ vectors with highest posterior probability among the visited models or on the γ_j's with largest marginal posterior probabilities.

5.5 Bayesian Variable Selection in Clustering via Dirichlet Process Mixture Models

Dirichlet process mixture (DPM) models have gained a lot of popularity in nonparametric Bayesian analysis and have particularly been successful in cluster analysis. Samples from a Dirichlet process are discrete with probability 1 and can therefore produce a number of ties, that is, form clusters.

A general DPM model is written as

$$\boldsymbol{x}_i|\boldsymbol{\theta}_i \sim F(\boldsymbol{\theta}_i)$$
$$\boldsymbol{\theta}_i|G \sim G \tag{5.15}$$
$$G \sim DP(G_0, \alpha),$$

where $\boldsymbol{\theta}$ is a vector of sample-specific parameters and DP is the Dirichlet process with concentration parameter α and base distribution G_0. Due to properties of the Dirichlet process, some of the $\boldsymbol{\theta}_i$'s will be identical and can be set to $\boldsymbol{\theta}_i = \boldsymbol{\phi}_{c_i}$, where c_i represents the latent class associated with sample i [2, 8].

5.5.1 Dirichlet Process Mixture Models

Mixture distributions with a countably infinite number of components can be defined in terms of finite mixture models by taking the limit as the number of components K goes to infinity

$$\boldsymbol{x}_i | c_i = k, \boldsymbol{\phi} \sim F(\boldsymbol{\phi}_k)$$
$$c_i | \boldsymbol{w} \sim \text{Discrete}(w_1, \ldots, w_K)$$
$$\boldsymbol{\phi}_k \sim G_0 \qquad (5.16)$$
$$\boldsymbol{w} \sim \text{Dirichlet}(\alpha/K, \ldots, \alpha/K).$$

As shown in [20], integrating over the mixing proportions $\boldsymbol{w}$ and letting K go to infinity leads to the following priors for the sample allocations:

$$p(c_i = c_l \text{ for some } l \neq i | \boldsymbol{c}_{-i}) = \frac{n_{-i,k}}{n - 1 + \alpha}$$
$$p(c_i \neq c_l \text{ for all } l \neq i | \boldsymbol{c}_{-i}) = \frac{\alpha}{n - 1 + \alpha}, \qquad (5.17)$$

where $\boldsymbol{c}_{-i}$ is the allocation vector $\boldsymbol{c}$ without the ith element and $n_{-i,k}$ is the number of $c_l = k$ for $l \neq i$. Thus, sample i is assigned to an existing cluster with probability proportional to the cluster size and it is allocated to a new cluster with probability proportional to α. As in the finite mixture case, we assume that samples in group k arise from a multivariate normal distribution with component parameters $\boldsymbol{\phi}_k = (\boldsymbol{\mu}_k, \boldsymbol{\Sigma}_k)$ and we use the latent indicator $\boldsymbol{\gamma}$ to identify discriminating variables as in (5.12).

5.5.2 Prior Setting and MCMC Implementation

We are interested in estimating the variable selection vector $\boldsymbol{\gamma}$ and the sample allocation vector $\boldsymbol{c}$. As in the finite mixture setting of Section 5.4, the other model parameters can be integrated out from the likelihood leading to a more efficient MCMC algorithm. We specify conjugate priors for the component parameters and take Bernoulli priors for the elements of $\boldsymbol{\gamma}$.

The variable selection indicator $\boldsymbol{\gamma}$ and the cluster allocation vector $\boldsymbol{c}$ are updated using the following MCMC steps:

(i) Update $\boldsymbol{\gamma}$ using a Metropolis algorithm.
(ii) Update $\boldsymbol{c}$ via Gibbs sampling using the following conditional posterior probabilities to assign each sample to an existing cluster or to a newly created one:

$$p(c_i = c_j \text{ for } l \neq i | \boldsymbol{c}_{-i}, \boldsymbol{x}_i, \gamma) \propto \frac{n_{-i,k}}{n - 1 + \alpha} \int F(\boldsymbol{x}_i; \boldsymbol{\phi}_{k(\gamma)}) \, dH_{-i,k}(\boldsymbol{\phi}_{k(\gamma)})$$
$$p(c_i \neq c_j \text{ for } l \neq i | \boldsymbol{c}_{-i}, \boldsymbol{x}_i, \gamma) \propto \frac{\alpha}{n - 1 + \alpha} \int F(\boldsymbol{x}_i; \boldsymbol{\phi}_{k(\gamma)}) \, dG_0(\boldsymbol{\phi}_{k(\gamma)}),$$

$$(5.18)$$

where $H_{-i,k}$ is the posterior distribution of $\boldsymbol{\phi}$ based on the prior G_0 and all observations $\boldsymbol{x}_l$ for which $l \neq i$ and $c_l = k$.

At each MCMC iteration, the number of clusters may decrease as components become empty, it may remain the same with possible changes in the sample allocations, or it may increase if new clusters are formed. The Gibbs sampler often exhibits poor mixing when dealing with mixture models. This can be improved by combining the MCMC algorithm with a split-merge method that essentially avoids local modes by separating or combining groups of observations based on a Metropolis–Hastings algorithm (see, for example, [14]). In addition, parallel tempering can be used to further improve the performance of the sampler. Details on the MCMC implementation can be found in [15].

Inference on the cluster structure and on the selected variables is performed using the MCMC output, similarly to what discussed in Section 5.4. In particular, the allocation vector $\boldsymbol{c}$ can be estimated by the MAP configuration, after removing the label switching, or it can be based on the posterior pairwise probabilities $p(c_i = c_j | \mathbf{X})$. For the variable selection vector $\boldsymbol{\gamma}$, inference can be drawn based on the vector with highest posterior probability or the elements γ_j with largest marginal posterior probabilities.

5.6 Example: Leukemia Gene Expression Data

We illustrate the variable selection methods both in the classification and the clustering settings using the widely analyzed leukemia microarray data of Golub et al. [11]. The data consists of 38 bone marrow samples collected from patients with two types of leukemia: 27 with acute lymphoblastic leukemia (ALL) and 11 with acute myeloid leukemia (AML). An independent data set of 24 ALL and 10 AML samples is also available for validation.

We pre processed the data following other investigators who have analyzed this particular data set (see, for example, [7]). The expression measures were truncated at 100 and 16,000, and probe sets with maximum and minimum intensities across samples such that max/min$\leq$ 5 or max$-$min$\leq$ 500 were excluded. This left 3,571 genes for analysis. The expression levels were then log-transformed and normalized across genes.

5.6.1 Illustration in a Classification Setting

We applied our multinomial probit model with $K = 2$. We chose Bernoulli priors for the variable selection indicators γ_j with the expected number of discriminating genes set to 5. We took normal and inverse-Wishart

Table 5.1. *Classification Results: GenBank Accession*
Numbers and Names of 20 Selected Genes

AccNum	Name
M27891	CST3 Cystatin C
Y00787	Interleukin-8 precursor
M28130	Interleukin-8 (IL8) gene
M84526	DF D component of complement (adipsin)
D88422	Cystatin A
X95735	Zyxin
M27783	ELA2 Elastatse 2, neutrophil
M96326	Azurocidin gene
M19507	MPO Myeloperoxidase
M57731	GRO2 oncogene
U46499	Glutathione S-transferase, microsomal
U05259	MB-1 gene
X82240	TCL1 gene (T-cell leukemia)
M57710	LGALS3 Lectin, galactoside-binding
M11722	Terminal transferase mRNA
J04615	SNRPN small nuclear ribonucleoprotein polypeptide N
U22376	C-myb gene extracted from human (c-myb) gene
Z69881	Adenosine triphosphatase, calcium
U02020	Pre-B cell enhancing factor (PBEF) mRNA
M63438	GLUL Glutamate-ammonia ligase (glutamine synthase)

priors for the parameters B and Σ in the regression model. See [25] for more insight on the choice of the hyperparameters. Nine MCMC chains with different starting γ vectors were run for 200,000 iterations each. We allowed ample burn-in time by discarding the first 100,000 iterations. Inference was done by pulling together the outcomes from the nine chains. We used marginal probabilities to locate sets of genes that can be of interest for further investigation by selecting genes with marginal posterior probabilities greater than a threshold. Interesting gene subsets can also be found by considering the models with highest posterior probabilities among those visited by the MCMC samplers. Table 5.1 lists the 20 genes selected at a threshold of .001 in decreasing order of their marginal posterior probabilities. These genes were also included in the 20 models with highest probabilities among those from the pooled output.

We assessed the predictive performance of the selected genes on the independent test data. The least squares prediction based on the single model with highest posterior probability misclassified 5/34 samples, while the prediction based on the 20 genes selected above led to a misclassification error of 2/34. These

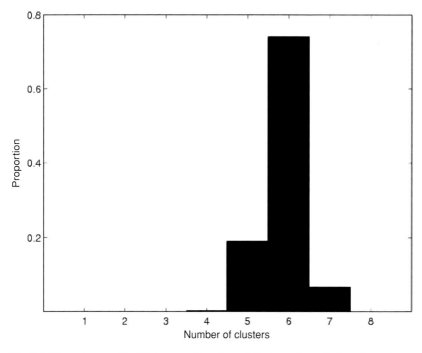

Fig. 5.1. Clustering results: Histogram of number of clusters of sampled configurations.

two misclassified samples are the same ones reported in [7] and [11] as difficult cases. In general, we noticed that good prediction can be obtained with one or two genes. For example, the model with adipsin alone gave a 1/34 misclassification error rate and cystatin alone misclassified 2 out of the 34 test samples.

5.6.2 Illustration in a Clustering Setting

We now exemplify the method for variable selection in the context of clustering using the DPM model formulation of Section 5.5. We assume that the leukemia subtypes for the 38 patients in the training data are not known and we try to cluster the samples into homogeneous groups. Thus, the goal is to uncover potential subclasses within the broadly defined leukemia group and simultaneously identify the discriminating genes.

We specified priors for the model parameters and chose the hyperparameters following the guidelines of Section 5.5. We assumed the gene selection indicators γ_j to be Bernoulli random variables and set the prior expected number of discriminating genes to 20. We ran several MCMC chains with different initial models for 200,000 iterations and used the first 100,000 as burn-in. Figure 5.1

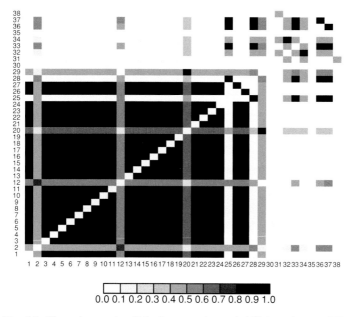

Fig. 5.2. Clustering results: Pairwise posterior probabilities $p(c_i = c_j | X)$.

shows an histogram of the number of clusters of the sampled configurations for one of the chains, after burn-in. We note that the sampler visits models with four to seven clusters. The sample allocation estimates based on the various approaches presented in Section 5.5 gave similar results. Figure 5.2 shows a heatmap of the pairwise posterior probabilities $p(c_i = c_j | X)$ that two samples are assigned to the same group. We note that the ALL patients were all, except for one sample, allocated to the same cluster with high posterior probabilities. The AML patients, on the other hand, exhibit less homogeneity. Thus, we were able to successfully separate the ALL and AML patients, and the results seem to suggest that there may be potential subtypes among the AML group.

As for the selected genes, we report some of them in Table 5.2. Several are known to be implicated with the differentiation and progression of leukemia cells. For example, caveolin-1 (CAV1), which is believed to be a useful marker for adult T-cell leukemia diagnosis, was selected. The model also picked the Charcot-Leyden crystal protein (CLC), which is involved in the differentiation of myeloid cell differentiation into specific lineages and is found to be downregulated in AML patients with high white blood cell count. Another interesting gene that was picked is the myeloid cell nuclear differentiation antigen (MNDA), which is correlated with myeloid and monocytic differentiation of acute leukemia but is absent in ALL.

Table 5.2. *Clustering Results: Some Selected Genes with
Known Association to Leukemia*

Gene	Description
AR	The amphiregulin gene is localized in chromosomal region 4q13-4q21, a common breakpoint for ALL.
CA2	Expressed in most patients with leukemic blast cells.
CAV1	Hematological cells express caveolin-1 in certain states of cell activation and are believed to be a useful marker for adult T-cell leukemia diagnosis.
CD14 antigen	Maps to a region of chromosome 5 that contains a cluster of genes encoding several myeloid-specific growth factors and frequently deleted in certain myeloid leukemias.
CLC	Believed to be associated with myeloid cell differentiation into specific lineage leukemias and found to be significantly down-regulated in AML patients with high white blood cell count.
CSTA	Cystein protease inhibitor that induces apoptosis of leukemia cells.
ELA2	Elastase 2 cleaves the fusion protein generated by the translocation associated with promyelocytic leukemia.
ID4	Putative tumor suppressor silenced by promoter methylation in the majority of human leukemias.
IL6 & IL8	These cytokines are elevated in activated T cells in large granular lymphocytic leukemia.
LTF	Lactoferrin can transactivate human T-cell leukemia virus type I, which causes adult T-cell leukemia and lymphoma.
MNDA	Correlated with myeloid and monocytic differentiation of acute leukemia, and expressed in M3 type leukemia but absent in ALL.
MT1G	The metalloprothionein gene cluster is mapped to 16p22, a breakpoint found in a subgroup of patients with AML.
PRAME	Expressed in acute leukemia samples, with highest association in AML tumors carrying t(8;21) or t(15;17) chromosomal abnormalities that have a relatively favorable prognosis.
THBS1	Methylation of THBS1 is associated with the absence of the Philadelphia chromosome and a favorable prognosis for ALL patients.
TRAIL	Induces apostolic cell death in most chronic myelogenous and acute leukemia derived Ph1-positive cell lines.

Among the selected genes, some were common to both the classification and clustering settings and have known association with leukemia. For instance, interleukin-8, which was identified in both cases, is a chemokine released in response to an inflammatory stimulus and is elevated in activated T cells in large granular lymphocytic leukemia. Cystatin A (CSTA), a cystein protease inhibitor that induces apoptosis of leukemia cells, and elastase 2, which cleaves the fusion protein generated by the translocation associated with promyeloctytic leukemia, were also found to discriminate leukemia subtypes in both models.

5.7 Conclusion

Bayesian variable selection techniques are well suited for the analysis of high-dimensional data. In this chapter, we have described methods to integrate the variable selection task into models for classification and clustering. The latter is a more complicated problem since the class discovery and gene selection are performed simultaneously. The methodologies were briefly illustrated on a DNA microarray data example.

The Bayesian approaches we have described offer a coherent framework in which variable selection and clustering or classification of the samples are performed simultaneously. Bayesian variable selection techniques can cope with a large number of regressors and have the flexibility of allowing the number of variables to exceed the number of observations. In addition, these methods allow the evaluation of the joint effect of sets of variables and the use of stochastic search techniques to explore the high-dimensional variable space. They provide joint posterior probabilities of sets of variables, as well as marginal posterior probabilities for the inclusion of single variables.

The methods we have described are not restricted to microarray data. Vannucci et al. [31], for example, describe adaptations of Bayesian variable selection methods for classification to the case of functional predictors. One of the applications discussed by the authors is to studies that involve proteomic mass-spectra. There the authors employ wavelet transforms as a tool for dimension reduction and noise removal, reducing spectra to wavelet components. The Bayesian variable selection mechanism built into the model allows the selection of those coefficients describing the discriminating features of the spectra.

Current developments of the Bayesian techniques we have described include extensions to the analysis of censored survival data. In Sha et al. [23] we propose a Bayesian variable selection approach for accelerated failure time (AFT) models under various error distributional assumptions. We use a data augmentation approach to impute the failure times of censored observations and mixture priors to perform variable selection. When applied to microarray data the proposed approach identifies relevant genes and provides a prediction of the survivor function.

Acknowledgments

Sha, Tadesse, and Vannucci are supported by NIH/NHGRI grant R01HG003319. Sha is also partially supported by BBRC/RCMI NIH grant 2G12RR08124 and Vannucci by NSF CAREER award DMS-0093208.

Bibliography

[1] Albert, J.H. and Chib, S. (1993) Bayesian analysis of binary and polychotomous response data, *Journal of the American Statistical Association*, **88**, 669–679.

[2] Antoniak, C.E. (1974) Mixtures of Dirichlet processes with applications to Bayesian nonparametric problems, *Annals of Statistics*, **2**, 1152–1174.

[3] Brown, P.J., Vannucci, M. and Fern, T. (1998) Multivariate Bayesian variable selection and prediction, *Journal of the Royal Statistical Society, Series B*, **60**, 627–641.

[4] Dahl, D.B. (2006). Model-based clustering for expression data via a Dirichlet process mixture model. In *Bayesian Inference for Gene Expression and Proteomics*, K. A. Do, P. Müller and M. Vannucci (Eds). Cambridge University Press, New York (this book).

[5] Dempster, A., Laird, N. and Rubin, D. (1977) Maximum likelihood for incomplete data via the EM algorithm (with discussion), *Journal of the Royal Statistical Society, Series B*, **39**, 1–38.

[6] Diebolt, J. and Robert, C.P. (1994) Estimation of finite mixture distributions through Bayesian sampling, *Journal of the Royal Statistical Society, Series B*, **56**, 363–375.

[7] Dudoit, S., Fridlyand, J. and Speed, T.P. (2002) Comparison of discrimination methods for the classification of tumors using gene expression data, *Journal of the American Statistical Association*, **97**, 77–87.

[8] Ferguson, T.S. (1983) Bayesian density estimation by mixtures of normal distributions. In *Recent Advances in Statistics*, H. Rizvi and J. Rustagi (Eds). New York: Academic Press.

[9] Fowlkes, E.B., Gnanadesikan, R. and Kettering, J.R. (1988) Variable selection in clustering, *Journal of Classification*, **5**, 205–228.

[10] Friedman, J.H. and Meulman, J.J. (2004) Clustering objects on subsets of attributes (with discussion), *Journal of the Royal Statistical Society, Series B*, **66**, 815–849.

[11] Golub, T.R., Slonim, D.K., Tamayo, P., Huard, C., Gassenbeek, M., Mesirov, J.P., Coller, H., Loh, M.L. Downing, J.R., Caligiuri, M.A., Bloomfield, C.D. and Lander, E.S. (1999) Molecular classification of cancer: Class discovery and class prediction by gene expression monitoring, *Science*, **286**, 531–537.

[12] George, E.I. and McCulloch, R.E. (1993) Variable selection via Gibbs sampling, *Journal of the American Statistical Association*, **88**, 881–889.

[13] Jain, A. and Dubes, R. (1988) *Algorithms for Clustering Data*. Englewood Cliffs, NJ: Prentice Hall.

[14] Jain, S., and Neal, R.M. (2004) A split-merge Markov chain Monte Carlo procedure for the Dirichlet process mixture model, *Journal of Computational and Graphical Statistics*, **13**, 158–182.

[15] Kim, S., Tadesse, M.G. and Vannucci, M. (submitted) Variable selection in clustering via Dirichlet process mixture models, *Biomerika*.

[16] Leamer, E.E. (1978) Regression selection strategies and revealed priors, *Journal of the American Statistical Association*, **73**, 580–587.

[17] McLachlan, G. and Basford, K. (1988) *Mixture Models: Inference and Applications to Clustering*. New York: Marcel Deckker.

[18] Miller, A. (1990) *Subset Selection in Regression*. London: Chapman & Hall.

[19] Mitchell, T.J. and Beauchamp, J.J (1988) Bayesian variable selection in linear regression, *Journal of the American Statistical Association*, **83**, 1023–1036.

[20] Neal, R.M. (2000) Markov chain sampling methods for Dirichlet process mixture models, *Journal of Computational and Graphical Statistics*, **9**, 249–265.

[21] Nguyen, D. and Rocke, D. (2002) Tumor classification by partial least squares using microarray gene expression data, *Bioinformatics*, **18**, 39–50.

[22] Richardson, S. and Green, P.J. (1997) Bayesian analysis of mixtures with an unknown number of components (with discussion), *Journal of the Royal Statistical Society, Series B*, **59**, 731–792.

[23] Sha, N., Tadesse, M.G. and Vannucci, M. (submitted). Bayesian variable selection for the analysis of microarray data with censored outcome.

[24] Sha, N., Vannucci, M., Brown, P.J., Trower, M.K., Amphlett, G. and Falciani, F. (2003) Gene selection in arthritis classification with large-scale microarray expression profiles, *Comparative and Functional Genomics*, **4**, 171–181.

[25] Sha, N., Vannucci, M., Tadesse, M.G., Brown, P.J., Dragoni, I., Davies, N., Roberts, T. C., Contestabile, A., Salmon, N., Buckley, C. and Falciani, F. (2004) Bayesian variable selection in multinomial probit models to identify molecular signatures of disease stage, *Biometrics*, **60**, 812–819.

[26] Stephens, M. (2000) Bayesian analysis of mixture models with an unknown number of components – An alternative to reversible jump methods, *Annals of Statistics*, **28**, 40–74.

[27] Stephens, M. (2000) Dealing with label switching in mixture models, *Journal of the Royal Statistical Society, Series B*, **62**, 795–809.

[28] Tadesse, M.G., Sha, N. and Vannucci, M. (2005) Bayesian variable selection in clustering high-dimensional data, *Journal of the American Statistical Association*, **100**, 602–617.

[29] Tibshirani, R. (1996) Regression shrinkage and selection via the lasso, *Journal of the Royal Statistical Society, Series B*, **58**, 267–288.

[30] Tibshirani, R., Hastie, T., Narashiman, B. and Chu, G. (2002) Diagnosis of multiple cancer types by shrunken centroids of gene expression, *Proceedings of the National Academy of Sciences*, **99**, 6567–6572.

[31] Vannucci, M., Sha, N. and Brown, P.J. (2005) NIR and mass spectra classification: Bayesian methods for wavelet-based feature selection, *Chemometrics and Intelligent Laboratory Systems*, **77**, 139–148.

[32] Vapnik, V. (1998) *Statistical Learning Theory*. New York: Wiley-Interscience.

[33] West, M. (2003) Bayesian factor regression models in large p small n paradigm. In *Bayesian Statistics 7*, J.M. Bernardo, M.J. Bayarri, J.O. Berger, A.P. David, D. Heckerman, A.F.M. Smith and M. West (Eds). Oxford: Oxford University Press.

6

Modeling Nonlinear Gene Interactions Using Bayesian MARS

VEERABHADRAN BALADANDAYUTHAPANI

The University of Texas M.D. Anderson Cancer Center

CHRIS C. HOLMES

University of Oxford and MRC Mammalian Genetics Unit

BANI K. MALLICK AND RAYMOND J. CARROLL

Texas A&M University

Abstract

DNA microarray technology enables us to monitor the expression levels of thousands of genes simultaneously, and hence helps to obtain a better picture of the interactions between the genes. In order to understand the biological structure underlying these gene interactions, we present here a statistical approach to model the functional relationship between genes and also between genes and disease status. We suggest a hierarchical Bayesian model based on multivariate adaptive regression splines (MARS) to model these complex nonlinear interaction functions. The novelty of the approach lies in the fact that we attempt to capture the complex nonlinear dependencies between the genes which otherwise would have been missed by linear approaches. Owing to the large number of genes (variables) and the complexity of the data, we use Markov Chain Monte Carlo (MCMC) based stochastic search algorithms to choose among models. The Bayesian model is flexible enough to identify significant genes as well as model the functional relationships between them. The effectiveness of the proposed methodology is illustrated using two publicly available microarray data sets: leukemia and hereditary breast cancer.

6.1 Introduction

DNA microarray technology has revolutionized biological and medical research. The use of DNA microarrays allows simultaneous monitoring of the expressions of thousands of genes (Schena et al. 1995; Duggan et al. 1999), and has emerged as a tool for disease diagnosis. This technology promises to monitor the whole genome on a single chip so that researchers can have a better picture of the interactions among thousands of genes simultaneously. In order to understand the biological structure underlying the gene interactions, that is, on what scale can we expect genes to interact with each other, we need to model the functional structure between the genes. However, due to the complexity of the data and the curse of dimensionality, it is not an easy task to find these structures. The purpose of this chapter is to present a statistical approach to model the functional relationship between genes and also between genes and disease status, with special focus on *nonlinear* relationships.

One of the key goals of microarray data is to perform classification via different expression profiles. In principle, gene expression profiles might serve as molecular fingerprints that would allow for accurate classification of diseases. The underlying assumption is that samples from the same class share expression profile patterns unique to their class (Yeang et al. 2001). In addition, these molecular fingerprints might reveal newer taxonomies that previously have not been readily appreciated. Several studies have used microarrays to profile colon, breast, and other tumors and have demonstrated the potential power of expression profiling for classification (Alon et al. 1999; Hedenfalk et al. 2001). Such problems can be classified as unsupervised, when only the expression data are available, and supervised, when a response measurement is also taken for each sample. In unsupervised problems (clustering) the goal is mainly to identify distinct sets of genes with similar expression profiles, suggesting that they may be biologically related. Both supervised and unsupervised problems also focus on finding sets of genes that relate to different kinds of diseases, so that future samples can be classified correctly. Classical statistical methods for clustering and classification have been applied extensively to microarray data (see Eisen et al. 1998 and Alizadeh et al. 2000 for clustering and Golub et al. 1999 and Hedenfalk et al. 2001 for classification). For this chapter we focus on classification and in doing so we also identify (select) the genes that are significantly more influential than the others, that is, variable selection.

A common objective in microarray studies is to highlight genes that (on average) coregulate with tissue type. This can be treated within a classification framework, where the tissue type is the response and the gene expressions are predictors. In this chapter we will consider rule-based classifiers to discover genes that coregulate and hence provide some of most explicit representations of the classification scheme. Rule-based classifiers use primitives such as IF A THEN B, where A relates to conditions on the value of a set of predictors (genes) $\mathbf{X}$ and consequence B relates to change in $\Pr(\mathbf{Y}|\mathbf{X})$. These type of rules are easy to interpret. The best known such models are Classification and Regression Trees (CART; Breiman et al. 1984), where decision trees provide a graphical order of the rules. The objective of this chapter is twofold: (1) find significant genes of interest and (2) find the underlying nonlinear functional form of the gene interaction. Related approaches in literature such as Lee et al. (2003) consider only linear functions of the genes, which may not be able to model such complex functional forms.

In this chapter we propose to use unordered rule sets based on a Bayesian nonparametric regression approach to model the high-dimensional gene expression data. In order to explore the complex nonlinear form of the expected responses without knowledge about the functional form in advance, it is imperative that we look to nonparametric techniques, since parametric models will not be flexible enough to model these complex functions. To capture the linear dependencies, and perhaps more crucially the nonlinear functional structures between the genes, we use a Bayesian version of multivariate adaptive regression splines (MARS), proposed by Friedman (1991) and extended in the Bayesian framework (BMARS) by Denison et al. (1998). MARS is a popular method for flexible regression modeling of high-dimensional data and has been extended to deal with classification problems (see, for example, Kooperberg et al. 1997).

In this chapter we treat the classification problem in a logistic regression framework. The logistic link has a direct interpretation of the log odds of having the disease in terms of the explanatory variables (genes). Since our model space is very large, that is, with p genes we have 2^p models, exhaustive computation over this model space is not possible. Hence Markov Chain Monte Carlo (MCMC; Gilks et al. 1996) based stochastic search algorithms are used. Our approach is to identify significant set(s) of genes over this vast model space, first to classify accurately and then to model the functional relationship between them. The flexible nonparametric setup creates a powerful predictive model, but unlike many black box predictive machines, our method identifies the significant genes as well as focuses on the interactions among them. In this sense, the method has the advantage that it combines scientific interpretation with accurate prediction.

In order to illustrate our methodology, we choose as examples two publicly available data sets: leukemia data (Golub et al. 1999) and hereditary breast cancer data (Hedenfalk et al. 2001). For each case we find sets of genes that have discriminating power. We also find the functional form of the main effect of dominant genes and the interaction function between genes that have significant interactions. Also, in data sets that we have investigated, our method shows equal ability to classify but uses far fewer genes to do so.

6.2 Bayesian MARS Model for Gene Interaction

For a binary class problem the response is usually coded as $Y_i = 1$ for class 1 and $Y_i = 0$ for the other class, where $i = 1, \ldots, n$ and where n is the number of samples (arrays). Gene expression data for p genes for n samples is summarized in an $n \times p$ matrix, $\mathbf{X}$, where each element x_{ij} denotes the expression level (gene expression value) of the jth gene in the ith sample, where $j = 1, \ldots, p$. The exact meaning of expression values may be different for different matrices, representing absolute or comparative measurements (see Brazma et al. 2001). Our objective is to use the training data $\mathbf{Y} = (Y_1, \ldots, Y_n)^T$ to estimate $p(\mathbf{X}) = \Pr(\mathbf{Y} = 1|\mathbf{X})$ or alternatively the logit function $f(\mathbf{X}) = \log[p(\mathbf{X})/(1 - p(\mathbf{X}))]$.

Assume that the Y_i's are independent Bernoulli random variables with $\Pr(Y_i = 1) = p_i$ so that $p(Y_i|p_i) = p_i^{Y_i}(1 - p_i)^{1-Y_i}$. We construct a hierarchical Bayesian model for classification as thus. Writing $p_i = \exp(\omega_i)/[1 + \exp(\omega_i)]$, wherein ω_i's are the latent variables introduced in the model to make Y_i's conditionally independent given the ω_i's. We relate ω_i to $f(\mathbf{X}_i)$ as

$$\omega_i = f(\mathbf{X}_i) + \epsilon_i, \tag{6.1}$$

where $\mathbf{X}_i$ is the ith row of the gene expression data matrix $\mathbf{X}$ (vector of gene expression levels of the ith sample) and ϵ_i are residual random effects. The residual random effects account for the unexplained sources of variation in the data, most probably due to explanatory variables (genes) not included in the study.

We choose to model f in nonparametric framework, primarily due to the fact that parametric approaches are not flexible enough to model such "rich" gene expression data sets. One of the most common choices for f is to use a basis function method of the form

$$f(\mathbf{X}_i) = \sum_{i=1}^{k} \beta_j B(\mathbf{X}_i, \theta_j),$$

where $\boldsymbol{\beta}$ are the regression coefficients for the bases $B(\mathbf{X}_i, \theta_j)$, which are nonlinear functions of $\mathbf{X}_i$ and θ. Examples of basis function include regression splines, wavelets, artificial neural networks, and radial bases. In this chapter we choose a MARS basis function proposed by Friedman (1991) to model f as

$$f(\mathbf{x}_i) = \beta_0 + \sum_{j=1}^{k} \beta_j \prod_{l=1}^{z_j} (x_{id_{jl}} - \theta_{jl})_{q_{jl}}, \tag{6.2}$$

where k is the number of spline basis, $\beta = \{\beta_1, \ldots, \beta_k\}$ is the set of spline coefficients (or output weights), z_j is the interaction level (or order) of the jth spline, θ_{jl} is a spline knot point, d_{jl} indicates which of the p predictors (genes) enters into the lth interaction of the jth spline, $d_{jl} \in \{1, \ldots, p\}$, and q_{jl} determines the orientation of the spline components, $q_{jl} \in \{+, -\}$ where

$(a)_+ = \max(a, 0)$, $(a)_- = \min(a, 0)$. We choose the MARS basis function as it can flexibly model the functional relationship between explanatory variables (genes) and gives interpretable models as compared to black box techniques such as artificial neural networks.

We illustrate this rather complex notation (6.2) through an example. Suppose a MARS model is of the following form (dropping the subscript i):

$$f = 2.5 + 3.2(x_{20} - 2.5)_+ + 4.1(x_{10} - 1.2)_-(x_{30} + 3.4)_+$$

Here we have $k = 2$ spline basis functions with $\beta = \{2.5, 3.2, 4.1\}$ as the spline coefficients. Gene 20 enters the model as a linear term (main effect) with interaction level $z_1 = 1$, knot point $\theta_{11} = 2.5$, and spline orientation $q_{11} = +$. We observe a bivariate interaction between genes 10 and 30, that is, $d_{21} = 10$, $d_{22} = 30$ with corresponding knots $= (1.2, -3.4)$ and spline orientation $= (-, +)$. See Friedman (1991) for a comprehensive illustration of the model.

Write (6.1) and (6.2) in matrix form as

$$\boldsymbol{\omega} = \Theta\beta + \epsilon, \tag{6.3}$$

where $\boldsymbol{\omega}$ is the vector of the latent variables and Θ is the MARS basis matrix,

$$\Theta = \begin{bmatrix} 1 & \prod_{l=1}^{z_1}(x_{1d_{1l}} - \theta_{1l})_{q_{1l}} & \cdots & \prod_{l=1}^{z_k}(x_{1d_{kl}} - \theta_{kl})_{q_{kl}} \\ 1 & \prod_{l=1}^{z_1}(x_{2d_{1l}} - \theta_{1l})_{q_{1l}} & \cdots & \prod_{l=1}^{z_k}(x_{2d_{kl}} - \theta_{kl})_{q_{kl}} \\ \vdots & \vdots & \ddots & \vdots \\ 1 & \prod_{l=1}^{z_1}(x_{nd_{1l}} - \theta_{1l})_{q_{1l}} & \cdots & \prod_{l=1}^{z_k}(x_{nd_{kl}} - \theta_{kl})_{q_{kl}} \end{bmatrix}. \tag{6.4}$$

In order to aid a Bayesian formulation we impose a prior structure on all the model parameters, $\mathcal{M} = \{\beta, \theta, q, d, z, \upsilon, k, , \lambda, \sigma^2\}$. The specific forms of the priors that we take are as follows. We assign a Gaussian prior to β with mean $\mathbf{0}$ and variance $\sigma^2 D^{-1}$, where $D \equiv \mathrm{diag}(\lambda_1, \lambda, \ldots, \lambda)$ is $(n+1) \times (n+1)$ diagonal matrix. We fix λ_1 to a small value, amounting to a large variance for the intercept term, but keep λ unknown. We assign an Inverse-Gamma (IG) prior to σ^2 and a gamma prior to λ with parameters (γ_1, γ_2) and (τ_1, τ_2) respectively. Note that the above model can be extended to have multiple prior variances on β as

$$p(\beta, \sigma) \sim \mathrm{N}_{n+1}(\beta|0, \sigma^2 D^{-1})\mathrm{IG}(\sigma^2|\gamma_1, \gamma_2),$$

where D is a diagonal matrix with diagonal elements $\lambda = (\lambda_1, \ldots, \lambda_{n+1})^T$. Once again λ_1 is fixed to a small value but all other λ's are unknown. We assign independent Gamma (τ_1, τ_2) priors to them.

The prior structure on the MARS model parameters are as follows. The prior on the individual knot selections θ_{jl} is taken to be uniform over the

n data points $p(\theta_{jl}|d_{jl}) = U(x_{1d_{jl}}, x_{2d_{jl}}, \ldots, x_{nd_{jl}})$, where d_{jl} indicates which of the genes enter our model and $p(d_{jl})$ is uniform over the p genes, $p(d_{jl}) = U(1, \ldots, p)$. The prior on the orientation of the spline is again uniform, $p(q_{jl} = +) = p(q_{jl} = -) = 0.5$. The interaction level in each spline has a prior, $p(z_j) = U(1, \ldots, z_{max})$, where z_{max} is the maximum level of interaction set by the user. Finally the prior on k, the number of splines, is taken to an improper one, $p(k) = U(1, \ldots, \infty)$, which indicates no a priori knowledge on the number of splines. Hence the model now has only one user defined parameter, z_{max}, the maximum level of interaction, for which we shall recommend a default setting in Section 6.5.

6.3 Computation

The information from the data are combined with the prior distributions on the parameters via Bayes' theorem and the likelihood function as

$$p(\omega, \theta, q, d, z, \beta, v, k, \lambda, \sigma^2|\mathbf{Y}) = p(\mathbf{Y}|\omega, \theta, q, d, z, \beta, v, k, \lambda, \sigma^2)$$
$$\times p(\omega, \theta, q, d, z, \beta, v, k, \lambda, \sigma^2).$$

For classification problems with binary data and logistic likelihood, conjugate priors do not exist for the regression coefficients. With the Bayesian hierarchical structure as in the previous section the posterior distributions are not available in explicit form, so we use MCMC techniques (Gilks et al. 1996) for inference. Conventional MCMC methods such as the Metropolis–Hastings (MH) algorithm (Metropolis et al. 1953; Hastings 1970) are not applicable here since the parameter (model) space is variable: we do not know the number of splines a priori. Hence we use the variable dimension reversible jump algorithm outlined in Green (1995).

In our framework, the chain is updated using the following proposals with equal probability:

(i) Add a new spline basis to the model.
(ii) Remove one of the k existing spline bases from the model.
(iii) Alter an existing spline basis in the model (by changing the knot points).

Following each move an update is made to the spline coefficients β. Note that the above three move steps are equivalent to adding, removing, and altering a column of Θ in (6.4). The algorithm is included in the appendix. The update to β is the critical step determining the efficiency of the algorithm. A poor proposal distribution for β results in the current state having low posterior probabilities and low acceptance rates. This is because adding, deleting, or altering a column of Θ in (6.4) would alter the remaining $\boldsymbol{\beta}$ parameters as they are now ill-tuned to the data.

We introduce the latent variables $\boldsymbol{\omega}$ to circumvent the problem. The idea is to introduce an extra set of parameters into the model that leave the original (marginal) model distribution unchanged, in order to improve the overall efficiency of the sampling algorithms. Therefore conditional on $\boldsymbol{\omega}$, all the other parameters are independent of $\mathbf{Y}$. This allows us to adopt conjugate priors for $(\boldsymbol{\beta}, \sigma^2)$ to perform the MCMC calculations as well as marginalize over the model space. Considerable computational advantage is gained from the fact that the posterior distribution of $\boldsymbol{\beta}$ given the other parameters is now known exactly, that is, normally distributed. The details of the procedure are given in the appendix.

6.4 Prediction and Model Choice

For a new sample with gene expression $\boldsymbol{x}_{\text{new}}$, the marginal posterior distribution of the new disease state, y_{new}, is given by

$$\Pr(y_{\text{new}} = 1 | \boldsymbol{x}_{\text{new}}) = \sum_{k=1}^{\infty} \int P(y_{\text{new}} = 1 | \boldsymbol{x}_{\text{new}}, \mathcal{M}_k) P(\mathcal{M}_k | Y) \, d\mathcal{M}_k, \quad (6.5)$$

where $\Pr(\mathcal{M}_k | Y)$ is the posterior probability and $\mathcal{M}_k$ indicates the MARS model with k splines. The integral given in (6.5) is computationally and analytically intractable and needs approximate procedures. We approximate (6.5) by its Monte Carlo estimate by

$$\Pr(y_{\text{new}} = 1 | \boldsymbol{x}_{\text{new}}) = \frac{1}{m} \sum_{j=1}^{m} P\left(y_{\text{new}} = 1 | \boldsymbol{x}_{\text{new}}, \mathcal{M}^{(j)}\right), \quad (6.6)$$

where $\mathcal{M}^{(j)}$ for $j = 1, \ldots, m$ are the m MCMC posterior samples of the MARS model parameters $\mathcal{M}$. The approximation (6.6) converges to the true value (6.5) as $m \to \infty$.

In order to select from different models, we generally use misclassification error. When a test set is provided, we first obtain the posterior distribution of the parameters based on training data, y_{trn} (train the model), and use them to classify the test samples. For a new observation from the test set $y_{i,\text{test}}$, we will obtain the probability $\Pr(y_{i,\text{test}} = 1 | y_{\text{trn}}, x_{i,\text{test}})$ by using the approximation to (6.5) given by (6.6). When this probability is greater than 0.5 we will classify it as 1 and when it is less than 0.5 we will classify it as 0. The number of misclassified samples from the test set is defined as the misclassification error.

If there is no test set available, we will use a hold-one-out cross-validation approach. We follow the technique described in Gelfand (1996) to simplify the computation. For the cross-validation predictive density, in general, let $\mathbf{Y}_{-i}$ be the vector of Y_j's without the ith observation Y_i,

$$P(Y_i|\mathbf{Y}_{-i}) = \frac{P(\mathbf{Y})}{P(\mathbf{Y}_{-i})} = \left[\int\{P(y_i|\mathbf{Y}_{-i}, \mathcal{M}_k)\}^{-1} P(\mathcal{M}_k|\mathbf{Y}) d\mathcal{M}_k\right]^{-1}.$$

The MCMC approximation to this is

$$\widehat{P}(Y_i|\mathbf{Y}_{-i,\mathrm{trn}}) = m^{-1}\sum_{j=1}^{m}\left\{P\left(y_i|\mathbf{Y}_{-i,\mathrm{trn}}, \mathcal{M}^{(j)}\right)\right\}^{-1},$$

where $\mathcal{M}^{(j)}$ for $j = 1, \ldots, m$ are the m MCMC posterior samples of the MARS model parameters $\mathcal{M}$. This simple expression is due to the fact that the Y_i's are conditionally independent given the model parameters $\mathcal{M}$.

6.5 Examples

We illustrate the Bayesian methodology with two microarray examples. For all the examples considered below we set the maximum level of interaction, $z_{\max} = 1$, that is, allow for only additive and bivariate interactions. The MCMC chain is run for 50,000 iterations of which the first 10,000 are discarded as burn-in.

6.5.1 Leukemia Data

This microarray data set is taken from Golub et al. (1999). The data set contains measurements corresponding to samples from Bone Marrow and Peripheral blood samples taken from 72 patients with either acute lymphoblastic leukemia (ALL) or acute myeloid leukemia (AML). As in the original paper we split the data into a training set of 38 samples (27 are ALL and 11 AML) and a test set of 34 samples (20 ALL and 14 AML). The data set contains expression levels for 7,129 human genes produced by Affymetrix high-density oligonucleotide microarrays.

In order to identify significant genes, we isolate those genes that enter our MARS model most frequently in the posterior samples; genes may enter the model either as a main effect or an interaction effect. The plots of the posterior mean main effect functions of the top six genes ranked in this manner are shown in Figure 6.1. These curves are estimated by

$$E\{f_i(X)\} = \frac{1}{T}\sum_{t=1}^{T}\sum_{\substack{j:z_j=1 \\ d_{jl}=i}}\beta_j^{(t)}\Theta_j^{(t)}(X), \qquad (6.7)$$

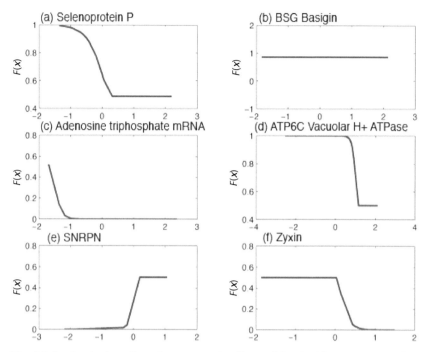

Fig. 6.1. Leukemia data: Posterior mean main effects of the significant genes entering the MARS model. The horizontal axis is the standardized expression level of the gene and the vertical axis is the mean main effect function.

where T is the number of models in the generated sample, indexed with the superscript. The second summation ensures that the curves are estimated by only considering the main effect basis functions involving the i gene (predictor), thus averaging over the basis functions relating to the desired gene main effect. These curves demonstrate the effect of individual genes on the odds of carrying a disease (ALL in this example). We can see that there is evidence that gene *BSG Basigin* shows little effect on the odds for all expression levels. As the expression level of gene *Adenosine triphosphatase mRNA* increases, the odds decrease linearly and are low for higher expression levels of this particular gene. For gene *Zyxin* the odds are unaffected over the negative expression values but decrease linearly for increasing positive expression values, while on the other hand exactly the opposite feature is found for gene *SNRPN Small nuclear ribonucleoprotein polypeptide N*, where the odds increase linearly for positive expression values and are unaffected in the negative range. Similar conclusions can be drawn for other genes too. This demonstrates how threshold basis functions such as MARS allow for insightful interpretation of the

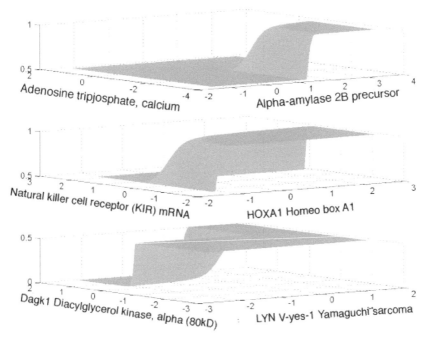

Fig. 6.2. Leukemia data: Posterior mean interaction functions of the significant genes entering the MARS model. The *x*- and *y*-axis are the standardized expression levels of the interacting genes and the vertical axis is the mean interaction function.

relationship between odds (response) and genes (predictors), with the added advantage being that MARS model automatically ignores genes that have little effect on the response.

Added to the effect of a single gene, our model also unearths gene pairs that have significant interactions along with the functional form of the interaction function. Figure 6.2 shows the bivariate interaction surface of the three gene pairs that have a significant interaction and appear in the posterior MCMC samples most number of times. This figure illustrates the joint contribution to the odds of having a disease of the two genes. The surface is estimated in a manner similar to (6.7), but now we only consider interaction terms involving the two genes desired in the second summation. This figure highlights the advantage of using flexible nonlinear MARS basis functions in discerning this complex interaction function between genes over linear approaches. In the top panel of Figure 6.2 we can see that high expression levels of gene *Alpha-Amylase 2B Precursor* combined with low (negative) expression levels of gene *Adenosine triphosphatase calcium* results in an increased level of response, which is unaffected for low levels of both genes. A similar feature is also detected observing

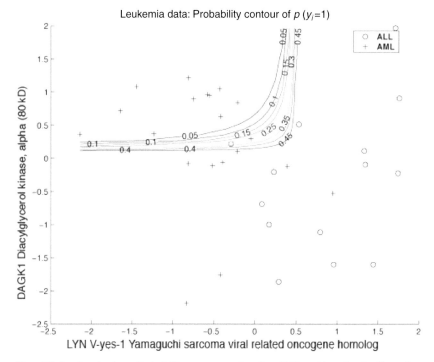

Fig. 6.3. Leukemia data: Probability contours showing $P(Y_i = 1)$ under the Bayesian MARS model. The circles and the crosses represent diseased/nondiseased respectively.

the interaction surface of genes *Natural killer cell receptor (KIR) mRNA* and *HOXA1 Homeo box A1*. From the bottommost panel we can observe that the odds increase as the expression level of gene *LYN V-yes-1 Yamaguchi sarcoma viral related oncogene homolog* increases and that of gene *DAGK1 Diacylglycerol kinase alpha* decreases.

Using two pairs of genes that discriminate between the two classes AML and ALL reasonably, we plot the probability contours, $\Pr(Y_i = 1)$ (Figure 6.3), to demonstrate the advantages of using a nonlinear model. Any linear approach would divide the predictor space into two regions separated by a straight line. Such a complex decision boundary can only be uncovered using a nonlinear model. Note that these predictive contours appear smooth even though individual MARS models have axis parallel nonsmooth contours. This is due to averaging over thousands of MARS models, thus marginalizing over the model space.

Golub et al. (1999) used a 50-gene predictor trained using their weighted voting scheme on the training samples. The predictor made strong predictions for 29 of the 34 test samples, declining to predict the other 5 cases. For the same case our misclassification error rate for the test set is 0.08, that is, we misclassify 3 out of the 34 test samples. Our results appear to be competitive to the results from Golub et al., but we use far fewer genes. Our mode for the distribution of $p(k|Y)$, the marginal density of the number of splines, is 2 basis terms, thus showing that we get competitive results by using considerably fewer genes.

6.5.2 Hereditary Breast Cancer

We use the microarray data set used in Hedenfalk et al. (2001) on breast tumors from patients carrying mutations in the predisposing genes, BRCA1 or BRCA2, or from patients not expected to carry a hereditary predisposing mutation. Pathological and genetic differences appear to imply different but overlapping functions for BRCA1 and BRCA2. They examined 22 breast tumor samples from 21 breast cancer patients, and all patients except one were women. Fifteen women had hereditary breast cancer, seven tumors with BRCA1 and eight tumors with BRCA2. For each breast tumor sample 3,226 genes were used. We use our method to classify BRCA1 versus the others (BRCA2 and sporadic).

Table 6.1 lists the top 50 genes that enter as main effects in the MARS model in posterior MCMC samples, along with the corresponding frequency of appearance. The "frequency" here is the proportion of number of times the given gene appears as a main effect in the MCMC posterior samples. Similarly, Table 6.2 shows the top 25 interacting genes that enter the MARS model. These genes enter our model most frequently while classifying BRCA1 versus BRCA2 and sporadic. A similar list of 51 genes which best differentiate among the types of tumor is also provided by Hedenfalk et al. (2001). We find quite a few overlapping genes (marked by an *) between the two lists like keratin 8 (KRT8), ODCantizyme, and ACTR1A. KRT8 is a member of the cytokeratin family of genes and cytokeratins are frequently used to identify breast cancer metastases by immunohistochemistry, and cytokeratin 8 abundance has been shown to correlate well with node-positive disease (Brotherick et al. 1998).

Figure 6.4 shows the posterior mean main effect function of the top six genes selected from the list. The vertical axis shows the odds of having BRCA1 mutation and the horizontal axis is the standardized expression level of that particular gene. An advantage of using a nonlinear approach is evident here as we can unearth a threshold expression level and its corresponding effect on the the odds of having a BRCA1 mutation. For example, for *polymerase (RNA) II*

Table 6.1. *Breast Cancer Data*

Image clone ID	Gene description	Frequency
767817	Polymerase (RNA) II (DNA-directed) polypeptide F	0.943
307843	ESTs (*)	0.932
81331	Fatty acid-binding protein, epidermal	0.921
843076	Signal transducing adaptor molecule (SH3 domain and ITAM motif) 1	0.917
825478	Zinc finger protein 146	0.895
28012	O-linked *N*-acetylglucosamine (GlcNAc) transferase	0.881
812227	Solute carrier family 9 (sodium/hydrogen exchanger), isoform 1	0.872
566887	Heterochromatin-like protein 1 (*)	0.856
841617	Ornithine decarboxylase antizyme 1 (*)	0.849
788721	KIAA0090 protein	0.833
811930	KIAA0020 gene product	0.822
32790	mutS (*E. coli*) homolog 2 (colon cancer, nonpolyposis type 1)	0.819
784830	D123 gene product (*)	0.811
949932	Nuclease sensitive element binding protein 1 (*)	0.807
26184	Phosphofructokinase, platelet (*)	0.801
810899	CDC28 protein kinase 1	0.795
46019	Minichromosome maintenance deficient (*S. cerevisiae*) 7 (*)	0.787
897781	Keratin 8 (*)	0.774
32231	KIAA0246 protein (*)	0.765
293104	Phytanoyl-CoA hydroxylase (Refsum disease) (*)	0.753
180298	Protein tyrosine kinase 2 beta	0.744
47884	Macrophage migration inhibitory factor (glycosylation-inhibiting factor)	0.732
137638	ESTs (*)	0.728
246749	ESTs, weakly similar to trg [*R. norvegicus*]	0.711
233365	HP1-BP74	0.695
815530	PAK-interacting exchange factor beta	0.680
123425	ESTs, moderately similar to AF141326 RNA helicase	0.642
22230	Collagen, type V, alpha 1	0.612
324210	Sigma receptor (SR31747 binding protein 1)	0.608
824117	Vaccinia related kinase 2	0.602
124405	Androgen induced protein	0.594
83210	Complement component 8, beta polypeptide	0.592
49788	Carnitine acetyltransferase	0.590
344352	ESTs	0.586
842806	Cyclin-dependent kinase 4	0.568
810734	Human 1.1 kb mRNA upregulated in retinoic acid treated HL-60	0.564
814701	MAD2 (mitotic arrest deficient, yeast, homolog)-like 1	0.554
36007	Zinc finger protein 133 (clone pHZ-13)	0.518
110503	FOS-like antigen-1	0.492
767784	jun D proto-oncogene	0.488

Image clone ID	Gene description	Frequency
486844	Gap junction protein, alpha 1, 43kD (connexin 43)	0.486
810408	Hypothetical 43.2 Kd protein	0.456
199381	vav 3 oncogene	0.446
509682	Histone deacetylase 3	0.446
43021	Histidyl-tRNA synthetase	0.438
212198	Tumor protein p53-binding protein, 2 (*)	0.418
840702	Selenophosphate synthetase; Human selenium protein (*)	0.402
666128	D component of complement (adipsin)	0.400
613126	Ubiquitin-specific protease 13 (isopeptidase T-3)	0.396
139705	ESTs	0.384

Note: Top 50 genes (predictors) entering MARS model as main effects ranked in descending order of the frequency of times they appear in posterior MCMC samples.

polypeptide it is seen that the odds are relatively high for negative expression levels while the odds decrease for higher expression levels of the gene. Figure 6.5 shows posterior mean interaction function of two pairs of genes that have significant interaction. This shows the combined effect of these two genes on the odds of carrying mutation of BRCA1. The top panel of Figure 6.5 shows that the odds decrease uniformly with expression levels of *BTG family, member 3* with higher odds when combined with low expression levels of *replication factor C (activator 1)* and lower odds when combined with higher expression levels of *replication factor C (activator 1)*. The bottom panel shows that there is evidence that higher expression levels of *Glycogenin* combined with low expression levels of *ornithine decarboxylase antizyme 1* lead to increased odds of carrying a mutation of BRCA1.

Since test data were not provided, to check our model adequacy we used full hold-one-out cross-validation. The results are summarized in Table 6.3. We compare our cross-validation results with other popular classification algorithms as in Lee et al. (2003). All the other methods use 51 genes for classification purposes while the MARS method selects far fewer genes; our mode of the distribution of $p(k|Y)$ is 3 showing that the number of splines basis terms (genes) used by the model adapts to the problem at hand and uses fewer genes with the results being competitive to any other method.

Table 6.2. *Breast Cancer Data*

Image clone ID	Gene description	Image clone ID	Gene description	Frequency
753285	Glycogenin	841617	Ornithine decarboxylase antizyme 1 (*)	0.950
134748	Glycine cleavage system protein H	137506	Dishevelled 2 (homologous to Drosophila dsh)	0.932
126412	Ring finger protein 14	282980	ESTs	0.922
784830	D123 gene product (*)	814270	Polymyositis/scleroderma autoantigen 1 (75kD)	0.906
823663	Fragile X mental retardation	377275	Ataxia-telangiectasia group D-associated protein	0.894
50754	Mitochondrial translational initiation factor 2	282980	ESTs	0.874
346117	Guanylate binding protein 2, interferon-inducible	786083	Ubiquitin-conjugating enzyme E2 variant 2	0.864
79898	Transducin-like enhancer of split 1	204179	Hypothetical protein FLJ20036	0.854
214537	Replication factor C (activator 1) 1 (145kD)	246304	BTG family, member 3	0.842
307843	ESTs (*)	199624	ESTs	0.744
136730	TATA box binding protein (TBP)-associated factor	32790	mutS (*E. coli*) homolog 2	0.708
711959	Polymerase (RNA) III (DNA directed) (62kD)	195947	ESTs, Weakly similar to [*H. sapiens*]	0.622
949932	Nuclease-sensitive element binding protein 1 (*)	38393	Connective tissue growth factor	0.616
756847	Suppressin	29054	ARP1 (actin-related protein 1, yeast) (*)	0.592
814054	KIAA0040 gene product	309045	Sarcolemmal-associated protein	0.576
51740	Hydroxyacyl-Coenzyme A	340644	Integrin, beta 8 (*)	0.566
823930	Actin-related protein 2/3 complex, subunit 1A (41 kD)	32609	Laminin, alpha 4	0.518
297392	Metallothionein 1L	366647	Butyrate response factor 1 (EGF-response factor 1)	0.504
73531	Nitrogen fixation cluster-like (*)	29063	Homo sapiens clone 23620 mRNA sequence	0.498
898123	Phosphoribosylglycinamide formyltransferase	32231	KIAA0246 protein (*)	0.480
194364	RNA binding motif protein 6	21652	Catenin (cadherin-associated protein), alpha 1	0.462
143227	ESTs	135381	Growth arrest and DNA-damage-inducible 34	0.442
249705	Deleted in split-hand/split-foot 1 region	344352	ESTs	0.408
771173	Hypothetical protein	784744	M-phase phosphoprotein 6	0.402
713647	Tetraspan 3	240033	Homo sapiens mRNA; cDNA DKFZp434L162	0.400

Note: Top 25 interacting genes entering MARS model ranked in descending order of the frequency of times they appear in posterior MCMC samples.

130

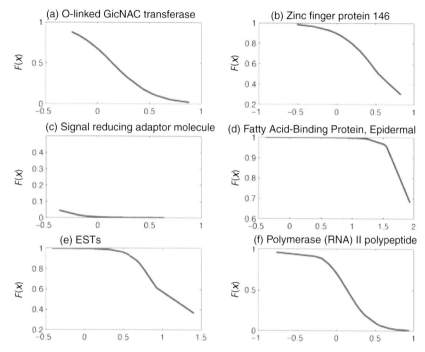

Fig. 6.4. Breast cancer data: Posterior mean main effects of the significant genes entering the MARS model. The horizontal axis is the standardized expression level of the gene and the vertical axis is the mean main effect function.

6.6 Discussion and Summary

We have presented an approach to model nonlinear gene interactions using a Bayesian MARS. Our method uses MCMC-based stochastic search algorithms to obtain the models. The advantage of our method is that we capture the nonlinear dependencies between the genes, dependencies that would have been missed by linear approaches. Our approach is not only flexible enough to model these complex interaction functions, but it also identifies significant genes of interest for further biological study. We illustrated our method using two microarray data sets which have been well analyzed in literature. In both cases we used far fewer genes and yet obtained competitive results to those reported in literature.

We have treated the binary case in detail in this chapter. When the response is not binary, such that the number of classes (C) is greater than two, then the problem becomes a multiclass classification problem. This can be handled in a manner similar to the binary classification approach, as follows. Let

Table 6.3. *Model Misclassification Errors Using
Hold-One-Out Cross-Validation for Breast Cancer Data*

Model	Number of misclassifies samples
Bayesian MARS	0
Feed-forward neural networks (3 hidden neurons, 1 hidden layer)	1.5 (average error)
Gaussian kernel	1
Epanechnikov kernel	1
Moving window kernel	2
Probabilistic neural network ($r = 0.01$)	3
kNN ($k = 1$)	4
SVM linear	4
Perceptron	5
SVM nonlinear	6

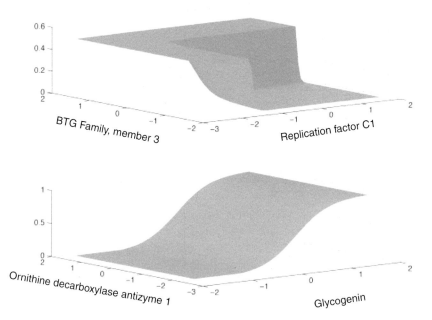

Fig. 6.5. Breast Cancer data: Posterior mean interaction functions of the significant genes entering the MARS model. The *x*- and *y*-axis are the standardized expression levels of the interacting genes and the vertical axis is the mean interaction function.

$\mathbf{Y}_i = (Y_{i1}, \ldots, Y_{iC})$ denote the multinomial indicator vector with elements $Y_{iq} = 1$ if the qth sample belongs to the qth class, and $Y_{ij} = 0$ otherwise. Let $\mathbf{Y}$ denote the $n \times C$ matrix of these indicators. The likelihood of the data given the MARS spline bases $(\Theta_1, \ldots, \Theta_C)$ is given by

$$P(Y_i = 1|\mathbf{X}_i) = p_1^{y_{i1}} p_2^{y_{i2}}, \ldots, p_C^{y_{iC}},$$

where p_q is the probability that the sample came from class q. This is modeled in a similar manner to the binary class case as in Section 6.2. The prior structure imposed on the parameters is also akin to that described in Section 6.2.

Acknowledgments

Holmes' research is supported by an e-science grant from the Medical Research Council, U.K. Carroll's research was supported by a grant from the National Cancer Institute (CA-57030), and by the Texas A&M Center for Environmental and Rural Health via a grant from the National Institute of Environmental Health Sciences (P30-ES09106). In addition, Mallick's research was supported in part by National Cancer Institute Grants CA-10462 and CA-57030.

Appendix: Technical Complements

Details of the Sampler

The algorithm for the MCMC is the following:

* Start with a constant intercept model with $k = 0$ and $\Theta = (1, \ldots, 1)'$.
* Set the initial values of the latent variables ω.
* Draw the intercept (β_0, σ^2) using the update for (β, σ^2) as given below.
* Start the MCMC sampler and iterate.
  - Draw latent variable ω given the current model.
  - Update prior precision λ on β as given below.
  - Update Θ using one of the following moves with equal probability.
    ○ Add a spline basis function.
    ○ Delete a spline basis function.
    ○ Alter a spline basis function.
  - Redraw (β, σ^2)
  - Accept the modifications to Θ and β with probability

$$Q = \min\left\{1, \frac{|\widehat{V}^*|^{1/2}}{|\widehat{V}|^{1/2}} \exp\left(\frac{a}{a^*}\right)\right\}, \tag{A.1}$$

   where $|\widehat{V}|$ is the determinant of the posterior variance covariance matrix of β and is given by $(\Theta'\Theta + D)^{-1}$, the superscript $*$ refers to the parameters of the proposed update model and a is the error term,

$$a = \omega'\omega - \widehat{\beta}'\widehat{V}^{-1}\widehat{\beta}. \tag{A.2}$$

  - Otherwise keep the current model.

The procedures for updating Θ, that is, adding, deleting, and modifying a spline base, and for updating $(\boldsymbol{\beta}, \sigma^2)$ are given below.

Adding a Spline
The steps to add a basis function to the model are as follows:

(i) Draw the interaction level of the spline $z_j \sim U(1, \ldots, z_{max})$.
(ii) Draw z_j elements $\{d_{j1}, \ldots, d_{jz_j}\}$ from $\{1, \ldots, p\}$ without replacement.
(iii) For each of the z_j interactions that make up the jth spline, select a data point at random from the data set, say x_i, and set the corresponding knot point $\theta_{jl} = x_{id_{jl}}$. Then draw the orientation of the spline from uniform $\{0, 1\}$, where 0 corresponds to $+$ (positive orientation) and 1 to $-$ (negative orientation).
(iv) Update $(\boldsymbol{\beta}, \sigma^2)$ as given below.

Deleting a Spline
Choose one of the k splines at random and remove it from the model and subsequently update the values of $(\boldsymbol{\beta}, \sigma^2)$ as shown below.

Modifying a Spline
The following is the procedure to modify a basis function to the model:

(i) Select at random one of the k splines, say the jth, to modify.
(ii) Select the lth of the z_j interactions at random and reset the knot point θjl by randomly drawing a data point x_i from the data set and fixing the value of $\theta_{jl} = x_{id_{jl}}$.
(iii) Update $(\boldsymbol{\beta}, \sigma^2)$ as given below.

Updating the Latent Variables $\boldsymbol{\omega}$
For the update to $\boldsymbol{\omega}$, we propose to update each ω_i in turn conditional on the rest. That is, we update $\omega_i | \boldsymbol{\omega}_{-i}, \mathbf{Y}, \mathcal{M}$ $(i = 1, \ldots, n)$, where $\boldsymbol{\omega}_{-i}$ indicates the $\boldsymbol{\omega}$ with the ith element removed.

The latent variables ω_i's conditional on the current model parameters $\mathcal{M}$ and the data Y_i do not have an explicit form. Thus we resort to the MH procedure with a proposal density $T(\omega_i^* | \omega_i)$ that generates the moves from the current state ω_i to a new state ω_i^*. The proposed updates are then accepted with probabilities,

$$\alpha = \min \left\{ 1, \frac{p(y_i | \omega_i^*) p(\omega_i^* | \boldsymbol{\omega}_{-i}, \Theta) T(\omega_i | \omega_i^*)}{p(y_i | \omega_i) p(\omega_i | \boldsymbol{\omega}_{-i}, \Theta) T(\omega_i^* | \omega_i)} \right\},$$

otherwise the current model is retained.
Finally, the full conditional for ω_i is,

$$p(\omega_i | \boldsymbol{\omega}_{-i}, \mathbf{Y}, \mathcal{M}) \propto \exp \left[\sum_{j=1}^{n} Y_i \omega_i - \sum_{j=1}^{n} \log(1 + \exp(\omega_i)) - \frac{1}{2\sigma^2} (\omega_i - \Theta_i' \boldsymbol{\beta})^2 \right],$$

where Θ_i is the ith row of MARS basis matrix Θ as given in (6.4).

It is convenient to take the proposal distribution $T(\omega_i^*|\omega_i)$ to be a symmetric distribution (e.g., Gaussian) with mean equal to the old value ω_i and a prespecified standard deviation.

Updating $(\boldsymbol{\beta}, \sigma^2)$ Conditional on Changes to the Spline Base and Latent Variables $\boldsymbol{\omega}$
Conditional on the latent variables $\boldsymbol{\omega}$ and the current MARS model, using Bayesian linear model theory we update the spline coefficients and the residual random effects, given the changes to the spline basis using their posterior distribution, so that

$$(\boldsymbol{\beta}, \sigma^2) \sim \mathrm{N}_{n+1}(\boldsymbol{\beta}|\boldsymbol{m}, \sigma^2 \mathbf{V})\mathrm{IG}(\sigma^2|\tilde{\gamma}_1, \tilde{\gamma}_2),$$

where $m = V(\Theta^*)'\boldsymbol{\omega}$, $V = [(\Theta^*)'\Theta^* + \boldsymbol{D}]^{-1}$, $\tilde{\gamma}_1 = (\gamma_1 + n/2)$, and $\tilde{\gamma}_2 = (\gamma_2 + (1/2)(\boldsymbol{\omega}'\boldsymbol{\omega} - m'Vm))$. Here Θ^* now is the $n \times (k + 1)$ matrix of outputs from k splines with the intercept and $\boldsymbol{D}$ is the prior precision on $\boldsymbol{\beta}$.

Updating prior precision $\boldsymbol{\lambda}$ conditional on the current model
We draw new values of λ_i using the conditional posterior distribution,

$$\lambda_i \sim \mathrm{Gamma}\left(\tau_1 + \frac{1}{2}, \tau_2 + \frac{\boldsymbol{\beta}'\boldsymbol{\beta}}{2}\right),$$

where k is the number of basis functions and $\boldsymbol{\beta}$ are the regression coefficients.

Bibliography

Alizadeh, A., Eisen, M., Davis, R. E., Chi Ma, Lossos, I., Rosenwald, A., Boldrick, J., Sabet, H., Tran, T., Yu, X.,Powell, J. I., Yang, L., Marti, G. E., Moore, T., Hudson, J. Jr., Lu, L., Lewis, D. B., Tibshirani, R., Sherlock, G., Chan, W. C., Greiner, T. C., Weisenburger, D. D., Armitage, J. O., Warnke, R., Levy, R., Wilson, W., Grever, M. R., Byrd, J. C., Botstein, D., Brown, P. O. and Staudt, L. M. (2000). Distinct Types of Diffuse Large B-cell Lymphoma Identified by Gene Expression Profiling. *Nature*, 403, 503–511.

Alon, U., Barkai, N., Notterman, D. A., Gish, K., Ybarra, S., Mack, D. and Levine, A. J. (1999). Broad Patterns of Gene Expression revealed by Clustering Analysis of Tumor and Normal Colon Tissues probed by Oligonucleotide Arrays. *Proc. Natl. Acad. Sci. U.S.A.*, 96, 6745–6750.

Brazma, A., Hingamp, P., Quakenbush, J., Sherlock, G., Spellman, P., Stoeckert, C., Aach, J., Ansorge, W., Ball C. A., Causton, H. C., Gaasterland, T., Glenisson, P., Holstege, F. C. P., Kim, I. F., Markowitz, V., Matese, J. C., Parkinson, H., Robinson, A., Sarkans, U., Schulze-Kremer, S., Stewart, J., Taylor, R., Vilo, J. and Vingron, M. (2001). Minimum Information about Micorarray Experiment (MAIME) – Towards Standards for Microarray Data. *Nat. Genet.*, 29, 365–371.

Breiman, L., Friedman, J. H., Olshen, R. and Stone, C. J. (1984). *Classification and Regression Trees.* Belmont, CA: Wadsworth.

Brotherick, I., Robson, C. N., Browell, D. A., Shenfine, J., While, M. D., Cunliffe, W. J., Shenton, B. K., Egan, M., Webb, L. A., Lunt, L. G., Young, J. R. and Higgs, M. J. (1998). Cytokeratin Expression in Breast Cancer: Phenotypic Changes Associated with Disease Progression. *Cytometry*, 32, 301–308.

Denison, D. G. T., Mallick, B. K. and Smith, A. F. M. (1998). Bayesian MARS. *Stat. Comput.*, 8, 337–346.

Duggan, D. J., Bittner, M. L., Chen, Y., Meltzer, P. S. and Trent, J. M. (1999). Expression Profiling Using cDNA Microarrays. *Nat. Genet.*, 21, 10–14.

Eisen, M. B., Spellman., P. T., Brown, P. O. and Botstein, D. (1998). Cluster Analysis and Display of Genome-wide Expression Patterns. *Proc. Natl. Acad. Sci. U.S.A.*, 95, 14863–14868.

Friedman, J. H. (1991). Multivariate Adaptive Regression Splines (with discussion). *Ann. Stat.* 19, 1–141.

Gelfand, A. (1996). Model Determination Using Sampling-Based Methods. In Gilks, W. R., Richardson, S. and Spiegelhalter, D. J. (Eds), *Markov Chain Monte Carlo in Practice*. London: Chapman and Hall.

Gilks, W. R., Richardson, S. and Spiegelhalter, D. J. (1996). *Markov Chain Monte Carlo in Practice*. London: Chapman and Hall.

Golub T. R., Slonim, D., Tamayo, P., Huard, C., Gaasenbeek., M., Mesirov, J., Coller, H., Loh, M., Downing, J., Caliguiri, M., Bloomfield, C. and Lender, E. (1999). Molecular Classification of Cancer: Class Discovery and Class Prediction by Gene Expression Monitoring. *Science*, 286, 531–537.

Green, P. J. (1995). Reversible Jump Markov Chain Monte Carlo Computation and Bayesian Model Determination. *Biometrika*, 82, 711–732.

Hastings, W. K. (1970). Monte Carlo Sampling Methods Using Markov Chains and Their Applications. *Biometrika*, 57, 87–109.

Hedenfalk, I., Duggan, D., Chen, Y., Radmacher, M., Bittner, M., Simon, R., Meltzer, P., Gusterson, B., Esteller, M., Kallioniemi, O. P., Wilfond, B., Borg, A. and Trent J. (2001). Gene Expression Profiles in Hereditary Breast Cancer. *N. Engl. J. Med.*, 344, 539–548.

Kooperberg, C., Bose, S. and Stone, C. J. (1997). Polychotomous Regression. *J. Am. Stat. Assoc.*, 93, 117–127.

Lee, K. Y., Sha N., Doughetry, E. R., Vanucci, M. and Mallick, B. K. (2003). Gene Selection: A Bayesian Variable Selection Approach. *Bioinformatics*, 19, 90–97.

Metropolis, N., Rosenbluth, A. W., Rosenbluth, M. N., Teller, A. H. and Teller, E. (1953). Equations of State Calculations by Fast Computing Machines. *J. Chem. Phys.*, 21, 1087–1091.

Schena, M., Shalon, D., Davis, R. and Brown, P. (1995). Quantitative Monitoring of Gene Expression Patterns with a Complementary DNA Microarray. *Science*, 270, 467–470.

Yeang, C. H., Ramaswamy, S., Tamayo, P., Mukherjee, S., Rifkin, R. M., Angelo, M., Reich, M., Lander, E., Mesirov, J. and Golub, T. (2001). Molecular Classification of Multiple Tumor Types. *Bioinformatics*, 17, 316–322.

7

Models for Probability of Under- and Overexpression: The POE Scale

ELIZABETH GARRETT-MAYER AND ROBERT SCHARPF
Johns Hopkins University

Abstract

The probability of expression (i.e., POE) scale was developed to achieve two main goals: (1) Microarray data are generated using a variety of measurement techniques that are not directly comparable. We sought to develop a common scale for which microarray data generated using differing methods could be converted and then compared. (2) In many cases, we are interested in defining whether genes and/or samples fall into one of three categories: overexpressed, underexpressed, or normally expressed. However, gene expression values are usually generated on a continuous scale. The scale that we have developed is categorical, assigning these continuous individual expression values probabilities of falling into one of these three categories. We describe the POE scale, several of its practical uses, and demonstrate its use on a lung cancer microarray data set.

7.1 POE: A Latent Variable Mixture Model

7.1.1 The Motivation and Practicality of POE

One reason for developing the probability of expression (POE) scale is to transform continuous expression values to a three-component categorical scale. Often the continuous expression values are displayed by image plots that use a red–green scale for over- and underexpression, respectively. The commonly used red and green image plots effectively display microarray data and generally have three main colors: red (overexpression), green (underexpression), and black (normal expression). The visual impact is that we see red, green, and black and not the "smooth-scale" that would blend from red to black to green as implied by continuous data. Our goal is to assign probabilities to each observed expression value where the probabilities correspond to the chance that an expression value should be called "red," "green," or "black."

The second goal is to provide a common gene expression metric. Our rationale for this stems from the problem that there are thousands of gene expression studies generated by multiple platforms that have been performed, many of which are publicly available. Due to the expense of microarray studies in recent years, many of these studies are quite small, some with fewer than 10 chips. Considered independently, the smaller studies provide insufficient evidence for identifying interesting genes. However, if multiple small studies of similar sample types (e.g., breast cancer and normal breast tissues) that address comparable biological hypotheses can be combined, then the power to detect interesting genes would increase significantly.

7.1.2 A Mixture Model Approach

Consider that we have measured gene expression for J genes and I samples, captured in a $J \times I$ matrix where elements in the gene expression matrix are represented by x_{ji}. Phenotypic information on sample i, such as indicators of whether the sample is cancerous or normal, the survival time of the individual from whom the sample was taken, or histologic subtype, if available, can be defined by y_i, which can take a vector form if more than one phenotype is of interest.

We present two types of POE estimation procedures: unsupervised and semisupervised. Both approaches use the same model framework, but the implementation is slightly different. The unsupervised approach assumes that no phenotype information is available, and the goal of the analysis is subtype discovery. The semi-supervised approach assumes that there is some relevant phenotypic information available and it is of interest to use this information as part of the scale development where a "reference" class is defined. One goal for an analysis using the semisupervised approach is to find differentially expressed genes, or, like the unsupervised approach, to discover subtypes.

7.2 The POE Model

7.2.1 The Latent Variable

The basic underlying assumption of the POE model is that a gene's expression across individuals follows a three-component mixture model. The components of the mixture are defined by e_{ji}:

$$e_{ji} = -1 \text{ gene } j \text{ is abnormally low in sample } i$$
$$e_{ji} = 0 \text{ gene } j \text{ is at a typical level in sample } i$$
$$e_{ji} = 1 \text{ gene } j \text{ is abnormally high in sample } i$$

The components e_{ji} provide a biologically meaningful interpretation for under-, over-, and normal expression. More motivation for this idea can be found in [10].

For each gene j, we define the under-, normally, and overexpressed distributions as $f_{-1,j}$, $f_{0,j}$, and $f_{1,j}$, respectively, where

$$x_{ji}|(e_{ji} = e) \sim f_{e,j}(\cdot), \qquad e \in \{-1, 0, 1\}. \tag{7.1}$$

The population proportion of samples that show overexpression in gene j is denoted by $\pi_j^+ = P(e_{ji} = 1)$, and the analogous parameter for underexpression is π_j^-. We assume that the latent variables e_{ji} are independent conditional on the πs and fs.

7.2.2 Model Assumptions

In Section 7.2.1, the distributions for the three components are generally defined by $f_{e,j}$ for $e \in -1, 0, 1$. Theoretically, there are many choices for these densities. In practice, issues of identifiability limit our choice. For instance, many data sets have relatively few samples (i.e., < 100) and so it is imperative to limit the number of parameters to be estimated. We have used uniform ($\mathcal{U}$) distributions for the over- and underexpression distributions, and a Gaussian ($\mathcal{N}$) distribution for normal expression. These choices have been successful in modeling the categorical nature of the data in both real and simulated data.

Our parameterization of POE is

$$f_{-1,j}(\cdot) = \mathcal{U}(-\kappa_j^- + \alpha_i + \mu_j, \alpha_i + \mu_j)$$
$$f_{0,j}(\cdot) = \mathcal{N}(\alpha_i + \mu_j, \sigma_j^2)$$
$$f_{1,j}(\cdot) = \mathcal{U}(\alpha_i + \mu_j, \alpha_i + \mu_j + \kappa_j^+).$$

Beginning with the Gaussian component (denoted by $f_{0,j}(\cdot)$), $\mu_j + \alpha_i$ is the expected expression for gene j in sample i, where μ_j represents the gene effect and α_i the sample effect, and σ_j is the standard deviation. We include a sample effect to account for different mean levels of expression across samples. In prenormalized samples where average expression per chip is standardized across chips, the sample effect readjusts the normalization so that it considers only the normally expressed values of x_{ji} and not those that are differentially expressed. The over- and underexpression distributions are nonoverlapping and each has a limit corresponding to the mean of the Gaussian distribution with widths of κ_j^- and κ_j^+ for the under- and overexpression components,

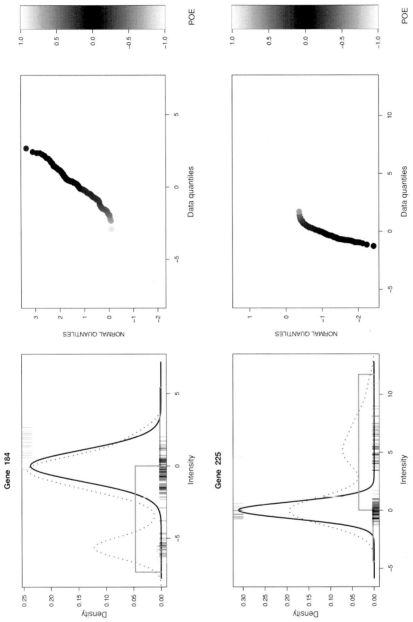

Fig. 7.1. Fit of the POE model for two genes. The figures on the left show the empirical density (dotted line) and the fitted mixture model (solid lines). Observed data are shown as tick marks above the figure (normal samples), and below the figure (tall ticks are squamous cell carcincmas, short ticks are adenocarcinomas). Figures on the right are quantile–quantile plots making evident deviations from normality. Shading of points shows the level of p_{ji}.

respectively. This particular three-component mixture model is depicted in Figure 7.1.

The parameterization described above is efficient because it requires relatively few parameters. For each gene, we estimate six parameters (μ_j, σ_j, κ_j^-, κ_j^+, π_j^-, π_j^+), but had we chosen a three-component Gaussian mixture model, we would have eight parameters to estimate (three means, three standard deviations, plus π_j^- and π_j^+). Our model is convenient in that stable estimates are provided even when the majority of the genes fall into the normal component of the mixture. Additionally, because of the flat shape of the uniform, no values are assigned very low densities. We have imposed an additional constraint that $\kappa_j^+ > r\sigma_j$ and $\kappa_j^- > r\sigma_j$ to ensure that the uniforms truly represent high and low values and do not have a large portion of their range overlapping with the Gaussian component. In our implementation, we generally choose a value of $r > 3$, which ensures relatively little overlap between the Gaussian and the uniform components.

In addition to efficiency in estimation, the chosen distributions are consistent with the nature of genomic and proteomic data. For example, it can be assumed in many cases that the error associated with measuring gene expression follows a Gaussian distribution, justifying our use of the Gaussian distribution for normal expression. In our applied setting, the uniform distribution naturally lends itself to the case of differential gene expression. In cancer applications, differential expression is often thought to be caused by the failure of biological mechanisms. As a result, the observed expression levels may take a broad range of values. Although we advocate the use of the three-component mixture model illustrated in Figure 7.1, other mixture models may be used.

Examples of normal/uniform mixtures for finding outliers and sparse clusters are discussed in [4]. For other examples of mixture modeling applied to microarray data, see [8, 9, 12].

7.2.3 Bayesian Hierarchical Model

A Bayesian hierarchical model is used for model estimation, as described by [10]. Inference is based on posterior distributions of the parameters defined in the previous sections. For the gene-specific parameters, we implement hierarchical modeling to borrow strength across genes. This is practical and reasonable due to the high gene-to-sample ratio which may make estimation of gene-specific parameters difficult. Additionally, there are likely to be artifacts associated with the technology that would affect all genes similarly. The hierarchical modeling that we have implemented is as follows:

$$\mu_j | \theta_\mu, \tau_\mu \sim \mathcal{N}(\theta_\mu, \tau_\mu)$$
$$\sigma_j^{-2} | \gamma, \lambda \sim \mathcal{G}(\gamma, \lambda)$$
$$\kappa_j^+ | \theta_\kappa^+ \sim \mathcal{E}(\theta_\kappa^+)$$
$$\kappa_j^- | \theta_\kappa^- \sim \mathcal{E}(\theta_\kappa^-)$$
$$\text{logit}(\pi_j^+) | \theta_\pi^+ \sim \mathcal{N}(\theta_\pi^+, \tau_\pi^+)$$
$$\text{logit}(\pi_j^-) | \theta_\pi^- \sim \mathcal{N}(\theta_\pi^-, \tau_\pi^-)$$

where $\mathcal{G}$ is the gamma distribution, and $\mathcal{E}$ is the exponential distribution. Gene-specific parameters are independent conditional on the hyperparameters on the right-hand side of the distributions above. Hyperparameters can be assigned dispersed, noninformative priors, as the large number of variables allows for data-driven estimation. For genes that show little or no evidence of high or low values (i.e., $\pi_j^- \approx \pi_j^+ \approx 0$), there is essentially no information in the data to estimate the parameters associated with the high and low distributions. The advantage of the hierarchical model is that the parameters for such genes are estimated by using information that is shared with other genes. In this parameterization, although we have not included a hierarchical distribution for α_i, the model could easily be modified to include a prior for α. Given the amount of information that is available to estimate α_i, such a parameterization may not be useful.

7.2.4 Model Estimation

A Markov chain Monte Carlo (MCMC) estimation procedure is used for model fitting. Data augmentation is used with an e_{ji} for each x_{ji} so that at each iteration of the chain, the latent variable was sampled [3, 11]. Sampling of the κ's is facilitated by marginalizing with respect to e when resampling κ. This results in the sampling sequence $[\kappa | \omega^*] \, [e | \kappa, \omega^*] \, [\omega^* | \kappa, e]$, where brackets indicate posterior distributions, ω denotes all the parameters, and ω^* denotes all the parameters excluding the κ's and the e's. As mentioned above, we include a constraint on the κ's, $\sigma_j r < \min(\kappa_j^+, \kappa_j^-)$, that improves identifiability. An additional constraint necessary for ensuring that all expression values assume positive probability in either the over- or underexpression distribution is $\kappa_j > \max_i(|x_{ji} - \mu_j - \alpha_i|)$ for each κ_j^+ and κ_j^-. Conditional on the e_{ji}, the full conditional distribution of π_j^+s and π_j^-s is Dirichlet, and the full conditional distribution of the normal component is conjugate (with the constraint relating the σ_j's and the κ's).

There are some ambiguities that need to be addressed as part of the estimation. The model attempts to find a three-component mixture for each gene. However, there will be many genes for which the gene expression values tend to follow a one-component Gaussian or bimodal distribution, and such genes have "empty" mixture components. In the case of unimodal data, the gene expression values will tend to fall into the Gaussian component, and the parameters defining the limits of the over- and underexpression distributions will be easily identified by the hierarchical distributions. A slightly less obvious situation is when the data appear to arise from a bimodal distribution, so that just one component of the mixture is empty. For this case, we have constrained the model so that $\pi_j^+ < 0.50$ and $\pi_j^- < 0.50$. Also, when the third component appears to have a very small fraction of samples (i.e., $\pi_j^+ < 1/I$ or $\pi_j^- < 1/I$), we collapse our three-component mixture into two components.

7.2.5 The POE Scale

After model estimation, the POE scale is created as a function of the posterior estimates of the model parameters. Using Bayes' rule, we estimate for each data point, x_{ji}, the probability that it is overexpressed (p_{ji}^+) and the probability that it is underexpressed (p_{ji}^-):

$$p_{ji}^+ = P(e_{ji} = 1 | x_{ji}, \omega) =$$
$$\frac{\pi_j^+ f_{1,j}(x_{ji})}{\pi_j^+ f_{1,j}(x_{ji}) + \pi_j^- f_{-1,j}(x_{ji}) + (1 - \pi_j^+ - \pi_j^-) f_{0,j}(x_{ji})} \quad (7.2)$$

$$p_{ji}^- = P(e_{ji} = -1 | x_{ji}, \omega) =$$
$$\frac{\pi_j^- f_{-1,j}(x_{ji})}{\pi_j^+ f_{1,j}(x_{ji}) + \pi_j^- f_{-1,j}(x_{ji}) + (1 - \pi_j^+ - \pi_j^-) f_{0,j}(x_{ji})}. \quad (7.3)$$

The POE scale is defined as the difference in these values, so that the POE scale ranges from -1 to 1. Genes with positive probability of underexpression have a POE value between -1 and 0 and those with positive probability of overexpression between 0 and 1. Because the under- and overexpression distributions do not overlap, any given value x_{ji} cannot have positive probability of both overexpression and underexpression (i.e., $\min(p_{ji}^+, p_{ji}^-) = 0$). Symbolically, we denote the POE value for gene j in sample i as

$$p_{ji} = p_{ji}^+ - p_{ji}^-. \quad (7.4)$$

An alternative useful scale uses an approximate Bayes' estimator to shrink the observed gene expression values. Here, an x_{ji} value that has strong evidence of being from the normal component (i.e., p_{ji} is close to 0) will have a shrunken value close to $\mu_j + \alpha_i$, while an x_{ji} value with strong evidence of differential expression will have a shrunken value close to the observed value, x_{ji}. These shrinkage estimates can be obtained by introducing latent quantitative expression values η_{ji} and defining $x_{ji} \sim \mathcal{N}(\eta_{ji}, \sigma_j)$ for the normal component, where $\eta_{ji} = \mu_j + \alpha_i$ with σ_j unknown. The over- and underexpressed classes are defined by $\eta_{ji} - \mu_j - \alpha_i \sim \mathcal{U}(0, \kappa_j^+)$ and $\eta_{ji} - \mu_j - \alpha_i \sim \mathcal{U}(-\kappa_j^-, 0)$, respectively. The posterior means z_{ji} of η_{ji} can be used as estimates of the shrunken expression values:

$$
\begin{aligned}
\mathcal{E}(\eta_{ji}) &= z_{ji} \approx \mu_j + \alpha_i + (x_{ji} - \mu_j - \alpha_i)p_{ji} \\
&= p_{ji}x_{ji} + (1 - p_{ji})(\mu_j + \alpha_i).
\end{aligned}
\tag{7.5}
$$

These can be thought of as multiple shrinkage estimates [6] and used as "denoised" versions of the original expression values.

7.3 Unsupervised versus Semisupervised POE

In the unsupervised setting, e_{ji} is a parameter to be estimated for each gene and each sample. This is a relatively straightforward latent variable problem and at each iteration of the MCMC, the e_{ji} values are sampled so that posterior estimates of probability of under- and overexpression can be easily estimated.

In the semi-supervised setting, we use the phenotypic information to assign e_{ji} to be "typical" for a relevant reference sample type:

$$
\begin{aligned}
&\text{if } y_i = 0 \quad \text{then} \quad e_{ji} = 0 \qquad \text{for } j = 1, \dots, J \\
&\text{if } y_i = 1 \quad \text{then} \quad e_{ji} \text{ is unknown} \quad \text{for } j = 1, \dots, J
\end{aligned}
$$

Assume that the phenotype of interest is disease and that $y_i = 0$ if sample i is normal and $y_i = 1$ if the sample is diseased. This parameterization assumes that all of the normal samples are from the normal component of the mixture, while the diseased samples are from the overexpression, underexpression, or normal components. Because only the e_{ji} of diseased samples can take values 1 and -1, the normal component of the mixture has the interpretation as the category that would be expected in normal samples. However, depending on the application of interest, the phenotypic category assigned to the normal component of the mixture may change. For example, assume that we have a heterogeneous set of lung cancer samples taken from patients with varying survival times. Our goal might be to identify genes that are relatively differentially expressed in long-surviving patients, or a subset of long-surviving patients. As such, we would want to define our reference to be samples who had short survival. In general, we are most likely to be interested in defining the reference to be a phenotype for which finding subgroups is not of interest: we want to use the hierarchical model to assign latent variable values of -1, 0, or 1 to genes in heterogeneous samples. This is consistent with the idea that there are multiple mechanistic pathways that can lead to cancer.

The assumption that the diseased samples can be from any of the three components yet the nondiseased samples are all from the normal components generates an asymmetry in the way that the unsupervised analysis is nested in the supervised analysis. However, it allows us to borrow strength from the utilized class information and adds efficiency and improved identifiability to model estimation. Implementation is almost identical to that for the unsupervised POE. The major difference is that the e_{ji} parameters are fixed for the reference category and are sampled for the other samples. Additionally, the constraints $\pi_j^+ < 0.50$ and $\pi_j^- < 0.50$ are removed.

7.4 Using POE Scale

Once the POE model has been estimated for a data set, then the POE transformed data can be used for a variety of purposes. Two that we describe here include evaluating the utility of genes for distinguishing between sample phenotypes, and mining for genes that are potentially related to subtypes.

7.4.1 Evaluating Diagnostic Criteria of Genes

We quantify diagnostic criteria of genes by their *sensitivity* (se) and *specificity* (sp). Considering a data set with normal and cancer samples, we define se and sp in the setting of normal and cancer samples as follows:

$se_j = P(\text{gene } j \text{ in sample } i \text{ is differentially expressed } | \text{ sample } i \text{ is cancer})$

$sp_j = P(\text{gene } j \text{ in sample } i \text{ is typically expressed } | \text{ sample } i \text{ is normal})$

The above definitions for se and sp are only applicable when using semi-supervised POE. Based on the estimated POE model for each gene, se_j and sp_j are easily calculated as a function of model parameters. For specificity of gene j we simply calculate 1 minus the average of $|p_{ji}|$ for the normal samples. For sensitivity, we estimate the average of $|p_{ji}|$ for the nonnormal samples. This procedure can be easily adapted to other subtypes.

Using gene-specific information, we can (1) identify genes that are related to phenotype or (2) filter genes that have low specificity and/or sensitivity from further analyses. In the context of normal and cancer diagnostics, we tend to place more emphasis on identifying genes with high specificity: this implies that the normal samples tend to have similar gene expression values (i.e., they all tend to fall within the normal component of the mixture). However, it is reasonable that we could be interested in genes with relatively low sensitivity (e.g., $se_j \approx 0.20$). For instance, sensitivities in the range of 0.20 and higher may imply that there is a subgroup of nonnormal samples that is differentially expressed. Genes with high specificity and at least moderate sensitivity may be useful for discriminating subclasses of cancer.

7.4.2 Mining for Genes

In both the semi-supervised and unsupervised POE approaches, we can apply methods to look for subsets of genes that define subtypes of cancers. We call this approach "gene mining" and the general idea is to find a set of genes with prespecified over- and underexpression profiles and to then look at the subgroups of samples based on gene expression profiles of a few chosen genes. This is an exploratory approach, as it is an unsupervised way of choosing interesting genes, and figures are provided for understanding how combinations of genes differentiate samples.

The gene mining approach hinges on two statistics: gene coherence, and gene agreement defined by

$$r_{jk} = \sum_{i=1}^{I}(p_{ji}^+ p_{ki}^+ + p_{ji}^- p_{ki}^- + (1 - p_{ji})(1 - p_{ki})), \qquad (7.6)$$

which ranges from 0 to I. r_{jj} is a measure of coherence of gene j, and r_{jk} is a measure of agreement for genes j and k for $j \neq k$. Intuitively, coherence measures how well a gene distinguishes between the components of the mixture when assigning class probabilities. The coherence will be high if the values of p_{ji} are close to -1, 0, or 1. Conversely, coherence will be low if many of the p_{ji}'s are near 0.50. Agreement is defined as the proportion of samples that "agree" across two genes in terms of their assignment to one of the components of the mixture.

For both coherence and agreement, we define thresholds of acceptable levels a priori. After the r_{jk} matrix has been calculated, we look at the the distribution of gene coherence (i.e., the diagonal of the matrix) to determine a reasonable threshold, typically based on a percentile of the distribution of coherences. Although high levels of coherence are preferable, the percentile chosen depends on the data set and whether a semisupervised or unsupervised estimation approach was used. For selecting a threshold for sufficient gene agreement, we have two approaches that we have used. The first approach chooses a fixed level of gene agreement (similar to that described for coherence), whereas the second approach sets a threshold for agreement as a proportion of coherence of the "seed" gene, described below. The latter approach may be more reasonable as gene coherence serves as an upper bound for a gene's agreement with other genes.

An algorithm has been developed for gene mining that utilizes user inputs to guide selection. As mentioned above, this is an exploratory approach for understanding gene expression across samples and as such there is no "best" set of genes provided by the algorithm. The way the algorithm works is that the user chooses a specific pattern of over- and underexpression (e.g., $\{0.20, 0.10\}$) and genes consistent with this pattern are identified. While it might seem difficult to choose an expression pattern, this is part of the flexibility of the mining approach: the procedure can be repeated for a variety of expression patterns and given the algorithm's speed, it will not be cumbersome or time-consuming. Additionally, the algorithm is not particularly sensitive to the choice of expression pattern. For example, the patterns $\{0.20, 0.10\}$ and $\{0.25, 0.05\}$ will likely choose very similar genes.

The algorithm is defined as follows, with more detail provided in [10] and [5].

(i) Choose an expression pattern that indicates the proportion of samples over- and underexpressed (e.g., $\{0.20, 0.05\}$ indicates 20% of samples are overexpressed, 5% underexpressed, and 75% are typically expressed).

(ii) For each gene, calculate the probability of exhibiting the over- and underexpression pattern defined in step i using the estimates of p_{ji}^{+} and p_{ji}^{-}. Then, sort genes based on this probability.

(iii) Choose the "seed gene": the gene with the highest probability from step ii that has sufficient coherence (according to the coherence threshold).

(iv) Identify genes that agree with the seed gene (using agreement threshold) and add these genes to the group seeded by the gene identified in step iii.

(v) Remove the seed gene and those that agree with it (in step iv) from consideration and repeat steps ii and iii to identify additional gene groups consistent with the expression pattern of interest.

For each implementation of the algorithm, we choose a different expression pattern of interest and identify homogeneous groups of genes (in terms of expression profiles). Because of the homogeneity, the genes can be considered statistically redundant. As such, when looking at molecular profiles, only one gene per gene group needs to be considered. It makes sense statistically to use the seed gene, because it is the most coherent. But, because an EST used as a seed gene may not be biologically interesting, users have the option to choose a gene from the gene group that is "familiar," in the sense that it is plausibly related to the biologic mechanism under investigation.

Once several interesting genes have been chosen based on the results of mining, molecular profiles can be created using the p_{ji} values. The profiles measure the probability of a particular sample having a profile, defined by under-, typical, and overexpression values for each of the genes being considered. For example, with only two genes defining a profile, we have nine (3^2) profiles: $(-1,-1), (-1,0), (-1,1), (0,-1), (0,0), (0,1), (1,-1), (1,0), (1,1)$. Profiles in this case will generally be most informative with relatively few genes, otherwise the number of profiles is unwieldy – even for only four genes, we have $3^4 = 81$ possible profiles. However, in practice, it is likely that many of the profiles will be "empty" in the sense that no samples will be very likely to fall into them. In that case, inference can be simplified by looking only at the profiles that have positive probabilities for one or more samples. A useful way of interpreting the profiles is via a heatmap, as we demonstrate in the example in the next section.

7.5 Example: POE as Applied to Lung Cancer Microarray Data

The methods described in the previous sections are demonstrated using microarray data on 177 lung tissue samples of three types: adenocarcinomas ($n = 139$), squamous cell carcinomas ($n = 21$), and normal lung tissue ($n = 17$) [1]. mRNA expression was measured using Affymetrix HGU95A oligonucleotide arrays, including 12,600 genes and ESTs, and the original .CEL files were available for analysis. The samples were collected from two different tumor banks, one at Brigham and Women's Hospital, and the other at Masschusetts General Hospital. Details of sample preparation and RNA extraction can be found in the Web supplement to [1], available at http://research.dfci.harvard.edu/meyerson/lungca. Data were preprocessed using RMA [7] for quantile normalization and to calculate expression values across probe sets. Initial screening of genes was performed to identify a subset of genes which show evidence of reproducibility using integrative correlation [2]. Using this approach, a total of 1,547 genes were kept for POE analysis.

Using the phenotype information (i.e., normal, squamous cell, or adenocarcinoma), the normal samples were chosen as a reference group and the semisupervised version of POE was fit to the data set. To understand the model, consider Figure 7.1 which shows the POE model fit to two genes. We see two genes, the first (gene 184) showing strong evidence of underexpression in the

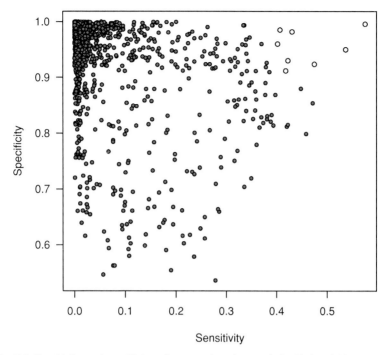

Fig. 7.2. Sensitivity and specificity of genes, where interest is in distinguishing cancers from normals.

squamous cell samples, and the second (gene 225) showing strong evidence of overexpression in some of both the squamous cell and adenocarcinomas.

For all of the genes in the analysis, sensitivity and specificity were estimated as described in Section 5.1 with the interest of distinguishing between cancers and normals. These values are plotted in Figure 7.2, where genes with high specificity (> 0.90) and relatively high sensitivity (> 0.40) are highlighted. Recall that in this application we would expect there might be subsets of cancerous samples and so we would not expect all of the cancer samples to fall into the differential expression components. As such, we tolerate seemingly low sensitivities, but we do prefer high specificity implying that the normal samples all tend to be included in the normal component of the mixture. In addition, we also considered which genes can distinguish between squamous and adenocarcinoma tumors. We do this by treating squamous cell carcinoma as the "reference" (i.e., the "normal" category), so that sensitivity represents the probability of a gene being differentially expressed given that it is adenocarcinoma, and specificity is the probability of a gene being typically expressed if it is squamous cell carcinoma. The results are not shown here for brevity.

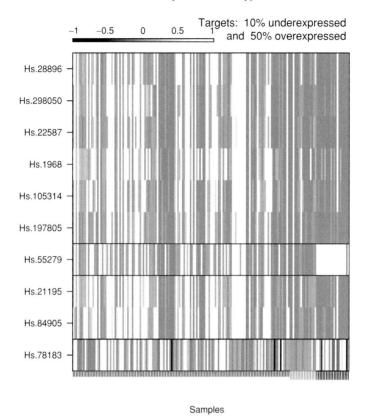

Fig. 7.3. POE mining plot, showing several gene groups found when mining for expression patterns of {0.10, 0.50}. Gene groups are separated by solid horizontal black lines. Seed genes are at the bottom of each gene group. Expression (as measured by POE) is shown in gray-scale, ranging from underexpression (black) to overexpression (white). Normal expression is gray. Unigene ID for each gene is shown on the y-axis. Samples are ordered according to phenotype, with adenocarcinomas indicated by short gray ticks, squamous cell carcinomas by black long ticks, and normal samples by gray long ticks.

At this point, we could use the sensitivity and specificity information to remove some genes from the analysis. We can also choose to keep the whole set of genes, and then consider the sensitivity and specificity of the genes when choosing which genes to include in our molecular profiling after mining. For this illustration, we will keep all genes and then refer back to their sensitivities and specificities when we perform profiling.

We applied the mining algorithm using the following expression patterns: {0.10, 0.25}, {0.10, 0.50}, {0.25, 0.10}. One of these is shown in Figure 7.3.

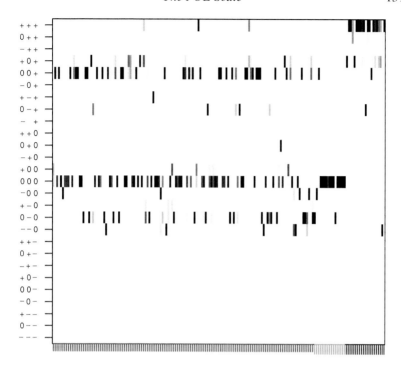

Samples

Fig. 7.4. Molecular profiles based on Hs.504115, Hs.518198, Hs.55279, respectively. Shading indicates probability of sample having a molecular profile ranging from white (probability of 0) to black (probability of 1). The vertical ticks on the horizontal axis are described in Figure 7.3.

There are several things to note. First, the normal samples have consistently "gray" expression across almost all of the selected genes, an expected result due to the semisupervised approach assigning normal samples to the Gaussian component. Rather it is more interesting that the patterns of differential expression are quite different in the gene groups. In particular, gene Hs.55279 is overexpressed in squamous cell carcinomas. For the other gene groups, the majority show normal to underexpression in the squamous cell samples.

Based on these gene mining procedures (the one shown in Figure 7.3 and the other two defined by the expression patterns described in the previous paragraph), three genes were chosen for creating molecular profiles. The molecular profiles of these genes are shown in Figure 7.4.

Hs.55279 (SERPINB5) is a gene encoding a serine protease inhibitor of the serpin family, termed maspin. Members of the maspin family have been reported to have tumor suppressor function. The sensitivity and specificity of SERPINB5 are 0.40, and specificity is 0.92, respectively.

Hs.504115 encodes a protein belonging to the TRIM protein family. This gene may function as a transcription factor involved in cancer, or in cell differentiation. The sensitivity of this gene was low (0.05), but discriminated well between the two types of cancer with specificity of 0.95.

Hs.518198 (Cystatin A) is known to be expressed in the lung and its protein product is an intracellular thiol proteinase inhibitor. Although it has not been reported to be involved in cancer, its sensitivity is 0.23 and specificity is 0.89.

7.6 Discussion

With the large number of gene expression studies published and publicly available, there is a great need for comparability of data and results. The POE scale was created to do just that: gene expression data from a variety of technologies can be transformed to the POE probability scale, allowing data to be combined and/or compared across studies. Two versions of POE are available. The unsupervised version of POE is used when there is no obvious reference category as defined by phenotype. The semisupervised POE is used when at least one subgroup (defined by phenotype) is defined and can be considered a reference category. For instance, in the example in Section 7.5 the phenotype was tissue type with categories adenocarcinoma, squamous cell carcinoma, and normal. The semisupervised POE was fit using the normal phenotype as the reference. As an alternative, the unsupervised POE model could have been used which would ignore phenotype information. In addition to using POE to transform the original data to a comparable scale, gene profiles and discrimination statistics can been derived using the POE-transformed data.

Our example demonstrates the POE approach on a lung cancer data set with 160 lung cancer and 17 normal lung tissue samples. After fitting POE, we evaluated each gene for its sensitivity and specificity, finding a handful of genes with high ($> 90\%$) specificity and relatively high ($> 40\%$) sensitivity. These genes could be further investigated and validated to determine if they are useful for distinguishing, in a clinical setting, between normal and malignant tissue. Additionally, the results were not presented, but we also estimated the sensitivity and specificity for discriminating between the squamous cell and the adenocarcinoma tissues, demonstrating that any phenotypic categories can be compared. However, the estimates of sensitivity and specificity are only meaningful in the context of the semisupervised POE: without declaring a reference category, we cannot assume that the normal component of the mixture will always represent the reference category. This is especially true in a situation such as we have in the lung cancer example where the majority of the samples are cancerous. Recall that in the unsupervised POE, the differential expression components are constrained so that $\pi_j^+ < 0.50$ and $\pi_j^- < 0.50$. For genes that show good separation between the cancers and normals (and there are far more cancer samples than normal samples), we would expect that the cancerous samples would be in the Gaussian component and the normal samples would be in the over- or underexpression components.

The gene mining techniques were also applied to find genes that show patterns for gene expression across phenotypes. This is particularly interesting when phenotype is unavailable and the goal is to describe new potential subtypes by molecular profiles. When phenotype is available, gene mining is a useful exploratory tool, but evaluating sensitivity and specificity is more useful for finding potentially interesting genes. For a detailed example of unsupervised POE for gene mining, see [10].

An important consideration is where to go from here. Using the sensitivities and specificities, and/or the gene mining tools, the POE user will find sets of genes of interest that look promising for describing cancer (or other phenotypic) subtypes. The critical next step is validation which can be achieved in several ways. One validation approach would be to apply these techniques to another comparable data set in regards to phenotype. For example, comparing sensitivities and specificities of genes across data sets would be a helpful way to investigate the reproducibility of results. Another approach would be to validate the interesting genes using more sensitive gene-specific approaches (e.g., RT-PCR for a small set of genes). This could be done using the same samples from the original data set, if they are available, or using newly collected tissues of the same subtypes (e.g., lung cancer and normal lung tissues).

POE is available as an R library and continues to be improved and expanded. It can be downloaded from http://astor.som.jhmi.edu/poe/.

Bibliography

[1] Bhattacharjee A, Richards WG, Staunton J, Li C, Monti S, Vasa P, Ladd C, Beheshti J, Bueno R, Gillette M, Loda M, Weber G, Mark EJ, Lander ES, Wong W, Johnson BE, Golub TR, Sugarbaker DJ, Meyerson M (2001). Classification of human lung carcinomas by mRNA expression profiling reveals distinct adenocarcinoma subclasses. *Proceedings of the National Academy of Sciences USA* 98:13790–13795.

[2] Cope L, Zhong X, Garrett-Mayer ES, Gabrielson E, Parmigiani G (submitted). Cross-study validation of the molecular profile of brca1-linked breast cancers.

[3] Diebolt J, Robert CP (1994). Estimation of finite mixture distributions through Bayesian sampling. *Journal of the Royal Statistical Society, Series B, Methodological* 56:363–375.

[4] Fraley C, Raftery AE (1998). How many clusters? Which clustering method? – Answers via model-based cluster analysis. *Computer Journal* 41:578–588.

[5] Garrett ES, Parmigiani G (2003). POE: Statistical tools for molecular profiling. In: G Parmigiani, ES Garrett, RA Irizarry, SL Zeger (eds.), *The Analysis of Gene Expression Data: Methods and Software*, 362–387. New York: Springer.

[6] George EI (1986). Minimax multiple shrinkage estimation. *The Annals of Statistics* 14:188–205.

[7] Irizarry RA, M BB, Collin F, Cope LM, Hobbs B, Speed TP (2003). Summaries of affymetrix genechip probe level data. *Nucleic Acids Research* 31:e15.

[8] Lee ML, Kuo FC, Whitmore GA, Sklar J (2000). Importance of replication in microarray gene expression studies: Statistical methods and evidence from repetitive cDNA hybridizations. *Proceedings of the National Academy of Sciences USA* 97(18):9834–9839.

[9] McLachlan GJ, Bean RW, Peel D (2002). A mixture model-based approach to the clustering of microarray expression data. *Bioinformatics* 18:413–422.

[10] Parmigiani G, Garrett ES, Anbazhagan R, Gabrielson E (2002). A statistical framework for expression-based molecular classification in cancer. *Journal of the Royal Statistical Society, Series B* 64:717–736.

[11] West M, Turner D (1994). Deconvolution of mixtures in analysis of neural synaptic transmission. *The Statistician* 43:31–43.

[12] Yeung K, Fraley C, Murua A, Raftery A, Ruzzo W (2001). Model-based clustering and data transformations for gene expression data. *Bioinformatics* 17:977–987.

8

Sparse Statistical Modelling in Gene Expression Genomics

JOSEPH LUCAS, CARLOS CARVALHO, QUANLI WANG,
ANDREA BILD, JOSEPH R. NEVINS, AND MIKE WEST

Duke University

Abstract

The concept of sparsity is more and more central to practical data analysis and inference with increasingly high-dimensional data. Gene expression genomics is a key example context. As part of a series of projects that has developed Bayesian methodology for large-scale regression, ANOVA, and latent factor models, we have extended traditional Bayesian "variable selection" priors and modelling ideas to new hierarchical sparsity priors that are providing substantial practical gains in addressing false discovery and isolating significant gene-specific parameters/effects in highly multivariate studies involving thousands of genes. We discuss and review these developments, in the contexts of multivariate regression, ANOVA, and latent factor models for multivariate gene expression data arising in either observational or designed experimental studies. The development includes the use of sparse regression components to provide gene-sample-specific normalisation/correction based on control and housekeeping factors, an important general issue and one that can be critical – and critically misleading if ignored – in many gene expression studies. Two rich data sets are used to provide context and illustration. The first data set arises from a gene expression experiment designed to investigate the transcriptional response – in terms of responsive gene subsets and their expression signatures – to interventions that upregulate a series of key oncogenes. The second data set is observational, breast cancer tumour-derived data evaluated utilising a sparse latent factor model to define and isolate factors underlying the hugely complex patterns of association in gene expression patterns. We also mention software that implements these and other models and methods in one comprehensive framework.

8.1 Perspective

A series of recent developments in Bayesian multivariate modelling has emphasised the relevance and utility of structured, sparsity-inducing hierarchical models in a variety of multivariate contexts and applied gene expression studies. We review and exemplify some of this methodology here, utilising two current cancer genomics projects to provide illuminating examples. The main methodological foci are as follows:

- A novel hierarchical "sparsity prior" for variable/effect selection in highly multivariate models, and its use and application in multivariate regression and ANOVA when many of the regression parameters and effects are expected to be zero [1];
- The use of such sparsity priors in connection with regressions for gene-sample-specific normalisation to correct for multiple components of nonbiological error and bias in expression intensity estimates – referred to as "assay artifacts" [1, 2]; and
- The use of such sparsity priors in Bayesian latent factor models for parsimonious representation of expression profiles and deconvolution of the complexities of patterns of covariation among genes that are potentially related to underlying pathway interactions as well as experimental influences [2, 3].

Over the last several years, the development of larger and richer genomic studies – both experimental and observational – has motivated a number of developments that underlie the current work. The decreasing costs of DNA microarray assays are leading to larger and richer data sets from observational studies in human cancers and other areas, and advances in molecular technologies such as siRNA are leading to rapid increase in the scale and complexity of designed experiments in which genome-scale gene expression (and other) data is the response variable. Across all such studies, the concepts of pattern profiling and expression signature identification are central: it is now common for analyses to utilise aggregate measures of gene expression on a selection of defined subsets of genes as characterising multiple aspects of either an underlying response to a biological intervention [4–7], or empirical prognostic markers in observational and clinical studies [8–17].

The two examples here provide specificity and context. The first data set comes from [6], where experiments using primary breast epithelial cells generate expression profiles that are used to identify subsets of genes that show transcriptional responses to the action of a known oncogenic activity. Each oncogene intervention is replicated several times and the responses are evaluated using Affymetrix U133+ DNA microarray data. Resulting selected subsets of genes – or metagenes, one for each oncogene response – are then explored in gene expression data sets from human tumours, where summary patterns of aggregate gene expression variations of these "oncogene signatures" may have prognostic or therapeutic significance. This study builds on the development of this general concept in biological pathway interrogation and disease studies [4, 5, 7]. The example highlights the need for sensitive evaluation of which of the thousands of genes are truly transcriptionally responsive, emphasises the need for care that false discovery be minimised, and promotes attention to questions of data quality, comparability, and the likely need for within-model correction for systematic, nonbiological biases and artifacts.

The second data set consists of expression profiles from human breast cancer tissues from a program with multiple clinical and basic pathway identification goals (e.g., [11, 15]). The example here concerns the complexity of structure in patterns of association among hundreds of genes connected to the key breast cancer hormonal and growth pathways linked to ER (oestrogen receptor) and HER2/ERB-B2 proteins, each of interest in connection with improved therapeutics in breast cancer. One interest is the potential for tumour-derived gene expression measures to provide increasingly accurate, and higher-resolution, evaluation of the status of these pathways, hence the interest in gene subsets related to transcriptional variation within these pathways. This links intimately with the prognostic interests in improved gene expression signatures as covariates in predictive models [15].

In the first example, the primary interest is ANOVA/regression modelling to identify gene subsets related to each of the interventions, and to account for artifactual effects in expression profiles across samples. The second example focuses on deconvolution of expression associations in a multivariate latent factor framework, again taking into account potential artifactual effects, and includes a predictive regression component to relate latent factors underlying gene expression across the ER and HER2 pathways to the (noisy) pathological measures of ER and HER2 status at the protein level using traditional immunohistochemistry. The overarching sparse factor regression model context subsumes both cases.

8.2 Sparse Regression Modelling

8.2.1 *General Framework and Notation*

Our data in these two examples, and many others, is generated from Affymetrix microarrays, and we utilise as a current standard the RMA expression intensity estimates on the log 2 (fold change) scale [18, 19]. In either example, write

$x_{g,i}$ for the expression of gene g on any sample i, assuming p genes and n independent samples. Then write x_i for the column p-vector of expression on sample i, and set $X = [x_1, \ldots, x_n]$. In notation, all vectors are column vectors, so that x_i' is the $1 \times p$ row vector, for example, and $\perp\!\!\!\perp$ denotes conditional independence.

In a regression or designed experiment context, we assume

$$x_i = \mu + Bh_i + v_i, \tag{8.1}$$

where μ is a p−vector of constant intercept terms, h_i is a known d-vector of covariates for sample i, with jth element $h_{j,i}$, B is the $p \times d$ matrix of regression parameters, v_i is a p−vector of assumedly normal error terms, and $v_i \sim N(0, \Psi)$ independently where Ψ is the $p \times p$ diagonal matrix of elements ψ_g $(g = 1, \ldots, p)$. Write μ_g for the gth element of μ, β_g' for the gth row of B, and $\beta_{g,j}$ for the jth element of β_g; the {gene g, sample i} univariate regression is then

$$x_{g,i} = \mu_g + \sum_{j=1}^{d} \beta_{g,j} h_{j,i} + v_{g,i}, \qquad v_{g,i} \perp\!\!\!\perp N(0, \psi_g). \tag{8.2}$$

The design vector h_i may include dummy variables representing the levels of experimental factors and the observed values of measured covariates.

Sparse regression modelling is defined by classes of priors on B. The other prior components are the prior for μ, typically taken as independent normals for the elements μ_g, and that for the unexplained components of variance ψ_g. The latter represent biological, technical, and measurement error that are idiosyncratic to each gene. With Affymetrix RMA data, experience with many data sets indicates technical variation in the range of about 0.1–0.5, with values around 0.2–0.3 being quite typical. For such data, then, values of ψ_g will typically range across 0.01–0.25 or thereabouts, so providing the basis for prior specification. A standard specification consistent with these guidelines – while rather diffuse – is used in the examples here; this is a common gamma prior with shape 5 and scale 1 for each of the ψ_g^{-1}.

8.2.2 Sparsity Priors

Sparsity modelling aims to induce (many) zeros in the high-dimensional ("tall and skinny") parameter matrix B, reflecting the view that the effects of covariates will be sparse. An intervention or measured covariate may relate to a number of genes – "downstream" genes in a pathway intervention experiment, for example – but many other genes will be unrelated. This complements the statistical view of parsimony in modelling – that is, we aim to identify as few parameters as the data and context require to adequately represent the observed patterns in the expression profiles. The traditional ideas underlying Bayesian "point-mass mixture" priors/models are then absolutely natural. Several groups have used this approach in expression genomics (e.g., [20–25]), as did [3] in the context of latent factor models.

Motivated by large-scale expression studies, this thinking and methodology has recently been extended with new hierarchical specifications for such "point-mass mixture" priors [1]. An example of the new class of general models is

$$\beta_{g,j} \sim (1 - \pi_{g,j})\delta_0(\beta_{g,j}) + \pi_{g,j}N(\beta_{g,j}|0, \tau_j), \tag{8.3}$$

conditionally independently over genes g and covariates j. Here $\delta_0(\cdot)$ is a point-mass at zero, $N(\cdot|m, t)$ is the normal prior of mean m and variance t, and the covariate-specific parameters τ_j control the levels of variation in the magnitudes of the nonzero $|\beta_{g,j}|$.

Importantly, this new model has individual {gene g, covariate j} association probabilities $\pi_{g,j}$; that is, $\pi_{g,j}$ is the probability gene g is associated with covariate j. Write $\Pi = \{\pi_{g,j}\}$ for these $p \times d$ probabilities. The new class of priors in [1] embodies the view that many genes will have *zero* (or very small) prior probability of association with any one covariate; we simply do not know which genes do, and which do not. The natural hierarchical model to reflect this view is

$$\pi_{g,j} \sim (1 - \rho_j)\delta_0(\pi_{g,j}) + \rho_j Be(\pi_{g,j}|sr, s(1 - r)), \tag{8.4}$$

where $Be(\cdot|sr, s(1 - r))$ is the beta prior (with mean r and variance $r(1 - r)/(1 + s)$) and the covariate-specific probabilities ρ_j are assumed to be drawn from a common specified prior $\rho_j \sim Be(\rho_j|av, a(1 - v))$. Note that while each gene-covariate pair now has its own *individual* probability $\pi_{g,j}$ of an effect, marginalising over these parameters shows that $r\rho_j$ is the implied *population* base-rate of nonzero effects for covariate j.

Posterior analysis leads to the evaluations of, among other things, the $p \times d$ posterior probabilities $\Pi^* = \{\pi_{g,j}^*\}$, where $\pi_{g,j}^* = Pr(\beta_{g,j} \neq 0|X)$; these reflect individual gene-covariate shrinkage effects, and may be used to rank and select genes showing association with covariate j. The model-based approach naturally shrinks $\pi_{g,j}^*$ toward zero for genes showing little evidence of association with covariate j, while estimating the ρ_j and "shrinking" the nonzero $\pi_{g,j}^*$ toward the estimated base-rate $r\rho_j$. This provides the automatic adaptation to the many inherent "point null (at zero) versus continuous alternative" hypotheses being evaluated – a key and critical strength of the Bayesian approach, obviating the need for any ad hoc (and post hoc) multiple testing/comparison consideration.

We stress that this hierarchical model is quite different to the traditional approach – it represents an hierarchical/random effects extension of the usual point-mass mixture prior approach, inserting an additional "layer" between the *individual* gene-covariate parameters $\pi_{g,j}$ and the implicit underlying population base-rate of nonzero $\beta_{g,j}$ effects. Now, by marginalisation over the $\pi_{g,j}$ in equation (8.3), we obtain

$$\beta_{g,j} \sim (1 - r\rho_j)\delta_0(\beta_{g,j}) + r\rho_j N(\beta_{g,j}|0, \tau_j). \tag{8.5}$$

This population-level model has the usual point-mass mixture form, with a base-rate $r\rho_j$ of nonzero covariate effects for covariate j. Critically, however, in the full model each gene-covariate combination also has its own prior "base-rate" $\pi_{g,j}$ that is estimated. Since equation (8.4) permits zero values, the posterior will then estimate the data-based support for $\pi_{g,j} = 0$ individually. This key feature, induced by the new hierarchical model component, can lead to practical improvements over the standard Bayesian approach in acting against false discovery, especially in contexts where the base-rate is likely to be relatively large. By inserting the additional hierarchical layer between the population base-rate of nonzero effects and the individual-level effects, the extended model is able to more adequately shrink toward zero through the induction of zeros under the prior, and hence posterior, for the $\pi_{g,j}$. As a result, the hierarchical model is more conducive to separation of the real signals from noise, and will act conservatively – reducing false discovery – relative to the traditional prior. An example in the next section, and displayed in Figure 8.1, very clearly highlights this.

The model of equations (8.3) and (8.4) is completed with priors for the variances τ_j, taken as conditionally conjugate inverse gamma distributions. Bayesian analysis is performed using Markov chain Monte Carlo (MCMC) methods to produce samples from the posterior distributions for all model parameters: μ, B, Ψ, and the τ_j. Full MCMC details are given in [1]. For our purposes here, MCMC analysis produces full posterior samples for all model parameters, now including the critical posterior "significance" parameters in the $p \times d$ matrix $\Pi^* = \{\pi^*_{g,j}\}$, as well as μ, B, Ψ, and the $\{\rho_j, \tau_j : j = 1, \ldots, d\}$. Additional important summaries involve posterior samples of the $(\beta_{g,j}|\beta_{g,j} \neq 0, X)$. Prior specification is completed through assignment of values to the beta prior hyperparameters (s, r) and (a, v), as well as prior hyperparameters for independent gamma priors for the ψ_g^{-1} for each $g = 1, \ldots, p$ as earlier mentioned; the examples here use $(s, r) = (10, 0.9)$ and $(a, v) = (200, 0.001)$ for these beta priors.

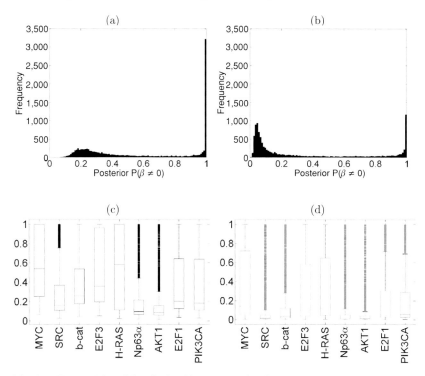

Fig. 8.1. Frames (a) and (b) display histograms of estimated posterior probabilities of nonzero effects on average expression of all genes based on the MYC oncogene intervention: (a) under the traditional shrinkage prior and (b) under the new hierarchical shrinkage prior. Frames (c) and (d) display boxplots of these estimated posterior probabilities of nonzero effects now for each of the nine experimental intervention groups: (c) under the traditional shrinkage prior and (d) under the new hierarchical shrinkage prior.

8.2.3 Example: Oncogene Intervention Experiments

The oncogene intervention data provides illumination. The experimental groups represent upregulation, using viral transfection, of key oncogenes MYC, SRC, b-catenin, E2F3, H-RAS, Np63α, AKT1, E2F1, and PIK3Ca. Several of these genes play transcriptional roles related to the complex Rb/E2F pathway [26, 27] that is pivotal in regulating cell cycle progression, cell proliferation, and cell death (apoptosis). The E2F family of transcription factors is particularly key in this complex of interacting pathways, and one interest relates to differential function for members of the E2F family. The design is a simple one-way classification: one control group with 15 samples (biological replicates), and 9 separate intervention groups with between 7 and 10 replicates per group, for a total of $n = 97$ samples. So μ_g is the average (log 2, RMA) expression for gene

g in the nonintervention control group, and the $d = 9$ parameters in β_g define changes in level relative to control in each of the 9 intervention groups. Across all genes, most of the $\beta_{g,j}$ parameters will be zero; the analysis aims to isolate gene-factor combinations with nonzero parameters to identify resulting groups of genes transcriptionally regulated via the cascade of activation initiated for each intervention.

Group $j = 2$ represents the MYC interventions, for example. Figure 8.1(b) displays a histogram of the MCMC-based estimates of the $\pi^*_{g,2}$ over all $p = 10,777$ genes used here. For comparison, Figure 8.1(a) shows the corresponding histogram under the traditional prior. The effect of the hierarchical model is clear: more shrinkage to zero or very small values of many probabilities, and improved isolation of significant effects consistent with the much reduced propensity for false discovery. Frames (c) and (d) of Figure 8.1 provide boxplots of these $\pi^*_{g,j}$ probabilities for each of the $j = 1 : 9$ intervention groups, again comparing the new hierarchical sparsity prior with the traditional, and even more clearly highlighting the impact. To verify and empirically validate the view that the traditional model typically fails to induce enough shrinkage – and overestimates the numbers of "significant" effects as a result – similar analyses have been performed in a series of simulation studies in which synthetic data have been generated from the model as defined. Pervasively, the numbers of inferred nonzero parameters – in terms of high values of the posterior probabilities of nonzero values gene-by-gene – are systematically overestimated under the traditional analysis and much more adequately estimated using the new sparsity prior.

8.3 Sparse Regression for Artifact Correction with Affymetrix Expression Arrays

8.3.1 Context and Model

Data from all microarray studies is contaminated by nonbiological noise from a multitude of sources. Low-level processing and normalisation methods aim to address and either correct for or model some of the issues of sample-to-sample, and in some cases gene-sample-specific, variation. However, high-throughput expression technologies are still effectively first-generation and the resulting data can often exhibit profound levels of artifactual noise and systematic experimental biases that are induced by small, random, and unpredictable changes and fluctuations in experimental controls (hybridisation temperatures, salinity, etc.), assay reagents, technician practices, equipment settings, and so forth. Complex patterns of such artifactual variations can impact on the resulting estimates of expression levels of many genes, but leave many others unchanged; variation in sequence structure (such as GC content) of oligonucleotides defining Affymetrix probe sets is just one reason for gene-sample-assay-specific variation in resulting expression intensities that require consideration. When a study on one microarray platform is performed over time, perhaps involving different technicians, stations/machines within a laboratory or even different laboratories, and almost surely different batches of arrays and reagents, the resulting differences across sample expression profiles will often have major time-of-study effects. Such effects will be reflected in many but not all genes, with a multidimensional complexity to the pattern of the effects across many genes that can dominate the inherent biological variation that is the target of the study. Issues of comparability of expression results are high-profile in discussions of the potential for microarrays in clinical testing (e.g., [28]), but in more routine applications the issues they generate can be easily underestimated. Low-level processing and normalisation partially corrects for such artifacts, but very often data will remain contaminated – often substantially so – by these "assay artifacts." Hence the need for follow-on statistical models to explicitly address assay artifacts as components of analysis.

Affymetrix arrays include probe sets for a number of housekeeping genes and also "maintenance" genes – genes that robustly show constant levels of expression over a diverse set of (in our case, human) tissue studies, and that serve as normalisation controls. Most studies ignore these normalisation controls and use data from the housekeeping genes as laboratory controls only to be informally checked as part of the overall quality assessment. These probe sets can provide read-outs of assay artifacts, and serve as covariate information to model out components of the complex artifactual distortions as a result. If substantial numbers of these normalisation control genes exhibit common patterns of systematic variation over samples at meaningful levels, and if patterns of similar form show up in levels of expression of subsets of other genes, then the normalisation gene set can provide regression-based corrections for those gene subsets. Assay artifacts will generally impact multiple subsets of genes in differing ways, but leave many genes uncontaminated. As a result, we need multiple such factors as regression covariates, and a model that allows for parsimonious – and sparse – estimation of the regression coefficients of these control factors across the thousands of genes on the array. Clearly, the sparse regression context here is ideal, and underlies an approach to gene-sample-specific, model-based artifact correction.

The model in [1] utilises multiple principal components of the set of normalisation control probes, and a selection of the housekeeping probes, as covariates; thus the regression vector h_i includes these "normalisation factors" as specified values, in addition to whatever other design and covariate structure is in the model. The analysis already described then applies directly to estimate the regression coefficients on these factors under the same sparsity prior; now, the rate π_j applying to any one (j) of the normalisation factors represents the proportion of genes showing association with that factor; a gene with a nonzero and higher value of $\pi_{g.j}^*$ is then identified as exhibiting variation over samples that is in part related to the assay artifact reflected in the normalisation factor j. The model thus provides the ability to isolate these effects from the other components of the regression. Evidently, if ignored, these effects may obscure underlying biological structure, leading to lost signals; potentially more perniciously, it may also generate false discovery through the suggestive appearance of significant effects that are in fact strongly associated with gene-study-specific artifacts. The oncogene experiment data provides useful examples.

8.3.2 Example: Oncogene Intervention Experiments

Figure 8.2 displays the first eight principal components from the normalisation control genes (in this case, 100 probe sets on the Affymetrix U133+ microarray). Systematic and stochastic assay artifacts are apparent in what should, in principle, be stable levels of expression of these summaries of control probes. The evident systematic differences between the two sets of replicate control samples in this data set (the initial black open and filled circles) provide information relevant to global gene-sample-specific normalisation in that many gene probe sets reflect similar systematic differences. These two different control samples were in fact generated and assayed several months apart, so that different assay conditions are surely why the two samples are different in terms of normalisation factors. The observations in purple represent the RAS intervention samples; clear distortions in the control probes are evident in the second normalisation factor for that group alone. The final set of 37 sample observations, coded yellow to blue, were intervention experiments performed and assayed several months after the first set, and the need for correction of samples is clear. Additional features representing apparent artifactual effects appear in additional principal components of the normalisation probes, as the image display in Figure 8.2(c) indicates. Figure 8.2(d) displays the (centered) expression levels of a selected gene, PEA-15 (PED), across samples. Though there may be real biological variation underlying some aspects of variation in expression of this gene (explored futher below), there is clear evidence of some systematic variation apparently related to structure in the patterns of artifactual variation of normalisation probes. The superimposed fitted values from the sparse ANOVA/regression model that incorporates the eight normalisation

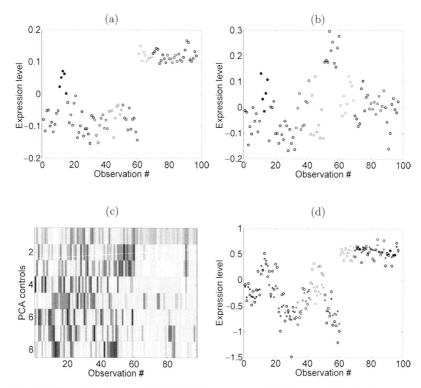

Fig. 8.2. First (a) and second (b) principal components in the expression levels across oncogene experiment observations of the set of normalisation control and housekeeping probe sets. The black symbols represent samples in the two control groups (10 initial control samples as open black circles, and 5 later control samples as filled black circles) that were assayed several months apart; the nine oncogene intervention groups are then color-coded for presentation. Frame (c) displays an image intensity plot of the first eight principal components across samples. Frame (d) displays the (centered) expression levels of gene PEA-15 (PED) plotted across samples (circles); superimposed (as crosses) are the (centered) fitted values from the sparse ANOVA/regression model with normalisation control factors. (See color plate 8.2.)

factors as regression terms highlight the artifacts in this gene. Many gene probe sets show little or no evidence of association with these assay artifact factors, though others are clearly contaminated; the sparse model approach can isolate and correct such cases within the formal shrinkage analysis.

The model fit to this gene is explored further in Figure 8.3. PEA-15 (PED) is a phosphoprotein that mediates apoptosis and plays roles in the molecular mechanisms of chemoresistance in cancer [29, 30]. The action of PEA-15 is known to depend on phosphorylation by AKT1, though AKT1 does not play a role in regulation of expression levels of PEA-15. On the other hand,

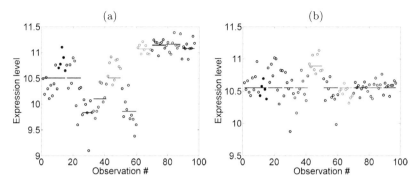

Fig. 8.3. Frame (a) displays expression levels of gene PEA-15 (PED) across samples; the horizontal lines superimposed represent the estimated levels of expression within each of the groups in the analysis that ignores the normalisation control factors. Frame (b) displays corrected expression levels from the sparse regression analysis using the control factors; the fitted effects of the control components have been subtracted from the samples displayed, and the horizontal lines superimposed represent the fitted parameters/levels for the intervention effects on expression within each group. (See color plate 8.3.)

PEA-15 is a direct target for regulation by members of the E2F family of transcription factors, with known promoter binding sequence for E2F (the E2F family members share a common binding site). Hence PEA-15 is anticipated to respond to one or more of the E2F interventions but to our knowledge should not show a transcriptional response as a result of any of the other interventions. As noted earlier, the data show strong association with the temporal sequence of the sample generation, real differences between the two sets of control samples, and structure related to the assay artifact patterns in the control components. Figure 8.3(a) displays the original RMA expression levels. Superimposed on frame (a) are horizontal lines representing the estimated levels of expression within each of the groups in the sparse ANOVA analysis that ignores the normalisation issue. Frame (b) displays corrected levels from the sparse analysis now including the normalisation factors; here the fitted effects of the normalisation factors have been subtracted from the samples displayed. Superimposed are horizontal lines representing the fitted parameters/levels for the intervention effects on expression within each group. This demonstrates the artifactual nature of the expression fluctuations in frame (a) and how the control factors correct those effects and are able to recover the apparent real transcriptional response of PEA-15 to the upregulation of E2F3 (the central group of samples, coloured cyan). That there is no corresponding effect in the E2F1 group (the penultimate group of samples, coloured red) is suggestive of differential function in transcriptional control of PEA-15 within the E2F family of transcription factors, consistent with the known diversity of functional roles across that family [7, 26]. Evidently, ignoring the assay artifact issue would, in this case, lead to substantial false discovery with frame (a) suggestive of multiple potential regulators of PEA-15 within the pathways downstream of several of this set of oncogenes, and also a false negative with respect to the role of E2F3. As with other examples, the artifactual differences between the two control sets in Figure 8.3(a), and the comparability of fitted values in Figure 8.3(b), provide support for the relevance of sparse gene-sample-specific normalisation component.

8.4 Sparse Latent Factor Models and Latent Factor Regressions

8.4.1 General Model Structure

Sparse latent factor models, as introduced to the statistics community in [3], represent a natural extension of the sparse regression modelling approach as well as a natural framework for more incisive development of approaches to pattern/signature profiling in expression genomics. The pilot gene expression study in [3] demonstrated the ability of latent factor models – under traditional Bayesian variable selection priors – to improve the identification and estimation of metagene groups and patterns related to underlying biological phenomena. Part of the motivation for that work was, again, directed at generating a more comprehensive statistical framework for flexible modelling of multiple, complex aspects of substructure in expression data, moving from the empirical methods (using singular value decomposition-based factors within multiple gene clusters, e.g., [8, 9, 11, 14]) into more formal models.

One of the key recent extensions and innovations in sparse factor modelling [2] is the application of the new hierarchical sparse prior modelling approach described and developed above. The extension of the sparse regression model framework of Sections 8.2.1 and 8.2.2 is immediate, as follows.

Extend the model of equation (8.1) with the addition of a latent factor component involving k latent factors. That is,

$$x_i = \mu + Bh_i + A\lambda_i + \nu_i, \tag{8.6}$$

where the k-vectors λ_i are independent random latent factors, distributed as

$$\lambda_i \sim N(0, I),$$

and A is a sparse $p \times k$ factor loadings matrix. As with B, the loadings matrix A will generally have many more rows than columns; the number of factors k will usually be very small compared to the number of genes. Structuring follows prior work with latent factor models in other contexts [31, 32]. The preferred structure for A has the upper right triangle of A set to zero, with positive diagonal elements $A_{i,i}$ for $i = 1, \ldots, k$. Sparse matrices A in fact lead to models that do not require identification constraints, but this specific structure is attractive as it permits the selection of the order of the first k variables (genes) in x_i as defining "names" for the latent factors.

One interpretation of the extended factor regression model is that of the regression $\mu + Bh_i$ with an extended "error" term $A\lambda_i + \nu_i$; this term has zero mean and variance matrix $\Sigma = AA' + \Psi$, so that the model represents a regression allowing complex patterns of correlation among the errors. In gene expression studies, especially involving observational data sets, this is particularly relevant since the structure of empirical patterns of covariation among genes across samples is generally rather elaborate, far more so than regression models will adequately describe. Complementing this view, in many applications we are interested in the latent factors as a statistical representation of groupings and cross-linkages of subsets of genes that may be biologically interpretable in terms of pathway interconnections. The notion of latent factor models as estimating and reflecting multiple interacting biological pathways through the associations observed in expression patterns is germane to some of our current studies.

Evidently, the sparsity prior strategy and resulting Bayesian analysis applies directly to this extended model. The sparsity prior of equation (8.3) is simply extended to also apply to the free elements of the factor loading matrix A, with a modification to constrain the diagonal elements to positivity. This then leads to an extension of the MCMC in which the latent factors themselves are also estimated: conditional on values of all latent factors $\Lambda = [\lambda_1, \ldots, \lambda_n]$, the analysis proceeds as in the straight regression model (with the minor change to add the positivity constraint on diagonal entries in A). Within each MCMC iteration, we then simply add in simulations from the complete conditional posterior of Λ given the data and all other parameters, and this is trivially a set of n conditionally independent k-variate normals for the columns of Λ, thereby neatly completing the MCMC setup. This extends the analysis in [3] to the hierarchical sparsity prior as well as to coupled ANOVA/regression and factor models.

8.4.2 Factor Regression Component

Many gene expression studies also involve explanatory associations between expression profiles and response variables (phenotypes). Following [3], we can couple response variables into the sparse regression and factor model framework to develop models in which the response is linked, via a separate regression model that itself may be subject to sparsity prior analysis, to the latent factors underlying gene expression. This again extends to a model-based context the notion of aggregate patterns in gene expression as predictors of outcomes; the latent factors λ_i are now the candidate predictors of phenotypic measures on sample/case i in the study. Additional generalisations of the initial framework of [3] are possible, but the example here adopts this approach.

Consider first the case of a continuous univariate response variable y_i on sample $i = 1, \ldots, n$. Linear regression on the latent factor structure underlying expression profiles is then simply incorporated as $y_i = \alpha + \theta' \lambda_i + \epsilon_i$ with independent normal errors. By simply prepending y_i to the expression vector x_i, we can clearly just extend the model of equation (8.6) to include α as a first entry in μ and the elements of θ as a first row of A. We may choose alternative prior specification for θ, or may just extend the sparsity prior directly. The latter approach is used for the example summarised below. This clearly extends trivially to include more than one response variable, and the example below has three such phenotypes, treated similarly. With such a model extension, analysis proceeds as before with minor changes to the MCMC.

Our example below involves three *binary* phenotypes, however, rather than continuous measurements. In the above example of a single response, suppose that we actually only observe a binary outcome $z_i = 0/1$. The linear regression framework maps onto this under a probit regression model, in which y_i is a latent variable and the errors $\epsilon_i \sim N(0, 1)$. This extension permits immediate analysis of binary phenotypes, simply extending the MCMC to iteratively impute samples of the "missing" latent $\{y_i\}$ together with all other model quantities in the standard manner for Bayesian binary regression (e.g., [3, 9, 33]).

8.4.3 Example: Breast Cancer Gene Expression Analysis

An analysis of expression profiles from primary breast tumours is illustrative of this framework, and also ties into current goals in breast cancer expression genomics. Some summaries of analysis of $n = 212$ samples appear in Figures 8.4–8.6. This data comes from a larger sample of expression profiles on breast tumours from the Sun-Yat Sen Cancer Center in Taipei [11, 15]. The analysis here involves $p = 500$ genes, many of which are related to key breast cancer hormonal and growth pathways – and the interactions of multiple such pathways – especially those linked to oestrogen through the ER (oestrogen receptor) pathway, the very strongly related PR (progesterone receptor) pathway, and the HER2/ERB-B2 proteins. ER and HER2 are each the target of current hormonal therapies in breast cancer. One interest in this application area is

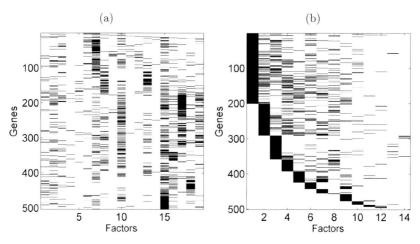

Fig. 8.4. Frame (a) displays a visual representation of the "skeleton" of the gene-factor association structure from the breast cancer expression example. The image is black for gene g (row)-factor j (column) combinations for which $\pi_{g,j}^* > 0.99$, for $g = 1, \ldots, 500$ and $k = 1, \ldots, 19$. The first 5 columns represent the normalisation control factors, and the final 14 columns represent the latent factors. Frame (b) provides a similar display but now restricting to the 14 latent factors alone, and reordering so that the most densely loaded factors come first; this provides a clearer visual display of the sparsity patterns and cross-talk between latent factors.

improved assays of levels of activation of these pathways, and this raises the question of gene-expression-based characterisation as alternatives, or adjuncts, to the traditional immunohistochemical (IHC) assays. For these samples, the IHC assays provide (imperfect and noisy) binary outcomes: 0/1 for each of ER+/−, PR+/−, and HER2+/−.

The example model for x_i is equation (8.6) with an intercept and the first five normalisation factors from this data set defining h_i so that $d = 5$. We then have $k = 14$ latent factors defining the dimensions of λ_i. Repeat analysis with more latent factors leads to the additional factors having very few loaded genes, so that the analysis essentially cuts back to that summarised. In addition, we couple in the three binary phenotypes as responses, using probit regression components as described above.

Figure 8.4(a) displays a binary representation of the posterior probabilities in Π^* across the $d = 5$ normalisation factors and the $k = 14$ latent factors; these 19 factors are indicated in that order horizontally, and genes represent rows of the image display. This gives a simple visual impression of the sparsity structure in both normalisation control and latent factor components.

It is evident that latent factor modelling has the capacity to adapt to artifactual as well as biological structure in patterns of covariation among genes, and this

(a)   (b)

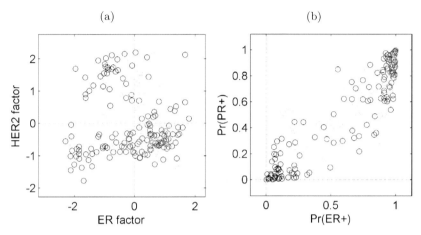

Fig. 8.5. Frame (a) is a scatter plot of the fitted values of 2 of the 14 latent factors – factor 1, the "HER2 factor," and factor 2, the primary "ER factor" – in the breast cancer example. The colour coding indicates IHC assay ER+ tumours (red), ER– cases (blue), and intermediate/indeterminate cases (cyan). The plot is concordant with the known association between HER2 and ER; HER2 overexpression generally occurs much more frequently in ER– tumours at a rate of about 30–40%. Frame (b) displays the fitted probabilities from the probit regression model linked to the latent factors as predictors of the IHC binary measures of ER and PR positivity, with colour coding as in frame (a). The positive correlation of ER and PR is evident in these factor-based probabilities, as is the discriminatory role of the estimated factors. (See color plate 8.5.)

is a common experience in a number of our studies. Here some of the latent factors, especially those with fewer significantly loaded genes, evidently reflect artifacts that the Affymetrix normalisation control genes are simply not picking up. The ability of the factor model to "soak up" such structure is a strength of the approach. The second frame in Figure 8.4 represents the same thresholded probabilities but now just for the $k = 14$ latent factors. Factors are reordered here to give a cleaner visual impression of the implied sparsity of the structure and the "cross-talk" between factors represented by genes significantly loaded on more than one factor.

Other factors very clearly reflect breast cancer biology and the ER/PR and HER2 pathways. This can be examined by listing genes most highly weighted on each factor, taking into account the absolute values of estimated $\beta_{g,j}$, and then examining these subsets of genes for known biological function. This analysis generates two factors replete with known ER-related genes, of which factor 2 is dominant in terms of exhibiting many ER-related genes and also strongly discriminating tumour samples based on the reported ER+/− IHC status (see Figure 8.5). One other factor, factor 1, significantly loads on the

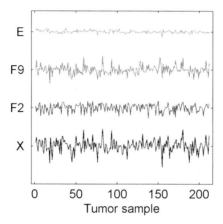

Fig. 8.6. Plot across breast tumour samples of levels of expression (X) of the gene Cyclin D1 (from the PRAD1/CCND1 probe set on the Affymetrix U95a microarray, one of three probe sets for Cyclin D1 on this array). Plots F2, F9, and E represent the estimated (posterior mean) effects of two of the latent factors and the fitted residual for this gene from the multivariate factor regression model. The four plots are on the same vertical scale, so indicating the breakdown of the expression fluctuations for Cyclin D1 according to contributions from, primarily, these two factors. Factor 2 is the primary ER factor, and factor 9 a factor defined by the three probe sets for Cyclin D1.

several probe sets for HER2/ERB-B2 as well as a small number of genes known to be regulated by or coregulated with HER2; this therefore defines a primary "HER2 factor." That these factors arise from the analysis, reflecting the major structure these pathways induce in gene expression patterns, indicates that there should be strong associations with the ER and HER2 IHC phenotypes through the coupled factor regression model component; this is evident in Figure 8.5. The relationship for PR is similarly well defined, as it is very highly correlated with ER and so well delineated by the factors that reflect ER pathway activation levels.

A final point relates to decompositions of gene expression. Figure 8.6 plots expression levels for one gene – a probe set representing Cyclin D1 on this microarray – across samples. Also plotted, on the same vertical scale, are the fitted effects of two factors for which $\pi^*_{g,j} > 0.99$ for this gene, factors 2 and 9, and the fitted residuals across the samples for this gene. The model represents a direct decomposition of the data into components contributed by the factors plus residual; the graph illustrates the key aspects of this decomposition for this gene. These two factors contribute comparably to the variations in expression of Cyclin D1 across the breast tumours. Factor 2 is an ER factor (discussed above). Cyclin D1 is a critical gene in cell cycle regulation, acting to phosphorylate the Rb protein and hence aid cell development and proliferation by relaxing inhibition of the E2F transcriptional machinery. Thus some component of expression variation reflects cell cycle activity unrelated to ER. However, Cyclin D1 is also known to be directly involved in the ER pathway; ER is a cell-type specific inducer of Cyclin D1, and Cyclin D1 antagonises repressors of ER. Hence we have a clear biological rationale and interpretation of the two factors arising from the statistical analysis. Indeed, factor 9 has only a very small number of significantly loaded genes, and the three most highly loaded (with estimated $\pi^*_{g,j}$ very close to 1, and the highest estimated loading parameters) are three Affymetrix probe sets representing Cyclin D1; that is, factor 9 is a cell cycle related "Cyclin D1" factor that is unrelated to ER.

8.5 Concluding Comments

Gene expression genomics is only one area of modern biotechnology in which the capacity to generate higher-resolution data on increasingly higher-dimensional variables continues to expand. In this and other areas, the concept of sparsity in mathematical and statistical models is central; the ability to induce sparse structure in increasingly high-dimensional and complex models will be more and more critical to scalability of statistical methods. The basic concepts and machinery of Bayesian hierarchical modelling are most relevant, and our theme here – hierarchical modelling with sparsity inducing priors – is highlighted by a number of gene expression genomic examples. Our references above include additional developments in sparse regression and factor modelling, with computational developments as well as applications. There are also close connections with sparse graphical modelling for display and interrogation of multivariate structure in gene expression contexts [34–36], a related area of current research interest in terms of both statistical methodology and genomic application.

The linkings of linear and binary/probit regression to factor models are of course just examples of broader classes of models for gene-expression-based prediction of clinical or physiological phenotypes. Similar extensions permit analysis of censored survival data, which is a central consideration in many genomic studies (e.g., [6, 15]). For example, latent variable imputation also easily leads to an approach to survival regression in which the underlying survival times (such as cancer recurrence or death, for example) are assumed conditionally log-normally (or log-T) distributed. Right-censored cases can then be treated by including the "missing" survival times as latent variables to be imputed, parallel to the treatment of the "missing" normal latent variables underlying binary data. Additional extensions utilising nonnormal survival models, including Weibull regression models [15] for example, are also amenable to treatment in this framework, though such developments will require customised extensions to the MCMC analysis.

Finally, executable code implementing the combined sparse factor regression models and methods presented here is freely available for interested researchers, and can be found at www.isds.duke.edu/~mw under the software link.

Acknowledgments

Components of the research reported here were supported under grants from the National Science Foundation (DMS 0102227 and 0342172) and the National Institutes of Health (NHBLI HL-73042, and CA-112952 from the NCI Integrated Cancer Biology Program).

Bibliography

[1] J. Lucas, Q. Wang, A. Bild, J.R. Nevins and M. West (submitted) Sparse Bayesian analysis and data synthesis in gene expression experiments. *ISDS Discussion Paper #05-14*, Duke University.
[2] C. Carvalho, Q. Wang, J. Lucas, J. Chang, J.R. Nevins and M. West (submitted) Sparse Bayesian factor analysis of gene expression data. *ISDS Discussion Paper #05-15*, Duke University.
[3] M. West (2003) Bayesian factor regression models in the "large p, small n" paradigm. *Bayesian Statistics 7* (eds. J.O. Bernardo et al.), Oxford: Clarendon Press, pp. 723–732.
[4] E. Huang, M. West and J.R. Nevins (2003) Gene expression phenotypes of oncogenic pathways. *Cell Cycle*, **2**, 415–417.
[5] E. Huang, S. Ishida, J. Pittman, H. Dressman, A. Bild, M. D'Amico, R. Pestell, M. West and J.R. Nevins (2003) Gene expression phenotypic models that predict the activity of oncogenic pathways. *Nature Genetics*, **34**, 226–230.
[6] A.H. Bild, G. Yao, J.T. Chang, Q. Wang, D. Harpole, J. Lancaster, A. Berchuk, J. Marks, M. West, H.K. Dressman and J.R. Nevins (2006) Patterns of oncogenic pathway deregulation in human cancers. *Nature*, **439**, 353–359.
[7] E.P. Black, T. Hallstrom, H.K. Dressman, M. West and J.R. Nevins (2005) Distinctions in the specificity of E2F function revealed by gene expression. *Proceedings of the National Academy of Sciences*, **102**, 15948–15953.
[8] R. Spang, H. Zuzan, M. West, J.R. Nevins, C. Blanchette and J.R. Marks (2001) Prediction and uncertainty in the analysis of gene expression profiles. *In Silico Biology*, **2**, 0033.
[9] M. West, C. Blanchette, H. Dressman, E. Huang, S. Ishida, R. Spang, H. Zuzan, J.R. Marks and J.R. Nevins (2001) Predicting the clinical status of human breast cancer utilizing gene expression profiles. *Proceedings of the National Academy of Sciences*, **98**, 11462–11467.
[10] E. Huang, M. West and J.R. Nevins (2002) Gene expression profiles and predicting clinical characteristics of breast cancer. *Hormone Research*, **58**, 55–73.
[11] E. Huang, S. Chen, H. Dressman, J. Pittman, M.H. Tsou, C.F. Horng, A. Bild, E.S. Iversen, M. Liao, C.M. Chen, M. West, J.R. Nevins and A.T. Huang (2003)

Gene expression predictors of breast cancer outcomes. *The Lancet*, **361**, 1590–1596.

[12] J.R. Nevins, E.S. Huang, H. Dressman, J. Pittman, A.T. Huang and M. West (2003) Towards integrated clinico-genomic models for personalized medicine: Combining gene expression signatures and clinical factors in breast cancer outcomes prediction. *Human Molecular Genetics*, **12**, 153–157.

[13] J. Pittman, E. Huang, J.R. Nevins and M. West (2003) Prediction tree models in clinico-genomics. *Bulletin of the International Statistical Institute*, **54**, 76.

[14] J. Pittman, E. Huang, Q. Wang, J. Nevins and M. West (2004) Binary analysis of binary prediction tree models for retrospectively sampled outcomes. *Biostatistics*, **5**, 587–601.

[15] J. Pittman, E. Huang, H. Dressman, C.F. Horng, S.H. Cheng, M.H. Tsou, C.M. Chen, A. Bild, E.S. Iversen, A.T. Huang, J.R. Nevins and M. West (2004) Integrated modeling of clinical and gene expression information for personalized prediction of disease outcomes. *Proceedings of the National Academy of Sciences*, **101**, 8431–8436.

[16] D.M. Seo, T. Wang, H. Dressman, E.E. Herderick, E.S. Iversen, C. Dong, K. Vata, C.A. Milano, J.R. Nevins, J. Pittman, M. West and P.J. Goldschmidt-Clermont (2004) Gene expression phenotypes of atherosclerosis. *Arteriosclerosis, Thrombosis and Vascular Biology*, **24**, 1922–1927.

[17] J. Rich, B. Jones, C. Hans, R. McClendon, D. Bigner, A. Dobra, J.R. Nevins and M. West (2005) Gene expression profiling and graphical genetic markers glioblastoma survival. *Cancer Research*, **65**, 4051–4058.

[18] R. Irizarry, B. Hobbs, F. Collin, Y. Beazer-Barclay, K. Antonellis, U. Scherf and T. Speed (2003) Exploration, normalisation, and summaries of high density oligonucleotide array probe level data. *Biostatistics*, **2**, 249–264.

[19] R. Irizarry, B. Bolstad, F. Collin, L. Cope, B. Hobbs and T. Speed (2003) Summaries of Affymetrix GeneChip probe level data. *Nucleic Acids Research*, **31**, e15.

[20] P. Broet, S.R. Richardson and F. Radvanyi (2002) Bayesian hierarchical model for identifying changes in gene expression from microarray experiments. *Journal of Computational Biology*, **9**, 671–683.

[21] H. Ishwaran and J. Rao (2003) Detecting differentially expressed genes in microarrays using Bayesian model selection. *Journal of the American Statistical Association*, **98**, 438–455.

[22] K.E. Lee, N. Sha, E.R. Dougherty, M. Vannucci and B.K. Mallick (2003) Gene selection: A Bayesian variable selection approach. *Bioinformatics*, **19**, 90–97.

[23] N. Sha, M. Vannucci, M.G. Tadesse, P.J. Brown, I. Dragoni, N. Davies, T.C. Roberts, A. Contestabile, N. Salmon, C. Buckley and F. Falciani (2004) Bayesian variable selection in multinomial probit models to identify molecular signatures of disease stage. *Biometrics*, **60**, 812–819.

[24] H. Ishwaran and J. Rao (2005) Spike and slab gene selection for multigroup microarray data. *Journal of the American Statistical Association*, **100**, 764–780.

[25] K.A. Do, P. Mueller and F. Tang (2005) A Bayesian mixture model for differential gene expression. *Journal of the Royal Statistical Society, Series C (Applied Statistics)*, **54**, 627–644.

[26] J.R. Nevins (1998) Toward an understanding of the functional complexity of the E2F and Retinoblastoma families. *Cell Growth and Differentiation*, **9**, 585–593.

[27] DICBP – Integration of Oncogenic Networks in Cancer Phenotypes, The Duke Univerity NCI Integrated Cancer Biology Program (ICBP), http://icbp.genome.duke.edu.

[28] E.P. Hoffman, T. Awad, A. Spira, J. Palma, T. Webster , G. Wright, J. Buckley, R. Davis, E. Hubbell, W. Jones, R. Tibshirani, R. Tompkins, T. Triche, W. Xiao, M. West and J.A. Warrington (2004) Expression profiling: Best practices for Affymetrix array data generation and interpretation for clinical trials. *Nature Reviews Genetics*, **5**, 229–237.

[29] F. Renault, E. Formstecher, I. Callebaut, M.P. Junier and H. Chneiweiss (2003) The multifunctional protein PEA-15 is involved in the control of apoptosis and cell cycle in astrocytes. *Biochemical Pharmacology*, **66**, 1581–1588.

[30] G. Stassi, M. Garofalo, M. Zerilli, L. Ricci-Vitiani, C. Zanca, M. Todaro, F. Aragona, G. Limite, G. Petrella and G. Condorelli (2005) PED mediates AKT-dependent chemoresistance in human breast cancer cells. *Cancer Research*, **65**, 6668–6675.

[31] O. Aguilar and M. West (2000) Bayesian dynamic factor models and portfolio allocation. *Journal of Business and Economic Statistics*, **18**, 338–357.

[32] H. Lopes and M. West (2003) Bayesian model assessment in factor analysis. *Statistica Sinica*, **14**, 41–67.

[33] V.E. Johnson and J.H Albert (1999) *Ordinal Data Modeling*. New York: Springer-Verlag.

[34] A. Dobra, B. Jones, C. Hans, J.R. Nevins and M. West (2004) Sparse graphical models for exploring gene expression data. *Journal of Multivariate Analysis*, **90**, 196–212.

[35] B. Jones and M. West (2005) Covariance decomposition in undirected Gaussian graphical models. *Biometrika*, **92**, 779–786.

[36] B. Jones, C. Carvalho, A. Dobra, C. Hans, C. Carter and M. West (2005) Experiments in stochastic computation for high-dimensional graphical models. *Statistical Science*, **20**, 388–400.

9

Bayesian Analysis of Cell Cycle Gene Expression Data

CHUAN ZHOU
Vanderbilt University

JON C. WAKEFIELD
University of Washington

LINDA L. BREEDEN
Fred Hutchinson Cancer Research Center

Abstract

The study of the cell cycle is important in order to aid in our understanding of the basic mechanisms of life, yet progress has been slow due to the complexity of the process and our lack of ability to study it at high resolution. Recent advances in microarray technology have enabled scientists to study the gene expression at the genome-scale with a manageable cost, and there has been an increasing effort to identify cell-cycle-regulated genes. In this chapter, we discuss the analysis of cell cycle gene expression data, focusing on model-based Bayesian approaches. The majority of the models we describe can be fitted using freely available software.

9.1 Introduction

Cells reproduce by duplicating their contents and then dividing into two. The repetition of this process is called the cell cycle, and is the fundamental means by which all living creatures propagate. On the other hand, abnormal cell divisions are responsible for many diseases, most notably cancer. Therefore, studying cell cycle control mechanisms and the factors essential for the process is important in order to aid in our understanding of cell replication, malignancy, and reproductive diseases that are associated with genomic instability and abnormal cell divisions.

For decades, biologists have been studying the cell cycle, using the model organism budding yeast *Saccharomyces cerevisiae*. This focus on budding yeast is due to the fact that it exists as a free living, single cell, which has the same general architecture and control pathways as the cells of its highly complex, multicellular relatives (e.g., humans). Moreover, a number of conditions have been identified that enable researchers to arrest yeast cells at a specific point in the cell cycle and then release them from that state in order to follow a population of cells that are progressing through the cell cycle in synchrony. Until technologies are available to follow the molecular events in individual cells, synchronizing populations of cells is our only means to follow and characterize the key events in the cell cycle.

Duplication of a complex structure like a living cell requires the organization and coordinated activity of thousands of components. These components are built from plans coded in the genes of the cell (DNA). This code is accessed and duplicated or transcribed into RNA and then read and translated to generate the components, which are called proteins. As with any assembly process, each component is required in different amounts and at different times. One universal strategy that has evolved to simplify this process is the regulation of transcription, which means that a gene is not transcribed (and translated) until the component is needed. It is believed that up to 20% of the genes of organisms as diverse as bacteria and humans may be transcriptionally regulated during the cell cycle and many of the components encoded by these genes participate in or control specific events in the cell cycle. For reviews of cell cycle regulation, see for example [10] and [15].

Recent breakthroughs in microarray technology have enabled biologists to measure the number of transcripts made from every gene in an organism's DNA. This microarray technology allows an unprecedented look at the state of a cell at a particular time within the cell cycle. Due to the importance of understanding the cell duplication process, studies of transcriptional regulation during the cell cycle of yeast were among the first experiments to be carried out using microarray technology. These pioneering efforts provided far more information than had been gleaned from the previous 20 years of research in the area. They also highlighted the need for computational methods for analyzing microarray data and for identifying statistically significant patterns in time series gene expression.

9.2 Previous Studies

As one of the first genome-wide gene expression studies, Cho et al. [4] used Affymetrix microarrays and visual inspection to identify 416 out of 6,000 yeast genes as cell-cycle-regulated. Spellman et al. [18] conducted a set of experiments using cDNA arrays and three different synchronization methods to obtain three more data sets. By fitting these profiles to sinusoidal functions and correlating those profiles with the profiles of transcripts already known to be cell-cycle-regulated, these authors identified 800 genes as cell-cycle-regulated. These data have further served as a testing ground for dozens of new computational methods; the earliest among these were a number of clustering algorithms [6, 16, 22].

Recently, there has been increasing interest in developing model-based approaches for analyzing gene expression data. The clustering algorithms are useful exploratory tools, but they lack the ability to model the variability at various levels of the microarray experiments, the structure to take into account covariates and external information, a distributional framework for formal statistical inference, and they also have difficulties with missing data. As a contrast, many of the problems associated with these ad hoc clustering algorithms can be overcome by assuming specific functional forms on the expression pattern or distributional assumptions on model parameters, leading to more informative analysis and principled inference. Zhao, Prentice, and Breeden [27] employed a single-pulse model (SPM) along with generalized estimating equation techniques to reexamine the three data sets by Spellman et al. [18]. Johansson, Lindgren, and Berglund [9] used a partial least-squares regression approach on the three data sets individually and in combination. Lu et al. [12] used a two-component mixture-Beta model with an empirical Bayesian method to detect periodic genes. Wakefield, Zhou, and Self [24] proposed a fully Bayesian hierarchical models for the analysis of cell cycle expression data, and their approach was subsequently extended by Zhou and Wakefield [28]. Other approaches using mixed-effect models and smoothing techniques have also been applied to these data (see, for example, [13]). However, the agreement between these methods is remarkably poor. As reported in a comparison study by Lichtenberg et al. [11], in total nearly 1,800 different genes have been proposed to be periodic – which is almost one-third of the *S. cerevisae* genome. These results suggest that more powerful statistical methods, more accurate data, or the incorporation of biological information are required to resolve these problems.

When applying model-based approaches to the time-course gene expression data, it is important to specify the model in such a way that it captures the systematic behavior of the regulation process as much as possible, otherwise important information might be missed. The incorporation of additional information is important due to the noise inherent in these time series data sets with no replicates, and also from the difficulties in comparing and combining the results from different data sets. The four experiments reported in [18] were carried out with different synchronization methods, in the hope that analysis of the combined data would minimize the effect of artifacts due to any one synchronization method. However, it is not clear how many periodic transcript profiles would be obscured by synchrony artifacts in any one data set, nor is it clear what other complexities would arise in combining them. In addition to the cycle lengths being different across experiments, the cycles themselves are slightly out of phase, because the points of arrest differ. Moreover, the synchrony at release is not perfect and it decays with time. An additional problem is that the arrested cells continue to grow and accumulate key cell components even during the arrest, so the first cycle after release may be shorter than the second one.

We emphasize that these experimental artifacts should be carefully considered in the analysis, as they are often systematically reflected in the expression levels throughout experiments course. Failure to recognize them may lead to unreliable results and erroneous conclusion. We have three major goals for this work: first, to extend and apply the model framework proposed in [24] to cell cycle time-course gene expression data with the characteristics described above; second, to provide a streamlined analysis of such data including evaluation of measurement error, filtering, and partitioning; third, to demonstrate that with carefully specified models, we can extract important biological information from such analysis.

9.3 Data

The working data is provided by Tata Pramila and Linda Breeden at the Fred Hutchinson Cancer Research Center. It was collected from cDNA microarrays and was normalized using GenePix software (Axon Instruments, Inc.) [1]. It has the advantages of refined microarray technology compared to that obtained 6 years earlier and a shorter sampling interval. Microarray experiments were also performed to directly assess measurement error. The three cell cycle data sets we used monitor all yeast transcripts and each involves the same α-factor method of synchronization; α-factor was used because it is a physiological arrest of wild-type cells from which cells recover rapidly. Since α-factor is a natural inhibitor of the cell cycle, we can assume that all cellular processes that might interfere with the viability or recovery of these cells from the arrest are stopped. The quality of the synchronous release can be inferred from the fact that periodic transcripts can be followed for up to four cell cycles after release from the arrest [3]. The timing of release is also highly reproducible, thus enabling multiple experiments to be compared.

The data was collected with the following design: cells were first synchronized by α-factor arrest; then the cells were released to progress through the cell cycle. Gene expression levels through the cell cycle relative to asynchronized cell samples were measured at 5-minute time intervals from $t = 0$ to $t = 120$ minutes. This length covers approximately two full yeast cell cycles. The 5-minute intervals offer finer resolution in time compared to those of Spellman et al. [18] and Cho et al. [4]. Two microarrays were performed with

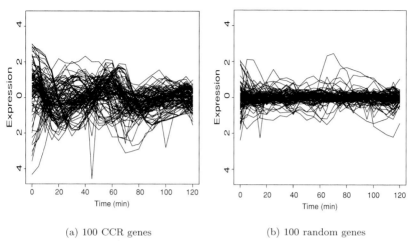

(a) 100 CCR genes   (b) 100 random genes

Fig. 9.1. Expression of 100 CCR genes and 100 randomly selected genes.

the RNA collected from this experiment. In the first case (referred to as 38 wt), the cell cycle transcripts were labeled with red dye, and the reference transcripts from asynchronous cells were labeled with green dye. A second microarray (30 wt) was then performed with the dyes swapped. This dye-swapped data set is treated as a replicated experiment. The duplicated experiment provided valuable additional information regarding the variability and magnitude of the expression patterns.

Another important data set consists of six arrays with expression measures of all transcripts relative to themselves to give a so-called self–self hybridization. Deviations from a ratio of 1 in these measurements indicate measurement error. Using the fully Bayesian-model-based approach, we were able to incorporate the additional information gathered from these data into our main analysis, using informative prior distributions.

All three data sets use the same 6,216 yeast transcripts, which cover the complete yeast genome. An initial exploratory analysis, which was confirmed by closer examination, revealed that the mRNA sample at 105 minutes was contaminated, and therefore the data generated from that array were dropped from subsequent analyses.

The left panel in Figure 9.1 shows expression of 100 genes which are known to be cell cycle regulated (CCR) from previous studies. It appears that they do demonstrate strong cyclic signals in our data set. As a contrast, a large portion of the genes do not show strong signals as we see from the random sample of 100 genes shown in the right panel of Figure 9.1.

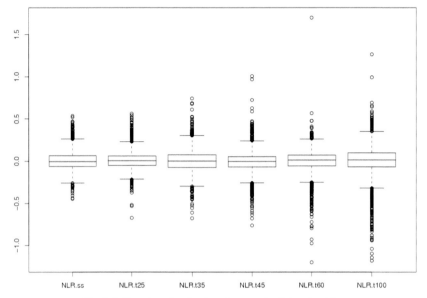

Fig. 9.2. Boxplots for the data from each of the six chips.

9.4 Bayesian Analysis of Cell Cycle Data

9.4.1 Measurement Error

There are various sources of variation involved in microarray experiments, and their identification and evaluation have proven to be crucial for making accurate inference. Other than variations which we can attribute to certain systematic sources, the remaining variability is often referred to as measurement error. To estimate measurement error, we use data from six microarrays with mRNAs collected at 0, 25, 35, 45, 60, and 100 minutes. These mRNAs were copied into cDNA, split, and then coupled to either Cy5 or Cy3 dyes. The two samples were mixed and hybridized to cDNA arrays. Fluorescence measured from each dye is expressed as a ratio and its deviation from unity provides an estimate of measurement error. This is often referred to as a same versus same measurement.

We now summarize the analysis of this reference data, based on which the prior distribution on the measurement error was specified. Figure 9.2 shows the boxplots of the data from these six chips; we can see that the average gene expressions of these asynchronized samples are close to zero. There were genes that exhibited large variations across time, but they did not appear to be cyclic under closer inspection. The samples appear to be more spread out at later times, suggesting that measurement error may increase with time. This observation supports our speculation that using only early data could underestimate the measurement error. Therefore we proceeded to carry out a Bayesian analysis using the pooled data from all six chips.

Let $y = \{y_1, \ldots, y_N\}$ denote the *pooled* reference data, and y_i denote the ith observation. We assume a simple normal model for the data

$$y_i \mid \mu, \sigma^2 \sim_{i.i.d.} \mathrm{N}(y_i \mid \mu, \sigma^2). \tag{9.1}$$

We assume a "noninformative" prior on (μ, σ^2) with $p(\mu, \sigma^2) \propto 1/\sigma^2$, which leads to the following posterior distribution:

$$p(\sigma^{-2} \mid y) = \mathrm{Ga}(\sigma^{-2} \mid a, b), \tag{9.2}$$

where $a = \frac{1}{2}(N - 1)$, $b = \frac{1}{2}ns^2$ with $ns^2 = \sum_{i=1}^{n}(y_i - \bar{y})^2$.

We could use the parameter values from this posterior analysis as a way of obtaining a prior specification for later analyses, but the large sample size from pooling the six chips leads to a highly concentrated posterior distribution on the standard deviation σ. The sampling posterior median of σ is 0.151, with 95% sampling interval (0.150, 0.153). To avoid being too restrictive, we calibrated a and b to allow larger variation. We set the modal value for σ to be 0.15, and an upper bound 0.5 so that $\mathrm{Pr}(0 < \sigma < 0.5) = 0.95$. Solving the resultant equations gave $a = 1.52$ and $b = 0.05$, under which the 95% sampling interval is (0.10, 0.68). These values were then used as priors in subsequent filtering and partitioning analysis.

9.4.2 Filtering

In cell cycle analysis, our main interest lies in identifying and characterizing genes that are cell-cycle-regulated. For those genes that show differential expression but do not coincide with cell cycle events, we do not consider them as cell-cycle-regulated, and consequently exclude them from later analysis. In this section, we apply a filtering procedure to cell cycle data. The aim is to first identify candidate periodic genes, and then perform more reliable analysis on these candidates, using a more sophisticated model tuned to the cell cycle nature of the data.

Let y_{ij} denote gene expression at time t_j for gene i, $i = 1, \ldots, n$, $j = 1, \ldots, T$. We assume a first order Fourier model for the data,

$$y_{ij} = R_i \cos 2\pi(f_0 t_j + \phi_i) + \epsilon_{ij}, \tag{9.3}$$

where $\epsilon_{ij} \sim_{i.i.d.} \mathrm{N}(0, \sigma_e^2)$ are the measurement errors and (R_i, ϕ_i) are gene-specific parameters, where R_i is the amplitude, that is, the magnitude of the cyclic signal, and ϕ_i is the phase, governing where the signal peaks. The cell cycle frequency is denoted by f_0, fixed at $1/58$ minute^{-1}, and assumed to be common to all genes. The cell cycle span is estimated to be 58 minutes using the known CCR genes [27].

For the purpose of filtering, we want to test the following hypothesis independently for each gene i:

$$M_0: R_i = 0 \; v.s. \; M_1: R_i \neq 0.$$

To carry out the filtering procedure, we need to specify the prior distributions. For measurement error, we assume $\sigma^{-2} \sim \text{Ga}(a, b)$, where a and b are determined from the reference data analysis described in Section 9.4.1.

We assume models M_0 and M_1 are equally probable a priori. Under M_0, the parameter ϕ_i is redundant. Under M_1, we assume R_i and ϕ_i are independent with the following prior distributions:

$$R_i \sim_{i.i.d.} \text{Exp}(\lambda) \tag{9.4}$$

$$\phi_i \sim_{i.i.d.} \text{Unif}(-0.5, 0.5) \tag{9.5}$$

Because the trigonometric functions in the Fourier model are periodic, ϕ_i is restricted to $(-0.5, 0.5)$ for identifiability, and so the uniform prior on ϕ_i is noninformative. We chose an exponential prior on the amplitude R_i because it has a simple form and reasonably reflects prior belief based on data. The parameter λ was based upon an exploratory analysis of the 100 known CCR genes. We have found that these 100 known CCR genes showed consistently strong signals in both the main and the dye-swapping experiments, and believed their expression levels were representative of genes with strong signals. So we extracted data for the 100 known CCR genes from the dye-swapping experiment and transformed them into the same format as the 38-wt data set by changing the signs of the log ratios. Model (9.3) can be reparameterized as

$$y_{ij} = A_i \cos(2\pi f_0 t_j) + B_i \sin(2\pi f_0 t_j) + \epsilon_{ij}, \tag{9.6}$$

with $A_i = R_i \cos 2\pi \phi_i$ and $B_i = R_i \sin 2\pi \phi$. Given f_0 and t_j, it is just a simple linear model, for which we can obtain least-squares estimates of (A_i, B_i) and transform them back to (R_i, ϕ_i). We chose λ to be 1.43 so that the mean amplitude is 0.7 with variance 0.5 on the basis of the least-squares estimates. We believe that amplitudes of these known CCR genes are within the upper range of the signals. We would expect many CCR genes to have smaller amplitude than these genes. Figure 9.3 shows the expression of the 100 CCR genes, with fitted curves based on the least-squares estimates. The distributional and

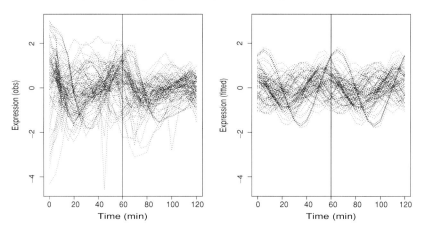

Fig. 9.3. Observed gene expression of 100 known CCR genes, and their fitted values based on least-squares estimates using model (9.3).

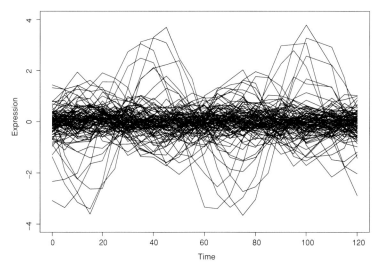

Fig. 9.4. $N = 100$ simulated gene expression time series based on the following priors: $R_i \sim \text{Exp}(1.43)$, $\phi_i \sim \text{Unif}(-0.5, 0.5)$, $\sigma_e^2 = 0.2^2$.

independence assumptions were checked by inspecting the histograms and scatter plots of the parameter estimates.

Figure 9.4 shows 100 simulated gene expression time series from the above priors including measurement error. It suggests our prior choices are reasonable, as we see patterns in the simulated data match quite closely to what we see in the main data (as seen in Figure 9.1).

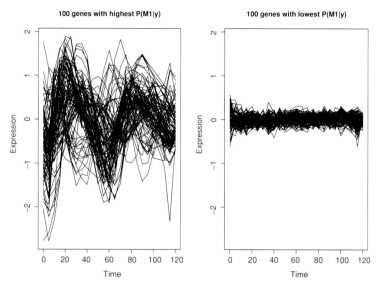

Fig. 9.5. Expression of the 100 highest ranked genes (left panel) and lowest ranked genes (right panel).

We sampled parameter values from the prior distributions and used importance sampling technique to estimate the posterior probabilities $p_i = \Pr(M_1 \mid y_i)$, and then ordered genes based on these probabilities. Figure 9.5 displays the 100 highest ranked genes and the 100 lowest ranked genes. It appears that the filter was able to pick out genes with large variations. Because the model (9.3) allows cyclic oscillation in the data, genes showing cyclic patterns tend to be ranked higher than genes that are not cyclic even though they may show differential expression. So the higher a gene is ranked by this filtering procedure, the more likely it is cyclic and thus a candidate for cell cycle regulation.

At this point, we can either pick a cutoff point subjectively, and proceed with genes above the threshold, or we can choose the cutoff point based on some more formal criteria, such as controlling the false discovery rate (FDR) and false negative rate (FNR). The concepts of FDR and FNR and the Bayesian procedures for controlling them have been discussed in [21]. Note FDR and FNR are two competing concepts; optimal results for minimizing both error rates cannot be achieved at the same time. We would miss nothing by rejecting all hypotheses and concluding that all genes are cell-cycle-regulated; so FNR $= 0$, but clearly FDR would be high in this case, and vice versa. Therefore some compromise has to be made, depending on the scientific question and our subsequent preference for making the two types of errors. In our analysis, we feel we are in a "discovery" mode, and therefore a certain amount of false discovery is tolerable as long as we do not miss too many cell cycle genes.

Figure 9.6 illustrates various thresholds from minimizing the loss function cFDR + FNR, where c is a positive number chosen to reflect our preference in controlling FDR and FNR. For example, if we are twice as concerned with FDR as with FNR, we could set $c = 2$ and consider the top 1,340 genes (bottom left panel). Of course, choosing an appropriate value c is not a trivial task.

As an alternative, Figure 9.7 shows the optimal number of rejections for minimizing Bayesian FNR while controlling Bayesian FDR at the 0.05 level. This is similar to the frequentist practice of maximizing the power while controlling the significance level. Based upon this result, we decided to identify the top 1,680 genes as candidates for cell cycle regulation, and the cutoff for marginal posterior probability $\Pr(M_1 \mid y_i)$ was set to be 0.78*. More sophisticated Bayesian methods for differential gene expression have been proposed (see, for example, [5]).

9.4.3 Model-Based Partitioning

This first-order Fourier model requires model refinement since it does not account for the attenuation in the cell cycle data. This synchronization causes an intrinsic difficulty in a cell cycle study. To effectively observe the cell cycles, yeast cells have to be initially synchronized. In addition, our ability to observe the true cell cycle span is impeded because the cell cycle can be altered by the synchronization. This fact has long been recognized by biologists, and has been addressed in gene expression analyses as well [12]. α-factor synchronization is considered as a better choice compared to other synchronization methods because of its relative ease, sensitivity, and gentleness to cells. α-factor is a mating pheromone that is secreted by haploid *S. cerevisiae* cells of the α mating type. It blocks cell division in G1 and induces mating-specific gene expression. Even when transcriptions are held at START,† during this time cell mass increases and cell wall growth continues, resulting in enlarged and frequently distorted cells. After the release the large size of cells leads to near elimination of the G1 phase and hence an abbreviated cell cycle. This is consistent with our observation that there tends to be shortened cell cycle span early on after release, but the difference decreases over time. Breeden [3]

---

* The discrepancy of 5 is due to the rounding error in 0.78.
† An important checkpoint in the eukaryotic cell cycle. Passage through START commits the cells to enter *S*-phase.

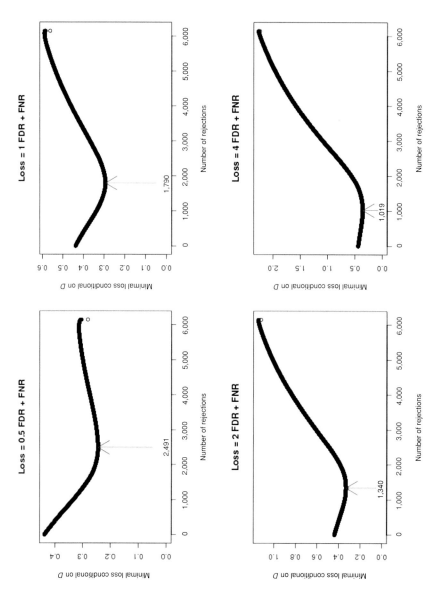

Fig. 9.6. Optimal solutions to different loss functions in the form of cFDR $+$ FNR.

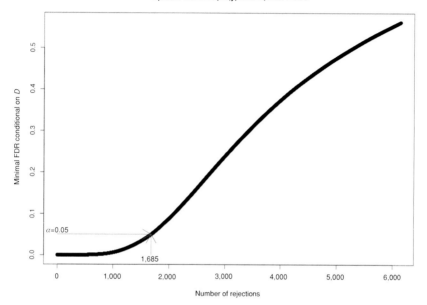

Fig. 9.7. Optimal solutions to minimizing FNR, subject to FDR ≤ 0.05.

recommends that with α-factor arrest, the first cycle after release should be considered a recovery cycle, which may differ from the normal mitotic cycle in specific ways. Any oscillating activity that persists through the second and third cycles after recovery is most likely to be a property of the normal mitotic cell cycle.

There are drug-induced cell cycle arrests, which are unnatural and potentially toxic and nonspecific. Genetically induced arrests using *cdc* mutants are more specific and two such arrests (*cdc28*, *cdc15*) have been used by Spellman et al. [18]. However, the arrests evoked by these mutations are abnormal in the sense that they are caused by the loss of a critical gene product. The cells arrest in an apparently uniform state, but it cannot be assumed that all cell-cycle-specific progresses are halted, or that recovery from the arrest occurs under balanced growth conditions. Even with the elutriation synchronization, which collects G1 cells based on size and introduces minimal perturbation, cells need some time before they resume normal mitotic cell cycles. With these synchronization methods, the first cell cycle should also be considered a recovery cycle, as with α-factor synchronization.

So if the first cycle cannot be trusted, why not run the experiments longer and only look at later cell cycles? This brings up a second point: the number of observable cell cycles is limited. Most of the time the cyclic signals dissipate after three or four cycles. There are several factors that could contribute to this phenomenon. One is how well the cells are synchronized. But even with a perfect synchrony, after two doublings only one of four of the cells experienced the initial conditions. This, in addition to random fluctuation in the transcription of each gene, means that soon the cells become asynchronous and we are unable to observe the cyclic patterns any more.

To make the matter even more complicated, certain signals we observe could be artifacts of the synchronization. Even with a perfect release from the arrest, this budding yeast divides asymmetrically yielding a new daughter cell that is smaller than the mother cell. This daughter cell must grow during the next G1 before it can enter *S*-phase. The mother cell has no growth requirement and as a result has a shorter G1 interval. This asymmetry precludes perfect synchronization. For example, in the case of α-factor synchrony, because α-factor is a mating pheromone, it will induce mating-specific gene expression. As a consequence, many mating-related genes will either be induced or repressed, leading to increased or decreased transcript levels. In some extreme cases, the changes in expression level are so dramatic that the cyclic signals are totally obscured.

In the following we extend the first-order Fourier model to allow variable frequency and time-dependent amplitude. Let y_{ij} denote the expression level of gene i measured at time t_j, and let $\boldsymbol{y}_i = (y_{i1}, \ldots, y_{iT_i})$ denote the expression profile for gene i measured across T_i time points, so that genes are allowed to be measured at different sets of time points or have missing values under our model.

- *Stage 1*: We assume each observed gene expression profile follow a multivariate normal distribution,

$$\boldsymbol{y}_i \mid \boldsymbol{\theta}_i, \boldsymbol{S}_i \sim \mathrm{N}_{T_i}(\boldsymbol{\theta}_i, \boldsymbol{S}_i), \tag{9.7}$$

where $\boldsymbol{\theta}_i$ is the $T_i \times 1$ mean vector and $\boldsymbol{S}_i$ is the $T_i \times T_i$ covariance matrix, for $i = 1, \ldots, n$.

- *Stage 2*: We introduce partition label z_i, which indicates the partition that gene i belongs to. We assume the mean vector is a context-specific function of covariates $\boldsymbol{X}_i$ and partition-specific parameter vector $\boldsymbol{\mu}_k$, with $\boldsymbol{\theta}_i = h(\boldsymbol{X}_i, \boldsymbol{\mu}_k)$ if $z_i = k$. For the cell cycle data, the covariate is time, and the mean structure has the form

$$h(t_j, \boldsymbol{\mu}_k) = e^{-\gamma_k t_j} \left\{ A_k \cos[2\pi f_{t_j}(\phi_k) t_j] + B_k \sin[2\pi f_{t_j}(\phi_k) t_j] \right\}, \tag{9.8}$$

where $f_{t_j}(\phi_k) = f_0\left(\frac{t_j}{t_{\max}}\right)^{\phi_k}$, with $\boldsymbol{\mu}_k = (A_k, B_k, \gamma_k, \phi_k)$ characterizing the mean trajectory, parameters A_k and B_k account for the amplitude and phase of the cyclic pattern, γ_k accounts for the attenuation in the amplitude, and ϕ_k is a time stretching factor for varying cell cycle length. We assume the covariance matrix is also characterized by partition-specific parameter(s) so that $S_i = S(\boldsymbol{\xi}_k)$ if $z_i = k$. If $T_i = T$ for all i, and there is no restriction on the covariance structure, we can assume $S_i = \boldsymbol{\Sigma}_k$, for example, $\sigma_k^2 \boldsymbol{I}$ given $z_i = k$.

- *Stage 3*: We assume the partition label z_i's are independent and identically distributed, conditional on the total number of partitions K and mixing proportion $\boldsymbol{\pi} = (\pi_1, \ldots, \pi_K)$,

$$\Pr(z_1, \ldots, z_n) = \prod_{i=1}^{n} \Pr(z_i \mid K, \boldsymbol{\pi}), \tag{9.9}$$

with

$$\Pr(z_i = k \mid K, \boldsymbol{\pi}) = \pi_k, \tag{9.10}$$

for $k = 1, \ldots, K$, and $i = 1, \ldots, n$.

- *Stage 4*: At this stage, we specify the prior distributions for the partition-specific parameters. Assume

$$\boldsymbol{\mu}_k \mid K, \boldsymbol{m}, \boldsymbol{V} \sim_{i.i.d.} \mathrm{N}_q(\boldsymbol{m}, \boldsymbol{V}), \tag{9.11}$$

$$\boldsymbol{\Sigma}_k^{-1} \mid K, g, \boldsymbol{R} \sim_{i.i.d.} \mathrm{Wishart}(g, (g\boldsymbol{R})^{-1}), \tag{9.12}$$

$$\boldsymbol{\pi} \mid K, \boldsymbol{\delta} \sim \mathrm{Dirichlet}(\boldsymbol{\delta}), \tag{9.13}$$

with priors on $\{\boldsymbol{\xi}_k\}$ if they are present in the model. We also include a "zero" partition with $A_k = B_k = 0$. Genes showing no cyclic pattern will be included in this partition.

- *Stage 5*: The hierarchy is completed with specification of prior constants and hyperpriors. Throughout the analysis, we choose $\boldsymbol{\delta}$ to be a K-vector of 1's for the Dirichlet prior. We assume the total number of partitions K follows a Poisson distribution with parameter λ if it is considered unknown. We choose $g = p$, the dimension of $\boldsymbol{\Sigma}_k$, for it is the least informative in the sense that the distribution is the flattest while being proper [25].

When K is known, this hierarchical model has a partitioning-by-features interpretation, and posterior computations can be carried out using standard Markov chain Monte Carlo (MCMC) software such as WinBUGS [19]. When K is unknown, it can be treated as a random variable and inferred from the data. More sophisticated techniques such as reversible-jump MCMC [17] or

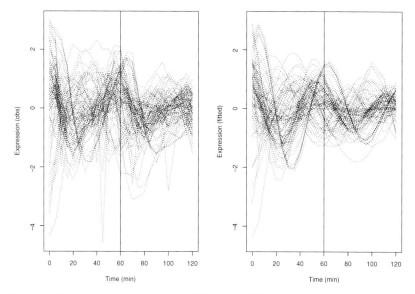

Fig. 9.8. Observed expression of the 100 known CCR genes, and their fitted values based on nonlinear least-squares estimates using model (9.8).

birth–death MCMC [20] are required to deal with the changing dimension. For more details on computation, see [24] and [28].

9.4.4 Results

We now report the results from applying our enhanced hierarchical mixture model to the cell cycle expression data.

Among all 6,309 genes (including controls) on each of the 24 microarrays ($t = 105$ was dropped due to mRNA contamination), 6,141 had no missing data across all chips, 75 had one missing value, 25 had two missing values, and 68 had three or more. A close inspection reveals that genes with many missing values tend to be highly unreliable, and thus genes with three or more missing values were dropped. Some of the measurements were flagged as unreliable at the data processing stage, but we still decided to include them in subsequent analysis because of the ad hoc nature of flagging.

We first identified 1,680 genes as candidates for cell cycle regulation using the filter described in Section 9.4.2. Next we evaluate the extension to the mean structure. Figure 9.8 shows the observed curves and the fitted curves based on nonlinear least-squares estimates from model (9.8). Compared to Figure 9.3, the improvement in the attenuation adjustment and time stretching is clear.

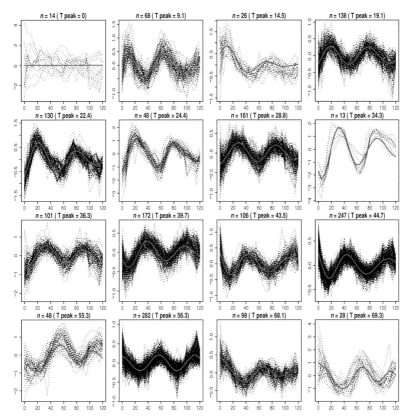

Fig. 9.9. Final partitioning with $K = 16$ fixed (note different vertical scales). (See color plate 9.9.)

We have found that the number of partitions K is highly sensitive to the prior specification, not only the Poisson prior, but also other priors on the variance parameters which could affect the size and shape of partitions. This is in agreement with Stephens [20]. In addition, our enhanced model allows genes to be classified at a finer scale (with more features), which lead to a large number of partitions. Given there is no clear definition regarding the underlying regulation pathways during the cell cycle, we found this number hard to interpret and highly variable depending on the prior choices, so we decided to restrict our attention to the analyses with K fixed. Figure 9.9 displays the classification and estimated mean profiles from fitting the enhanced model to the 38-wt data with K fixed at 16. There is an inherit unidentifiability problem with Bayesian mixture modeling so that relabeling needs to be carried out, (see [20]) for discussion). Here we relabeled the partitions on the basis of time to the first peak. This decision is based on the fact that the cell cycle events are regulated in an orderly fashion. The early activation or deactivation of transcription factors are often responsible for the next wave of gene expression, so this relabeling has an appealing biological interpretation.

Our model was able to identify some interesting cell cycle gene partitions, and the effect of model enhancement is obvious. From Figure 9.9, we can see that partitions 3, 6, 8, 13, and 16 are partitions with strong cyclic signals, and they all show the dissipation of synchrony over time. In particular, partition 3 has a greatly heightened first peak, which is large enough to obscure the later cyclic pattern. Without the improvement to the model, we may not be able to identify this group of genes. We suspect these genes are related to the mating process, so their expression is induced by the pheromone. Several partitions appear to have shortened first cycles, such as partition 2, 3, and 11. These are G_1 or G_2 phase genes, confirming our speculation that the synchronization may shorten the growth phase. At least 9 out of the 13 genes classified into partition 8 are the S-phase histone coding genes. The products of these genes form a single complex that is used for DNA condensation. These genes are coordinately regulated and have been well characterized. A closer inspection reveals that many genes in partition 2 are $M–G_1$ genes and share a promoter element called ECB; many genes in partitions 5 and 6 are late G_1 genes and share MCB and/or SCB promoter elements; partition 9 consists of G_2-phase genes and many of them also share the MCB/SCB promoter elements; and many genes in partition 13 appear to share MCM1 and FKH sites. Partition 11 contains many genes involved in ribosome biogenesis. Their promoters are enriched for two sequence motifs referred to as PAC and RRPE [8, 23]. Our data indicate that these transcripts are modestly periodic and peak 10 minutes after the histones peak.

Note that the time to first peak in partition 16 is larger than 58 minutes, the normal cell cycle span we used. This is because the attenuation at the beginning of the experiment is so large that the first peak of this partition is obscured. If we shift the time to peak by 58 minutes, we can see that this group actually coincide with partition 2, except with much larger amplitude.

Under the Bayesian mixture models, specific partitions are susceptible to the relabeling problem. But as suggested in [24], we can examine the probabilities of *coexpression* $p(z_i = z_{i'} \mid y)$, which are invariant to relabeling. A good visual display of coexpression is the heatmap. Due to space limitation, we select a subsample of the partitions to display. Figure 9.10 shows the coexpression, with dark areas indicating high coexpression, and, as expected, shaded areas are close to the diagonal, suggesting strong coexpression within partitions.

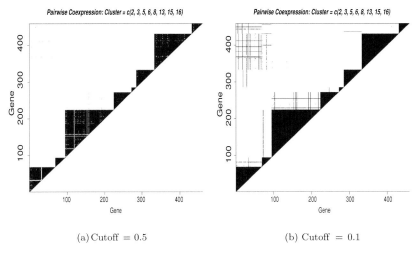

(a) Cutoff $= 0.5$ (b) Cutoff $= 0.1$

Fig. 9.10. Heatmap of probabilities that two genes share a common label, for partitions 2, 3, 5, 6, 8, 13, 15, and 16. Shaded blocks correspond to pairwise probabilities larger than the chosen cutoff.

There is some overlap between partitions 1 and 2, which is not surprising given our previous discussion.

The posterior classification probability of each gene $p(z_i = k \mid \mathbf{y})$ provides a natural measure of uncertainty concerning the partitioning of each individual gene. However, it is also of interest to measure the strength of the partitions, such as how tight genes are *within* a partition, and how much overlap there is *between* different partitions. So we examine the sensitivity and specificity of the partitions, where *sensitivity* is the probability of coexpression, given labeling in the same partition, and *specificity* is the probability of noncoexpression, given labeling in different partitions. Such functions cannot be evaluated with traditional partitioning approaches.

The sensitivity of partition k is estimated by

$$\text{Sensitivity} = \sum_{i,i' \in C_k} p(z_i = z_{i'} = k \mid \mathbf{y})/N_{k1}, \qquad (9.14)$$

where C_k denotes partition k, and N_{k1} is the number of distinct gene pairs classified into C_k. The specificity of partition k is estimated by

$$\text{Specificity} = \sum_{i \in C_k, i' \in C_{k'}, k' \neq k} p(z_i = k, z_{i'} = k' \mid \mathbf{y})/N_{k2}, \qquad (9.15)$$

where C_k and $C_{k'}$ are different partitions, and N_{k2} is the number of distinct gene pairs with only one gene classified into C_k. The sensitivity and specificity

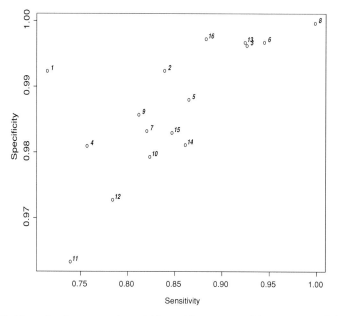

Fig. 9.11. Strength of coexpression within and between partitions, measured through sensitivity and specificity.

of the 16 partitions are shown in Figure 9.11. Partition 1 is the "zero" partition for noncyclic genes, so it is not surprising to see it has the lowest sensitivity. Partitions 11 and 12 only have weak signals and there is overlap between genes in these partitions, hence their sensitivity and specificity are low. Partition 8 contains a tight group of histone genes that have strong cyclic signals, and it is ranked the highest in terms of sensitivity and specificity. Other high-quality partitions include partitions 3, 6, 13, and 16, as was evident from Figure 9.9. The sensitivity and specificity estimates provide a natural quantitative measure of the quality of partitions, based on which we can focus on the high-quality partitions, and proceed with validation or more sophisticated analysis such as motif discovery.

Studying the coexpression can also provide important information about relationship between partitions. For example, Figure 9.12 shows several genes identified from the heatmap that had high coexpression with genes in partition 16 though they were classified into partition 2. Examination of the mean trajectories reveals that the peaks of one trajectory appear to coincide with the other, suggesting these two partitions could be coregulated, although the magnitude of the signals differs. Some would argue that these genes should be considered coregulated as long as the peaks and troughs of their oscillations

Genes classified in cluster 2, and coexpression with cluster 16

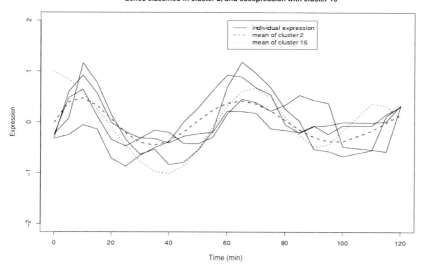

Fig. 9.12. Selected genes partitioned into group 2, but with coexpression with partition 16.

concur, regardless of their magnitude. Here we distinguish these genes, for we speculate that genes with higher amplitude may contain more promoting elements, or some other element(s) responsible for increased expression levels, or the low amplitude profiles may be from genes with unstable mRNAs. In fact, a sequence search reveals that partition 16 and partition 2 do share common MCM1 elements. The relevant motif is TTTCCNNNNNNGGAAA, a flanking palindrome to which two MCM1 proteins bind (N = A or C or G or T). Such binding is required for transcriptional activation at the M/G_1 boundary. And as we thought, the partition 16 genes have multiple elements and a larger consensus sequence, and the partition 2 genes have only one site. Many partition 2 genes do not have the MCM1 site at all. This causes us to suspect that there may be new element(s) in partition 2 genes which have similar properties as MCM1. We will continue investigation of these speculatives.

9.5 Discussion

As explained above, the changing cell cycle span and magnitude of signals are systematic and correspond to actual biological phenomena. Although a large number of research papers have been published on the topic of cell cycle gene expression, few have taken these systematic variations into account. Zhao et al. [27] considered the issue of decreasing signals in their SPM, in which they allowed the precision to decrease over time. Bar-Joseph [2] mentioned both issues, but used semiparametric models instead of directly modeling the phenomena. Here we advocate a science-motivated, model-based approach toward cell cycle gene expression analysis. We believe that it is less appropriate to rely totally on data-driven approaches, regardless of the biological context and scientific questions waiting to be addressed.

Because every synchronization protocol has its limitations, a prudent strategy for determining whether a specific process is cell-cycle-regulated is to employ at least two different synchrony methods. If the oscillation can be observed through two or more mitotic cycles in two different synchrony experiments, it is unlikely the oscillation is induced by the arrest [3]. But combining analyses from different experiments is a difficult task, and has not been fully addressed by researchers. We leave it as future research, and do not attempt this problem here.

Our approach of assuming a mixture model with flexible mean structures is crucially different from the "model-based" clustering approach of Yeung et al. [26], who analyzed similar data but simply assumed that the data arose from a mixture of T-dimensional normal distributions and hence did not acknowledge the time ordering of the data (the analysis would be unchanged if the time ordering were permuted). In particular, it would be desirable to allow serial dependence, within such an approach, but the MCLUST software [7] that is used by Yeung et al. [26] does not allow for this possibility, and it does not perform well when the dimension T gets large. In their approach, missing data and unbalanced design also cause complications, whereas in our model no such problems arise. Medvedovic and Sivaganesan [14] also proposed a Bayesian hierarchical model for clustering microarray data, but again they failed to take the time ordering into account in their approach.

We have demonstrated that our enhanced model can provide further insight into our understanding of cell cycle transcription programs. In our enhanced model, each partition is characterized by a set of four parameters. Intuitively speaking, the finer we characterize the mean model, the easier to distinguish different features and we see more partitions. So we were not surprised to find that a large number of partitions were being identified under our refined model. Although many numerical methods for detecting underlying clusters based on gene expression data have been published, none of them are satisfactory. From our experience we have found that without plausible interpretation and biological validation, the number of partitions produced by numerical analysis is highly unreliable, and sometimes even misleading. The partitions are defined by the model, which in turn is motivated by the biology. The ultimate validation of the partitioning should be based on scientific investigation, with data analysis providing numerical support and further hypotheses. In other words, the conclusion should be based on science, not just on data analysis.

Bibliography

[1] Axon Instruments, Inc. (2005). *GenePix Pro. 6.0 User's Guide & Tutorial – Microarray Acquisition and Analysis Software for GenePix Microarray Scanners.* Axon Instruments, Inc.

[2] Bar-Joseph, Z., Gerber, G., Gifford, D. K., and Jaakkola, T. S. (2002). A new approach to analyzing gene expression time series data. *Proceedings of the Sixth Annual International Conference on Research in Computational Molecular Biology*, 39–48.

[3] Breeden, L. L. (1997). α-factor synchronization of budding yeast. *Methods in Enzymology*, **283**, 332–341.

[4] Cho, R. J. et al. (1998). A genome-wide transcriptional analysis of the mitotic cell cycle. *Molecular Cell*, **2**, 65–73.

[5] Do, K., Müller, P., and Tang, F. (2005). A Bayesian mixture model for differential gene expression. *Journal of the Royal Statistical Society C*, **54**, 627–644.

[6] Eisen, M. B., Spellman, P. T., Brown, P. O., and Botstein, D. (1998). Cluster analysis and display of genome-wide expression patterns. *Proceedings of the National Academy of Sciences USA*, **95**, 14863–14868.

[7] Fraley, C. and Raftery, A. E. (1998). How many clusters? Which clustering method? Answers via model-based cluster analysis. *Computer Journal*, **41**, 578–588.

[8] Hughes, J. D., Estep, P. W., Tavazoie, S., and Church, G. M. (2000). Computational identification of Cis-regulatory elements associated with groups of functionally related genes in *Saccharomyces cerevisiae*. *Journal of Molecular Biology*, **296**, 1205–1214.

[9] Johansson, D., Lindgren, P., and Berglund, A. (2003). A multivariate approach applied to microarray data for identification of genes with cell cycle-coupled transcription. *Bioinformatics*, **19**, 467–473.

[10] Kelly, T. J. and Brown, G. W. (2000). Regulation of chromosome replication. *Annual Review of Biochemistry*, **69**, 829–880.

[11] de Lichtenberg, U., Jensen, J., Fausbøll, A., Jensen, T. S., Bork, P., and Brunak, S. (2005). Comparison of computational methods for the identification of cell cycle-regulated genes. *Bioinformatics*, **21**, 1164–1171.

[12] Lu, X., Zhang, W., Qin, Z. S., Kwast, K. E., and Liu, J. S. (2004). Statistical resynchronization and Bayesian detection of periodically expressed genes. *Nucleic Acids Research*, **32**, 447–455.

[13] Luan, Y. and Li, H. (2004). Model-based methods for identifying periodically expressed genes based on time course microarray gene expression data. *Bioinformatics*, **20**, 332–339.

[14] Medvedovic, M. and Sivaganesan, S. (2002). Bayesian infinite mixture model based clustering of gene expression profiles. *Bioinformatics*, **18**, 1194–1206.

[15] Morgan, D. O. (1997). Cyclin-dependent kinases: Engines, clocks, and microprocesses. *Annual Review of Cell Developmental Biology*, **13**, 261–291.

[16] Quackenbush, J. (2002). Microarray data normalization and transformation. *Nature Genetics Supplement*, **32**, 496–501.

[17] Richardson, S. and Green, P. (1997). On Bayesian analysis of mixtures with unknown number of components (with discussion). *Journal of the Royal Statistical Society, Series B*, **59**, 731–792.

[18] Spellman, P. T., Sherlock, G., Zhang, M. Q., Iyer, V. R., Anders, K., Eisen, M. B., Brown, P. O., Botstein, D., and Futcher, B. (1998). Comprehensive identification of cell cycle-regulated genes of the yeast *Saccharomyces cerevisiae* by microarray hybridization. *Molecular Biology of the Cell*, **9**, 3273–3297.

[19] Spiegelhalter, D. J., Thomas, A., Best, N. G., and Lunn, D. (2002). *WinBUGS User Mannual, Version 1.4.*, Medical Research Council Biostatistics Unit, Institute of Public Health, Cambridge University.

[20] Stephens, M. (2000). Bayesian analysis of mixture models with an unknown number of components – An alternative to reversible jump methods. *Annals of Statistics*, **28**, 40–74.

[21] Storey, J. D. (2002). A direct approach to false discovery rates. *Journal of the Royal Statistical Society, Series B*, **64**, 479–498.

[22] Tamayo, P., Slonim, D., Mesirov, J., Zhu, Q., amd Kitareewan, S., Dmitrovsky, E., Lander, E., and Golub, T. (1999). Interpreting patterns of gene expression with self-organizing maps: Methods and application to hematopoietic differentiation. *Proceedings of the National Academy of Sciences USA*, **96**, 2907–2912.

[23] Wade, C., Shea, K. A., Jensen, R. V., and McAlear, M. A. (2001). EBP2 is a member of the yeast RRB regulon, a transcriptionally coregulated set of genes that are required for ribosome and rRNA biosynthesis. *Molecular and Cellular Biology*, **21**, 8638–8650.

[24] Wakefield, J., Zhou, C., and Self, S. (2003). Modelling gene expression over time: Curve clustering with informative prior distributions. In Bernardo, J., Bayarri, M., Berger, J., Dawid, A., Heckerman, D., Smith, A., and West, M., editors, *Bayesian Statistics 7, Proceedings of the Seventh Valencia International Meeting*, Clarendon Press, Oxford, 721–733.

[25] Wakefield, J. C., Smith, A. F. M., Racine-Poon, A., and Gelfand, A. E. (1994). Bayesian analysis of linear and non-linear population models by using the Gibbs sampler. *Applied Statistics*, **43**, 201–221.

[26] Yeung, K., Fraley, C., Murua, A., Raftery, A., and Ruzzo, W. (2001). Model-based clustering and data transformations for gene expression data. *Bioinformatics*, **17**, 977–987.

[27] Zhao, L. P., Prentice, R., and Breeden, L. (2001). Statistical modeling of large microarray data sets to identify stimulus-response profiles. *Proceedings of the National Academy of Sciences USA*, **98**, 5631–5636.

[28] Zhou, C. and Wakefield, J. (in press). A Bayesian mixture model for partitioning gene expression data. *Biometrics*.

10

Model-Based Clustering for Expression Data via a Dirichlet Process Mixture Model

DAVID B. DAHL

Texas A&M University

Abstract

This chapter describes a clustering procedure for microarray expression data based on a well-defined statistical model, specifically, a conjugate Dirichlet process mixture model. The clustering algorithm groups genes whose latent variables governing expression are equal, that is, genes belonging to the same mixture component. The model is fit with Markov chain Monte Carlo and the computational burden is eased by exploiting conjugacy. This chapter introduces a method to get a point estimate of the true clustering based on least-squares distances from the posterior probability that two genes are clustered. Unlike ad hoc clustering methods, the model provides measures of uncertainty about the clustering. Further, the model automatically estimates the number of clusters and quantifies uncertainty about this important parameter. The method is compared to other clustering methods in a simulation study. Finally, the method is demonstrated with actual microarray data.

10.1 Introduction

The main goal of clustering microarray data is to group genes that present highly correlated data; this correlation may reflect underlying biological factors of interest, such as regulation by a common transcription factor. A variety of heuristic clustering methods exist, including k-means clustering (MacQueen 1967) and hierarchical agglomerative clustering. These methods have had an enormous impact in genomics (Eisen et al. 1998) and are intuitively appealing. Nevertheless, the statistical properties of these heuristic clustering methods are generally not known. Model-based clustering procedures have been proposed for microarray data, including (1) the MCLUST procedure of Fraley and Raftery (2002) and Yeung et al. (2001), and (2) the Bayesian mixture model based clustering of Medvedovic and Sivaganesan (2002) and Medvedovic et al. (2004). Model-based techniques offer advantages over heuristic schemes, such as the ability to assess uncertainty about the resulting clustering and to formally estimate the number of clusters.

This chapter describes a model-based clustering procedure for microarray expression data based on a well-defined statistical model, specifically, a conjugate Dirichlet process mixture (DPM) model. In the assumed model, two genes come from the same mixture component if and only if their relevant latent variables governing expression are equal. The model itself, known as BEMMA for Bayesian Effects Model for Microarrays, was first introduced by Dahl and Newton (submitted) as a means of exploiting the clustering structure of data for increased sensitivity in a battery of correlated hypothesis tests (e.g., finding differentially expressed genes). The focus of this chapter is not finding differential expression, but rather identifying the underlying clustering structure of expression data.

Computations for Bayesian mixture models can be challenging. Unlike the finite and infinite mixture models of Medvedovic and Sivaganesan (2002) and Medvedovic et al. (2004), the proposed method is, however, conjugate. This conjugacy permits the latent variables to be integrated away, thereby simplifying to state space over which the Markov chain is run. The model is fit using Markov chain Monte Carlo (MCMC), specifically using the conjugate Gibbs sampler (MacEachern 1994; Neal 1992) and the merge–split algorithm of Dahl (2003). Each iteration of the Markov chain yields a clustering of the data.

Providing a single point estimate for clustering based on the thousands of clusterings in the Markov chain has been proven to be challenging (Medvedovic and Sivaganesan 2002). One approach is to select the observed clustering with the highest posterior probability; this is called the maximum a posteriori (MAP) clustering. Unfortunately, the MAP clustering may only be slightly more probable than the next best alternative, yet represent a very different allocation of observations. Alternatively, Medvedovic and Sivaganesan (2002) and Medvedovic et al. (2004) suggest using hierarchical agglomerative clustering based on a distance matrix formed using the observed clusterings in the Markov chain. It seems counterintuitive, however, to apply an ad hoc clustering method on top of a model which itself produces clusterings.

This chapter proposes a method to form a clustering from the many clusterings observed in the Markov chain. The method is called least-squares model-based clustering (or, simply, least-squares clustering). It selects the observed clustering from the Markov chain that minimizes the sum of squared deviations from the pairwise probability matrix that genes are clustered. The least-squares clustering has the advantage that it uses information from all the clusterings (via the pairwise probability matrix) and is intuitively appealing because it selects the "average" clustering (instead of forming a clustering via an external, ad hoc algorithm).

Section 10.2 presents the details of the proposed model, including the likelihood, prior, and how to set the hyperparameters. Section 10.2.3 describes the model fitting approach and how the conjugate nature of the model aids in its fitting. Section 10.3 details the new least-squares clustering estimator using draws from the posterior clustering distribution. Section 10.4 presents a simulation study showing that the method compares well with other clustering methods. Finally, the model is demonstrated in Section 10.5, using a microarray data set with 10,043 probe sets, 10 treatments conditions, and 3 replicates per treatment condition. This section also introduces the effects intensity plot which displays the clustering of all genes simultaneously. The chapter ends with a discussion in Section 10.6.

10.2 Model

The model-based clustering procedure presented here is based on the Bayesian Effects Model for Microarrays (BEMMA) of Dahl and Newton (submitted). The model was originally proposed as a means to gain increased sensitivity in a battery of correlated hypothesis tests by exploiting the underlying clustering structure of data. In their application, Dahl and Newton (submitted) were interested in identifying differentially expressed genes. In this chapter, we apply their model to the task of clustering highly correlated genes that may reveal underlying biological factors of interest.

10.2.1 Likelihood Specification

The model assumes the following sampling distribution:

$$y_{gtr} \,|\, \mu_g, \tau_{gt}, \lambda_g \sim N(y_{gtr} \,|\, \mu_g + \tau_{gt}, \lambda_g), \qquad (10.1)$$

where y_{gtr} is a suitably transformed expression of replicate r ($r = 1, \ldots, R_t$) of gene g ($g = 1, \ldots, G$) at treatment condition t ($t = 1, \ldots, T$) and $N(z|a, b)$ denotes the univariate normal distribution with mean a and variance $1/b$ for the random variable z. The parameter μ_g represents a gene-specific mean, the gene-specific treatment effects are $\tau_{g1}, \ldots, \tau_{gT}$, and λ_g is a gene-specific sampling precision.

The model assumes that coregulated genes have the same treatment effects and precision. That is, genes g and g' are in the same cluster if

$(\tau_{g1}, \ldots, \tau_{gT}, \lambda_g) = (\tau_{g'1}, \ldots, \tau_{g'T}, \lambda_{g'})$. The clustering can be encoded with cluster labels $c_1, \ldots, c_G$, where $c_g = c_{g'}$ if and only if genes g and g' are in the same cluster.

The gene-specific means $\mu_1, \ldots, \mu_G$ are nuisance parameters; they are not related to differential expression across treatments and they are not used to define clusters. Indeed, there can exist constant differences in expression from probe sets known to be coregulated. These constant differences may be due to the biology (e.g., mRNA degradation) or the microarray technology (e.g., hybridization differences between probes or labeling efficiency). Whatever the reason, constant differences between probe sets may naturally exist in microarray experiments, yet they are not of interest. Indeed, two genes having a constant difference across treatments is the essence of coregulation.

The nuisance parameters $\mu_1, \ldots, \mu_G$ could be handled by specifying a prior over them and integrating the likelihood implied by (10.1) over this prior. The resulting model would be nonconjugate since the prior specification (detailed in the next subsection) induces mixing with respect to both the treatment effects $\tau_{g1}, \ldots, \tau_{gT}$ and the sampling precision λ_g. (If the mixing were only with respect to the treatment effects, conjugacy would remain intact when integrating over the nuisance parameters $\mu_1, \ldots, \mu_G$.) Fitting this nonconjugate model would be computationally challenging in the presence of thousands of genes.

The following pragmatic approach is used to address the nuisance parameters $\mu_1, \ldots, \mu_G$. Select a reference treatment (taken here to be the first treatment for notational convenience). Let d_g be a vector whose elements are $y_{gtr} - \overline{y}_{g1}$ for $t \geq 2$, where $\overline{y}_{g1}$ is the mean of the reference treatment. Further, let $\tau_g = (\tau_{g2}, \ldots, \tau_{gT})$ be a treatment effect vector and $N = \sum_{t=2}^{T} R_t$ be the dimension of d_g. Simple calculations reveal that d_g is independent of the nuisance parameters $\mu_1, \ldots, \mu_G$ and distributed:

$$d_g \mid \tau_g, \lambda_g \sim N_N(d_g \mid X\tau_g, \lambda_g M), \qquad (10.2)$$

where $N_c(z \mid a, b)$ is a c-dimensional multivariate normal distribution with mean vector a and covariance matrix b^{-1} for the random vector z. Also, M is an $N \times N$ matrix equal to $(I + \frac{1}{R_1}J)^{-1}$, where I is the identify matrix and J is a matrix of ones. Finally, X is an $N \times (T-1)$ design matrix whose rows contain all zeros except where the number 1 is needed to pick off the appropriate element of τ_g. If one prefers, the model could equivalently be written in terms of sample averages from each treatment. This would, for example, reduce the dimension of d_g from N to T.

10.2.2 Prior Specification

Clustering based on equality of τ's and λ's across genes is achieved by using a Dirichlet process prior for these model parameters, resulting in a Dirichlet process mixture (DPM) model. See Müller and Quintana (2004) and references therein for a review of the DPM model literature. The model assumes the following prior:

$$\tau_g, \lambda_g \,|F(\tau_g, \lambda_g) \sim F(\tau_g, \lambda_g)$$
$$F(\tau, \lambda) \sim DP(\eta_0 F_0(\tau, \lambda)), \tag{10.3}$$

where $DP(\eta_0 F_0(\tau, \lambda))$ is the Dirichlet process having centering distribution $F_0(\tau, \lambda)$ for the random variables τ and λ and mass parameter η_0. The centering distribution $F_0(\tau, \lambda)$ is a joint distribution for τ and λ having the following conjugate density:

$$p(\tau, \lambda) = p(\tau \,|\lambda)p(\lambda)$$
$$= N_{T-1}(\tau \,|0, \lambda\Psi_0)Ga(\lambda \,|\alpha_0, \beta_0), \tag{10.4}$$

where $Ga(z \,|a, b)$ is the gamma distribution with mean a/b for the random variable z and α_0, β_0, and Ψ_0 are fixed hyperparameters set based on either prior experience or current data.

10.2.3 Sampling from the Posterior Distribution

Quintana and Newton (2000) and Neal (2000) have good reviews and comparisons of methods for fitting DPM models. We suggest fitting the proposed model using MCMC. The centering distribution $F_0(\tau, \lambda)$ in (10.4) is conjugate to the likelihood for τ_g and λ_g in (10.2). Thus, the model parameters may be integrated away, leaving only the clustering of the G genes. As a result, the stationary distribution of a Markov chain for the model is $p(c_1, \ldots, c_G|d_1, \ldots, d_g)$, the posterior distribution of the clustering configurations. This technique was shown by MacEachern (1994) and MacEachern et al. (1999) to greatly improve the efficiency of Gibbs sampling and sequential importance sampling, respectively. Efficiency is very important if the model is to be useful in practice.

It should be noted that the technique of integrating away the model parameters is merely a device used for model fitting. Inference on the model parameters $\tau_1, \ldots, \tau_G$ and $\lambda_1, \ldots, \lambda_G$ can still be made by sampling from posterior distribution of the model parameters (i.e., (10.6) in next subsection) after having obtained samples from the posterior clustering distribution.

The Gibbs sampler can be used to sample from the posterior clustering distribution of conjugate DPM models (MacEachern 1994; Neal 1992). The Gibbs sampler repeatedly takes a gene out of the clustering and draws a new cluster label from the full conditional distribution. Because the Gibbs sampler only moves one gene at a time, it may explore the posterior clustering distribution rather slowly. Jain and Neal (2004) and Dahl (2003) present merge–split algorithms that attempt to update more than one cluster label at a time. The Gibbs sampler and both of these merge–split samplers require the evaluation of the posterior predictive distribution. The next subsection gives the full conditional distribution and the posterior predictive distribution for the proposed model.

10.2.4 Full Conditional and Posterior Predictive Distributions

The full conditional distribution is essential for fitting the model using the Gibbs sampler. Let c_{-i} denote the collection of all cluster labels except that corresponding to gene i. For notational convenience, let the cluster labels in c_{-i} be numbered from 1 to k and let $k + 1$ be the label of an empty cluster. Finally, let n_c be the number of cluster labels equal to c (not counting c_i), unless cluster c is empty, in which case, n_c is set to the mass parameter η_0. The full conditional distribution is a multinomial distribution given by

$$p(c_i = c \,|\, c_{-i}, d_1, \ldots, d_G) \propto n_c \int B(d_i | \tau, \lambda) p(\tau, \lambda | D_c) \, d\tau \, d\phi, \quad (10.5)$$

for $c = 1, \ldots, k + 1$, where $B(d_i | \tau, \lambda)$ is the normal distribution in (10.2), and $p(\tau, \lambda | D_c)$ is the density of the posterior distribution of τ and λ based on the prior $F_0(\tau, \lambda)$ in (10.4) and all differences d_j for which $j \neq i$ and $c_j = c$. In the case of an empty cluster, $p(\tau, \lambda | D_c)$ is just the density of the prior $F_0(\tau, \lambda)$ and n_c is set to the mass parameter η_0 instead of 0; otherwise, it is rather straightforward to show that

$$\begin{aligned} p(\tau, \lambda | D_c) &\propto p(\tau | \lambda, D_c) p(\lambda | D_c) \\ &= N_{T-1}(\tau \,|\, \Psi_{n_c}^{-1} S_1, \lambda \Psi_{n_c}) Ga(\lambda \,|\, \alpha_{n_c}, \beta_1), \end{aligned} \quad (10.6)$$

where

$$\begin{aligned} \Psi_{n_c} &= \Psi_0 + n_c X' M X, \\ \alpha_{n_c} &= \alpha_0 + \frac{n_c N}{2}, \\ \beta_1 &= \beta_0 + \frac{1}{2} S_2 - \frac{1}{2} S_1' \Psi_{n_c}^{-1} S_1, \\ S_1 &= \sum_{d \in D_c} X' M d, \quad \text{and} \\ S_2 &= \sum_{d \in D_c} d' M d. \end{aligned} \quad (10.7)$$

The integral in (10.5) refers to the posterior predictive distribution of d belonging to cluster c. For conjugate DPM models, this distribution can usually be found in closed form. In the present model, the posterior predictive distribution for a new difference vector d^* evaluated at d (when its cluster label c^* is c and given the data D_c having cluster label c) has the following density:

$$p(d^* = d \mid c^* = c, D_c) = c_n \frac{\beta_1^{\alpha_{n_c}}}{\beta_2^{\alpha_{n_c}+1}}, \tag{10.8}$$

where

$$\beta_2 = \beta_0 + \frac{1}{2} S_2 + \frac{1}{2} d' M d - \frac{1}{2} (X' M d + S_1)' \Psi_{n_c+1}^{-1} (X' M d + S_1)$$

$$c_n = \frac{\Gamma(\alpha_{n_c}+1)}{\Gamma(\alpha_{n_c})} \sqrt{\frac{\mid \Psi_n \mid\mid M \mid}{\mid \Psi_{n_c+1} \mid (2\pi)^N}}. \tag{10.9}$$

It is interesting to note that (10.8) is not the usual multivariate Student t-distribution.

10.2.5 Setting the Hyperparameters

Lacking strong prior belief about the hyperparameters $\eta_0, \alpha_0, \beta_0$, and Ψ_0, an empirical Bayes procedure can be used. Notice that (10.7) implies that $\Psi_{n+1} = \Psi_n + X' M X$ and $\alpha_{n+1} = \alpha_n + \frac{N}{2}$. That is, for each additional observation, Ψ_n and α_n are incremented by $X' M X$ and $\frac{N}{2}$, respectively. It is natural, therefore, to set the hyperparameter Ψ_0 to $n_0 X' M X$ and the hyperparameter α_0 to $n_0 \frac{N}{2}$, for $n_0 > 0$ representing the number of observations that prior experience is worth. By default, we recommend $n_0 = 1$.

As shown in (10.1) and (10.4), the hyperparameters α_0 and β_0 are, respectively, the shape and rate parameters of the gamma prior distribution for the precision of an observation in a given cluster. We recommend setting α_0 and β_0 such that the mean of this distribution, α_0/β_0, matches a data-driven estimate of the expected precision for a cluster. Equivalently, in terms of the standard deviation, choose α_0 and β_0 so that $\sqrt{\beta_0/\alpha_0}$ matches the estimated standard deviation for a cluster. The software implementation of BEMMA uses the median standard deviation across all probe sets if no value is specified by the user. Since $\alpha_0 = n_0 \frac{N}{2}$ (from the previous paragraph), specifying the expected standard deviation implies a value for β_0.

The final hyperparameter to consider is the mass parameter η_0, which affects the distribution on the number of clusters. The mass parameter in DPM models has been well studied (Escobar 1994; Escobar and West 1995; Liu 1996;

Medvedovic and Sivaganesan 2002). From Antoniak (1974), the prior expected number of clusters is

$$K(G) = \sum_{g=1}^{G} \frac{\eta_0}{\eta_0 + g - 1}.$$

In some DPM model applications, the mass parameter is set to 1.0. This seems overly optimistic for microarray experiments since, for example, it implies a prior belief that there are less than 12 clusters in data set with 50,000 genes. We use an empirical Bayes approach which sets η_0 such that the posterior expected number of clusters equals the prior expected number of clusters. The software implementation of BEMMA provides this option.

10.3 Inference

Draws $c_1, \ldots, c_B$ from the posterior clustering distribution can be obtained using MCMC, where B is a number of sampled clusterings. Several methods have been used to arrive at a point estimate of the clustering using draws from the posterior clustering distribution. Perhaps the simplest method is to select the observed clustering that maximizes the density of the posterior clustering distribution. This is known as the maximum a posteriori (MAP) clustering. Unfortunately, the MAP clustering may only be slightly more probable than the next best alternative, yet represent a very different allocation of observations.

For each clustering c in $c_1, \ldots, c_B$, an association matrix $\delta(c)$ of dimension $G \times G$ can be formed whose (i, j) element is $\delta_{i,j}(c)$, an indicator of whether gene i is clustered with gene j. Element-wise averaging of these association matrices yields the pairwise probability matrix of clustering, denoted $\widehat{\pi}$. Medvedovic and Sivaganesan (2002) and Medvedovic et al. (2004) suggest forming a clustering estimate by using the pairwise probability matrix $\widehat{\pi}$ as a distance matrix in hierarchical agglomerative clustering. It seems counterintuitive, however, to apply an ad hoc clustering method on top of a model which itself produces clusterings.

We introduce the least-squares model-based clustering (or, simply, least-squares clustering), a new method for estimating the clustering of observations using draws from a posterior clustering distribution. As with the method of Medvedovic and Sivaganesan (2002), the method is based on the pairwise probability matrix $\widehat{\pi}$ that genes are clustered together. The method differs, however, in that it selects one of the observed clusterings in the Markov chain as the point estimate. Specifically, the least-squares clustering c_{LS} is the observed clustering c which minimizes the sum of squared deviations of its association matrix $\delta(c)$ from the pairwise probability matrix $\widehat{\pi}$:

$$c_{LS} = \underset{c \in \{c_1, \dots, c_B\}}{\arg\min} \sum_{i=1}^{G} \sum_{j=1}^{G} (\delta_{i,j}(c) - \widehat{\pi}_{i,j})^2. \qquad (10.10)$$

The least-squares clustering has the advantage that it uses information from all the clusterings (via the pairwise probability matrix) and is intuitively appealing because it selects the "average" clustering (instead of forming a clustering via an external, ad hoc clustering algorithm).

Uncertainty about a particular clustering estimate can be accessed from the posterior clustering distribution. For example, one can readily estimate the probability that two genes are clustered together by computing the relative frequency of this event among the clusterings in the Markov chain. Also, the posterior distribution of the number of clusters is easily obtained.

10.4 Simulation Study

This section provides a simulation study comparing the proposed clustering method to several standard methods. To assess the robustness of the clustering methods, four degrees of clustering are considered:

Heavy clustering: Data with 12 clusters of 100 genes per cluster.
Moderate clustering: Data with 60 clusters of 20 genes per cluster.
Weak clustering: Data with 240 clusters of 5 genes per cluster.
No clustering: Data with no clustering of the genes.

Each data set has 1,200 genes. The simulated experimental design is a time-course experiment (with three time points) and two groups, making in all $T = 6$ treatments.

Each cluster may be classified as either containing genes that are differentially expressed or equivalently expressed. Clusters that are equivalently expressed have equal treatment effects for the two treatments within a time point. Clusters that are differentially expressed have independently sampled treatment effects at one or more of the time points. In all cases, the precision λ for a cluster is a draw from a gamma distribution with mean 1 and variance $1/10$, the treatment effects $\tau_1, \dots, \tau_6$ for a cluster are drawn independently from a normal distribution with mean 0 and variance $(9\lambda)^{-1}$, and the gene-specific shift μ is drawn from a normal distribution with mean 7 and variance 1.

Regardless of the degree of clustering, each data set contains 300 genes that are differentially expressed. A third of the differentially expressed clusters have unequal treatment effects at only one time point, a third have unequal treatment effects at two time points, and the remaining third have unequal treatment effects at all three time points. Finally, the observed data is drawn as specified in (10.1), with the first time point having five replicates per treatment and the other time points having three replicates.

10.4.1 Simulation Results

The MAP and least-squares clusterings based on the BEMMA model (as described in Section 10.3) were computed for each simulated data set and are labeled "BEMMA(map)" and "BEMMA(least-squares)," respectively. To compare the performance of BEMMA, the MCLUST procedure (Fraley and Raftery 1999, 2002) and hierarchical clustering (Hartigan 1975; Ihaka and Gentleman 1996) were applied to the simulated data. Specifically, the following methods were used:

MCLUST: The Mclust( ) function of the mclust package of R (Ihaka and Gentleman 1996)

HCLUST(correlation,average): Hierarchical clustering where the distance between genes was one minus the square of the Pearson correlation of the sample treatment means and using the "average" agglomeration method

HCLUST(correlation,complete): Hierarchical clustering using correlation distance and using the "complete" agglomeration method

HCLUST(effects,average): Hierarchical clustering where the distance between genes was the Euclidean distance between the sample treatment effects and using the "average" agglomeration method

HCLUST(effects,complete): Hierarchical clustering using effects distance and using the "complete" agglomeration method

Hierarchical clustering is a heuristic clustering procedure, while BEMMA and MCLUST are model-based clustering procedures. The number of clusters in the data is unspecified in the proposed model. For simplicity, the number of clusters for the other clustering methods was set to the true number of clusters.

There are many indices for measuring the agreement between two clusterings. In a comprehensive comparison, Milligan and Cooper (1986) recommend

Table 10.1. *Adjusted Rand Index for BEMMA and Other Methods*

Degree of clustering	Clustering method	Adjusted Rand index w/95% C.I.	
Heavy	MCLUST	0.413	(0.380, 0.447)
	BEMMA(least-squares)	0.402	(0.373, 0.431)
	BEMMA(map)	0.390	(0.362, 0.419)
	HCLUST(effects,average)	0.277	(0.247, 0.308)
	HCLUST(effects,complete)	0.260	(0.242, 0.279)
	HCLUST(correlation,complete)	0.162	(0.144, 0.180)
	HCLUST(correlation,average)	0.156	(0.141, 0.172)
Moderate	BEMMA(least-squares)	0.154	(0.146, 0.163)
	MCLUST	0.144	(0.136, 0.152)
	BEMMA(map)	0.127	(0.119, 0.135)
	HCLUST(effects,complete)	0.117	(0.111, 0.123)
	HCLUST(effects,average)	0.101	(0.095, 0.107)
	HCLUST(correlation,average)	0.079	(0.075, 0.083)
	HCLUST(correlation,complete)	0.073	(0.068, 0.078)
Weak	MCLUST	0.050	(0.048, 0.052)
	HCLUST(effects,complete)	0.045	(0.043, 0.048)
	BEMMA(least-squares)	0.042	(0.040, 0.043)
	HCLUST(effects,average)	0.037	(0.035, 0.038)
	BEMMA(map)	0.031	(0.030, 0.033)
	HCLUST(correlation,average)	0.029	(0.027, 0.030)
	HCLUST(correlation,complete)	0.027	(0.025, 0.029)

Note: Large values of the adjusted Rand index indicate better agreement between the estimated and true clustering.

the adjusted Rand index (Hubert and Arabie 1985; Rand 1971) as the preferred measure of agreement between two clusterings. Large values for the adjusted Rand index mean better agreement. That is, an estimated clustering that closely matches the true clustering has a relatively large adjusted Rand index.

Table 10.1 shows the adjusted Rand index for BEMMA and the other clustering methods. Under heavy, moderate, and weak clustering, the MCLUST does very well. BEMMA too performs well. Notice that the newly proposed least-squares clustering method of Section 10.3 performs better than the MAP clustering method. The hierarchical clustering procedures generally do not perform very well, especially those based on the correlation distance matrix.

In summary, the simulation study suggests that the least-squares clustering is able to estimate the true clustering relatively well. It does about as well as MCLUST and much better than hierarchical clustering, even though

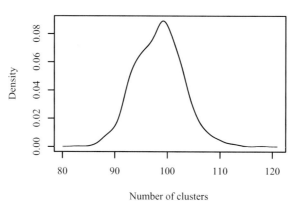

Fig. 10.1. Posterior distribution of the number of clusters.

BEMMA does not have the benefit of knowing the true number of clusters. Further, the model-based nature of BEMMA allows one to readily assess the variability in the estimated clustering. Finally, when information on differential expression is desired, BEMMA is also shown by Dahl and Newton (submitted) to be a very sensitive method for detecting differentially expressed genes.

10.5 Example

The proposed method was implemented on a replicated, multiple treatment microarray experiment. Researchers were interested in the transcriptional response to oxidative stress in mouse skeletal muscle and how that response changes with age. Young (5-month-old) and old (25-month-old) mice were treated with an injection of paraquat (50 mg/kg). Mice were sacrificed at 1, 3, 5, and 7 hours after paraquat treatment or were sacrificed having not received paraquat (constituting a baseline). Thus, $T = 10$ experimental conditions were under consideration. Edwards et al. (2003) discuss the experimental details. All treatments were replicated three times. Gene expression was measured on $G = 10{,}043$ probe sets using high-density oligonucleotide microarrays manufactured by Affymetrix (MG-U74A arrays). The data was background-corrected and normalized using the Robust Multichip Averaging (RMA) method of Irizarry et al. (2003) as implemented in the affy package of BioConductor (Gentleman et al. 2004). For a review of the issues and procedures for background-correction and normalization, see Irizarry et al. (2003) and Dudoit et al. (2002)

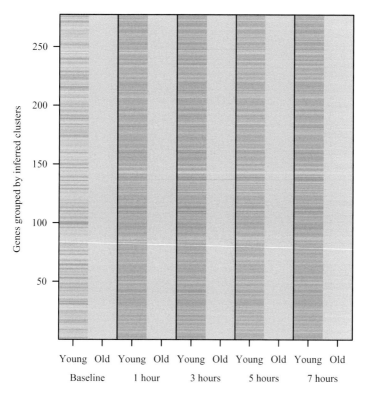

Fig. 10.2. Effects intensity plot for genes clustered with the probe set of interest. This effects intensity plot shows the estimated treatment effects for the other probe sets that were clustered with the probe set of interest in the least-squares clustering. Rows correspond to the genes in this cluster. The reference treatment is old at baseline and is shaded gray. Lighter shades indicate underexpression relative to the reference, whereas darker shades indicate overexpression.

10.5.1 Burn-in and Posterior Simulation

The model was fit using MCMC. The hyperparameters α_0, β_0, Ψ_0, and η_0 were set according to Section 10.2.5, resulting in the prior and posterior expected number of clusters being 98 (i.e., mass parameter $\eta_0 = 15$).

Two Markov chains were run from one of two extreme starting configurations: (1) all genes belonging to a single cluster, or (2) each gene belonging to its own cluster. One iteration of the Markov chain consisted of a Gibbs scan (accounting for more than 97% of the CPU time) and five sequentially allocated merge–split proposals of Dahl (2003). The moving average (of size 50) of the number of clusters was monitored. When these averages crossed, the chains were declared to be burned-in. Trace plots of various univariate

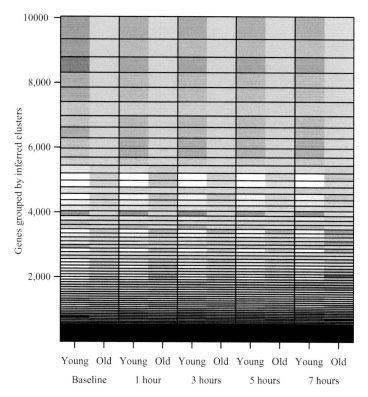

Fig. 10.3. Effects intensity plot for all probe sets. This figure, based on the least-squares clustering, shows the estimated treatment effects of all the clusters simultaneously and sorts the clusters based on size.

summaries of the chains support this burn-in procedure. Two desktop computers independently implemented this burn-in procedure and then sampled from the posterior for less than four days. To reduce disk storage requirements, the sample was thinned by saving only one in 100 states, leaving a total of 1,230 nearly independent draws from the posterior distribution.

10.5.2 Inference

The least-squares clustering (described in Section 10.3) of the expression data had 105 clusters, ranging in size from 1 to 700 probe sets. Pairwise probabilities of coregulation can readily be obtained by examining the relative frequency that genes are clustered together in states of the Markov chain. The posterior distribution of the number of clusters is given in Figure 10.1.

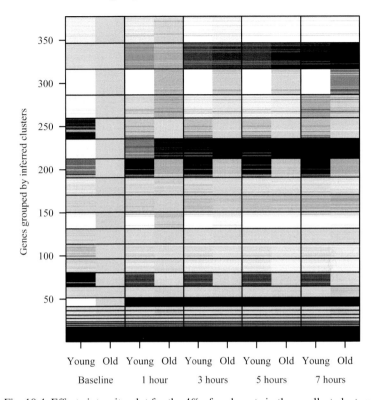

Fig. 10.4. Effects intensity plot for the 4% of probe sets in the smallest clusters.

Probe set 92885_at was identified as scientifically interesting based on another analysis. Biologists may be interested in the other probe sets that are clustered with probe set 92885_at. The proposed clustering procedure provides this information. Figure 10.2 graphically shows the treatment effects for the other probe sets that were clustered with probe set 92885_at in the least-squares clustering. The columns represent the 10 different treatment conditions and the rows correspond to the probe sets in this cluster. The reference treatment is old at baseline and is shaded gray. At other treatments, lighter shades are used to indicate underexpression relative to the reference and the darker shades indicate overexpression.

This chapter introduces the effects intensity plot which displays the entire clustering in one plot. An effects intensity plot is produced by making a plot like Figure 10.2 for each cluster and then stacking them in order of size. Figure 10.3 shows an effects intensity plot for the least-squares clustering. Since some of the clusters are very small, the smaller clusters are difficult to see. To better see the small clusters, Figure 10.4 shows only 4% of the probe sets corresponding to the smallest clusters. Notice that the smaller clusters exhibit more variation from the reference treatment than do the larger clusters. The effects intensity plot can help researchers visualize a clustering and identify clusters for additional study.

10.6 Conclusion

This chapter describes a model-based clustering procedure for microarray expression data based on a conjugate Dirichlet process mixture model. The model was first proposed by Dahl and Newton (submitted) to exploit clustering for increased sensitivity in a battery of correlated hypothesis tests. This chapter shows how the model can also be used as a clustering procedure. The model is fit with MCMC and the computational burden of the DPM model is eased by exploiting conjugacy. This chapter also introduced least-squares model-based clustering in which a point estimate of the true clustering is based on squared distances for the pairwise probability matrix. Unlike ad hoc clustering methods, the model provides measures of uncertainty about the clustering. Further, the model automatically estimates the number of clusters and quantifies uncertainty about this parameter. The method compares well to other clustering methods in a simulation study and the demonstration shows its feasibility using a large microarray data set.

Bibliography

Antoniak, C. E. (1974), "Mixtures of Dirichlet processes with applications to Bayesian nonparametric problems," *The Annals of Statistics*, 2, 1152–1174.

Dahl, D. B. (2003), "An improved merge-split sampler for conjugate Dirichlet Process mixture models," Technical Report 1086, Department of Statistics, University of Wisconsin – Madison.

Dahl, D. B. and Newton, M. A. (submitted), "Using clustering to enhance hypothesis testing."

Dudoit, S., Yang, Y. H., Luu, P., Lin, D. M., Peng, V., Ngai, J., and Speed, T. P. (2002), "Normalization for cDNA microarray data: A robust composite method addressing single and multiple slide systematic variation," *Nucleic Acids Research*, 30, e15.

Edwards, M., Sarkar, D., Klopp, R., Morrow, J., Weindruch, R., and Prolla, T. (2003), "Age-related impairment of the transcriptional responses to oxidative stress in the mouse heart," *Physiological Genomics*, 13, 119–127.

Eisen, M. B., Spellman, P. T., Brown, P. O., and Botstein, D. (1998), "Cluster analysis and display of genomic-wide expression patterns," *Proceedings of the National Academy of Sciences (USA)*, 95, 14863–14868.

Escobar, M. D. (1994), "Estimating normal means with a Dirichlet process prior," *Journal of the American Statistical Association*, 89, 268–277.

Escobar, M. D. and West, M. (1995), "Bayesian density estimation and inference using mixtures," *Journal of the American Statistical Association*, 90, 577–588.

Fraley, C. and Raftery, A. E. (1999), "MCLUST: Software for model-based cluster analysis," *Journal of Classification*, 16, 297–306.

Fraley, C. and Raftery, A. E. (2002), "Model-based clustering, discriminant analysis, and density estimation," *Journal of the American Statistical Association*, 97, 611–631.

Gentleman, R. C., Carey, V. J., Bates, D. M., Bolstad, B., Dettling, M., Dudoit, S., Ellis, B., Gautier, L., Ge, Y., Gentry, J., Hornik, K., Hothorn, T., Huber, W., Iacus, S., Irizarry, R., Li, F. L. C., Maechler, M., Rossini, A. J., Sawitzki, G., Smith, C., Smyth, G., Tierney, L., Yang, J. Y. H., and Zhang, J. (2004), "Bioconductor: Open software development for computational biology and bioinformatics," *Genome Biology*, 5, R80.

Hartigan, J. A. (1975), *Clustering Algorithms*, John Wiley & Sons, New York.

Hubert, L. and Arabie, P. (1985), "Comparing partitions," *Journal of Classification*, 2, 193–218.

Ihaka, R. and Gentleman, R. (1996), "R: A language for data analysis and graphics," *Journal of Computational and Graphical Statistics*, 5, 299–314.

Irizarry, R., Hobbs, B., Collin, F., Beazer-Barclay, Y., Antonellis, K., Scherf, U., and Speed, T. (2003), "Exploration, normalization, and summaries of high density oligonucleotide array probe level data," *Biostatistics*, 4, 249–264.

Jain, S. and Neal, R. M. (2004), "A split-merge Markov chain Monte Carlo procedure for the Dirichlet process mixture model," *Journal of Computational and Graphical Statistics*, 13, 158–182.

Liu, J. S. (1996), "Nonparametric hierarchical Bayes via sequential imputations," *The Annals of Statistics*, 24, 911–930.

MacEachern, S. N. (1994), "Estimating normal means with a conjugate style Dirichlet process prior," *Communications in Statistics, Part B – Simulation and Computation*, 23, 727–741.

MacEachern, S. N., Clyde, M., and Liu, J. S. (1999), "Sequential importance sampling for nonparametric Bayes models: The next generation," *The Canadian Journal of Statistics*, 27, 251–267.

MacQueen, J. (1967), "Some methods for classification and analysis of multivariate observations," in *The 5th Berkeley Symposium on Mathematical Statistics and Probability,* Vol. 1, eds. Cam, L. M. L. and Neyman, J., University of California Press, Barkeley, pp. 281–297.

Medvedovic, M. and Sivaganesan, S. (2002), "Bayesian infinite mixture model based clustering of gene expression profiles," *Bioinformatrics*, 18, 1194–1206.

Medvedovic, M., Yeung, K., and Bumgarner, R. (2004), "Bayesian mixture model based clustering of replicated microarray data," *Bioinformatrics*, 20, 1222–1232.

Milligan, G. W. and Cooper, M. C. (1986), "A study of the comparability of external criteria for hierarchical cluster analysis," *Multivariate Behavioral Research*, 21, 441–458.

Müller, P. and Quintana, F. (2004), "Nonparametric Bayesian data analysis," *Statistical Science*, 19, 95–110.

Neal, R. M. (1992), "Bayesian mixture modeling," in *Maximum Entropy and Bayesian Methods: Proceedings of the 11th International Workshop on Maximum Entropy and Bayesian Methods of Statistical Analysis*, eds. Smith, C. R., Erickson, G. J., and Neudorfer, P. O., Kluwer Academic Publishers, Dordrecht, pp. 197–211.

Neal, R. M. (2000), "Markov chain sampling methods for Dirichlet process mixture models," *Journal of Computational and Graphical Statistics*, 9, 249–265.

Quintana, F. A. and Newton, M. A. (2000), "Computational aspects of nonparametric Bayesian analysis with applications to the modeling of multiple binary sequences," *Journal of Computational and Graphical Statistics*, 9, 711–737.

Rand, W. M. (1971), "Objective criteria for the evaluation of clustering methods," *Journal of the American Statistical Association*, 66, 846–850.

Yeung, K. Y., Fraley, C., Murua, A., Raftery, A. E., and Ruzzo, W. L. (2001), "Model-based clustering and data transformations for gene expression data," *Bioinformatics*, 17, 977–987.

11

Interval Mapping for Expression Quantitative Trait Loci

MENG CHEN AND CHRISTINA KENDZIORSKI

University of Wisconsin at Madison

Abstract

Efforts to identify the genetic loci responsible for variation in quantitative traits have traditionally focused on one or at most a few phenotypes. With high-throughput technologies now widely available, investigators can measure thousands of phenotypes for quantitative trait loci (QTL) mapping. Gene expression measurements are particularly amenable to QTL mapping and the results from these expression QTL (eQTL) studies have proven utility in addressing a number of important biological questions. Although useful in many ways, the results are limited by lack of statistical methods designed specifically for this problem. Most studies to date have applied single QTL trait analysis methods to each expression trait in isolation. Doing so can reduce the power for eQTL localization since information common across transcripts is not utilized; furthermore, false discovery rates can be inflated if relevant multiplicities are not considered. To maximize the information obtained from eQTL mapping studies, new statistical methods are required. We here review the eQTL mapping problem and commonly used approaches, and we propose a new method to facilitate eQTL interval mapping. Results are demonstrated using simulated data and data from a study of diabetes in mouse.

11.1 Introduction

Although efforts to identify the genetic loci responsible for variation in quantitative traits have been going on for over 80 years [36], the vast majority of studies have taken place in the last two decades. This is due largely to two major advances in the 1980s: the advent of restriction fragment length polymorphisms (RFLPs) [1] making it possible to genotype markers on a large scale and the advent of statistical methods for the related data analysis [25].

219

A recent advance of comparable significance has been made in the area of phenotyping. With high-throughput technologies now widely available, investigators can measure thousands of phenotypes at once. Gene expression measurements are particularly amenable to QTL mapping and much excitement abounds for this field of "genetical genomics" [3, 8, 17, 18]. These so-called expression QTL (eQTL) studies have been used to identify candidate genes [5, 10, 13, 15, 20, 37, 42], to infer not only correlative but also causal relationships among modulator and modulated genes [2, 37, 44], to better define traditional phenotypes [37], to serve as a bridge between genetic variation and traditional complex traits of interest [37], and perhaps most importantly, to identify "hot spot" regions – genomic regions where multiple transcripts map [2, 31]. These regions are particularly attractive for follow-up studies as they are likely to contain master regulators that affect transcripts of common function and serve as potential targets of gene therapies [8, 37].

Although successful in many ways, the methods used in eQTL studies to date are limited. In the earliest studies, each transcript was considered separately as a phenotype for QTL mapping, and single trait QTL analysis was then carried out thousands of times. This allowed for eQTL identification at and in between markers. However, although adjustments for multiple tests across genome locations were considered, no adjustments were made for multiple tests across transcripts. This can lead to a potentially serious multiple testing problem and an inflated false discovery rate (FDR). Kendziorski et al. [21] proposed a Bayesian approach that combined data across both markers and transcripts, facilitating simultaneous localization of eQTL while controlling an overall expected posterior FDR. Their approach, the mixture over markers (MOM) model, allows for the identification and rank ordering of eQTL and hot spots. The disadvantage is that no information is provided between markers.

In this chapter, we review the eQTL mapping problem and commonly used approaches, and we propose a new method to facilitate eQTL interval mapping. Section 11.2 provides a brief background on the data collected and questions addressed in eQTL mapping experiments. The data and questions are very similar to those observed in traditional QTL mapping studies and, not surprisingly, so too are early methods of analysis. Section 11.3 provides a brief summary of the early analysis methods, with subsequent developments for eQTL mapping methods reviewed in Section 11.4. As we discuss, the methods currently available for eQTL mapping either allow for interval mapping of eQTL but do not properly account for multiplicities across transcripts, or they account for multiplicities but do not allow for interval mapping. Section 11.5 provides the details of our interval mapping approach designed so that inferences between markers can be made while at the same time relevant error rates can be controlled. Results are demonstrated on simulated data and data from a study of diabetes in mouse. Our perspectives on this problem are discussed in Section 11.6.

11.2 eQTL Mapping Experiments

The general data collected in an eQTL mapping experiment consists of a genetic map, marker genotypes, and microarray gene expression data (phenotypes) measured on a set of individuals. A genetic marker is a region of the genome of known location. These locations make up the genetic map. The distance between markers is given by genetic distance, measured in centimorgans (cM; the expected percentage of crossovers between two loci during meiosis). At each marker, genotypes are obtained. Expression QTL mapping studies take place in both human and experimental populations. We focus on the latter. For these populations, the marker genotype structure is simplified.

For example, studies with experimental populations most often involve arranging a cross between two inbred strains differing substantially in some trait of interest to produce F1 offspring. Segregating progeny are then typically derived from a backcross ($F_1 \times$ Parent) or an F_2 intercross ($F_1 \times F_1$). Repeated intercrossing ($F_n \times F_n$) can also be done to generate so-called recombinant inbred (RI) lines. For simplicity of notation, we focus on a backcross population. Consider two inbred parental populations P_1 and P_2, genotyped as AA and aa, respectively, at M markers. The offspring of the first generation (F_1) have genotype Aa at each marker (allele A from parent P_1 and a from parent P_2). In a backcross, the F_1 offspring are crossed back to a parental line, say P_1, resulting in a population with genotypes AA or Aa at a given marker. For notational simplicity, we denote AA by 0 and Aa by 1. Each individual in an eQTL study is genotyped as 0 or 1 at the M markers.

Phenotypes for each individual are obtained via microarrays, which allow us to snapshot the expressions of thousands of genes at the same time. The oligonucleotide and spotted cDNA microarrays are the two types of technology that are most widely used. A nice review of these two commonly used microarray technologies can be found in [33]. We present a very brief, by no means complete review here.

Affymetrix is one company that produces oligonucleotide chips that contain tens of thousands of probe sets, or DNA sequences related to a gene. We will refer to these sequences throughout this chapter as "transcripts." Each probe set contains some number (usually 11) of perfect match (PM) and mismatch (MM) probe pairs. A PM probe is a sequence of 25 nucleotides exactly matched to a particular gene and thus measures the expression of that gene.

The MM probe differs from the PM probe by a single base substitution at the center base (i.e., 13th) position. The MM was designed in an effort to estimate the background and nonspecific hybridization that contributes to the signal measured for the PM. There are a number of methods for processing and normalization (DNA-Chip Analyzer (dChip) [26, 27]; Robust Multiarray Analysis (RMA) [16] Positional-Dependent-Nearest-Neighbor (PDNN) [45]). RMA is currently the most widely used.

In a spotted cDNA array experiment, a gene is represented by a long cDNA fragment. The experimental sample of interest is labeled with fluorescent tags of some color (often red), and a reference sample with another color (often green). The amount of cDNA hybridized to each probe is approximated by measuring the amount of fluorescence emitted by excitation of the tags. Yang et al. [43] propose useful methods for cDNA array data preprocessing and normalization. With proper preprocessing and normalization, from either technology (or alternative technologies), a single summary score of expression for each transcript on each array is obtained. These summary scores are the phenotypes used for eQTL mapping.

11.3 QTL Mapping Methods

The literature on QTL mapping methods is quite large. We here review only those methods relevant to eQTL mapping and refer the interested reader to [9] or [29] for more information.

11.3.1 Single Phenotype Mapping

Consider a backcross with n progeny and univariate phenotypes y_i measured on ith individual, $i = 1, \ldots, n$, together with genotypes for a set of M markers. Let $g_{im} = 0$ or 1 according to whether the individual i has genotype AA or Aa at the mth marker, $m = 1, \ldots, M$. The model most commonly used to test for a single segregating QTL at location l, between markers m and $m + 1$, is

$$y_i = \mu + \beta^* g_{il}^* + e_i, \qquad (11.1)$$

where g_{il}^* is the genotype at the test position for individual i [25], taking value 0 or 1 with probability depending on the genotypes of the flanking markers and the test position; β^* is the effect of the putative QTL and e_i's are assumed independent and identically distributed (iid) as Normal $(0, \sigma^2)$. The logarithm base 10 of the likelihood ratio, the so-called LOD score, is calculated to test

$$H_0: \beta^* = 0 \quad \text{vs.} \quad H_1: \beta^* \neq 0. \qquad (11.2)$$

This is repeated across the genome. We refer to this interval mapping approach as QTL-IM. Much effort has been expended to derive the appropriate genome-wide LOD score threshold [7, 11, 12, 14, 25, 34, 35]. Each of these methods is designed to account for the multiple tests across genome locations. For traditional QTL mapping studies, a QTL is inferred at locations where the LOD profile exceeds the chosen threshold. Generally, the genome-wide threshold is obtained using the 95th percentile of the distribution of the maximum genome-wide LOD scores, under the null hypothesis of no segregating QTL.

11.3.2 Multiple Phenotype Mapping

In many QTL mapping studies, there are multiple traits being measured. Performing single trait analysis repeatedly is not optimal since information in the correlation structure among the traits is not utilized. It is well known that accounting for the correlation structure can increase the power of QTL detection [19, 23]. For this reason, QTL methods designed specifically to address the multi-trait case are very attractive (for a review of multi-trait QTL mapping methods, see [28] and references therein). However, as the number of traits gets large, so too does the number of parameters that need to be estimated. In some cases, this can be prohibitive.

11.4 Currently Available eQTL Mapping Methods

The earliest eQTL mapping studies applied single phenotype–single QTL mapping methods repeatedly to every transcript in isolation [2, 37]. Multitrait QTL mapping methods have not been used as investigators recognize that estimation of a phenotype covariance matrix with thousands of phenotypes is not feasible. In [37], transcript-specific LOD score profiles were obtained using standard QTL-IM. A common genome-wide LOD score threshold was chosen to account for the potential increase of type I error induced by testing across multiple markers. Brem et al. [2] conducted a Wilcoxon-Mann-Whitney rank sum test for every transcript at every marker. Nominal p values were reported and the number of linkages expected by chance was estimated by permutations. Transcript-specific LOD profiles were also obtained in [6] and [15]. In these studies, permutations were used to obtain empirical p-values associated with the maximum LOD score; q values [39, 40] were then used to adjust for multiplicities across transcripts.

These methods provide a straightforward approach to the identification of eQTL, and they have been used to ascertain important biological results.

However, the theoretical properties of these approaches in the presence of thousands of transcripts are not known and the operating characteristics have not been studied. Preliminary results from simulations such as those described in [21] suggest that for many of these approaches, FDR is not consistently controlled and power is often compromised. This is consistent with the results of [6], where the FDR threshold was increased to 25% so that a reasonable transcript list size could be obtained. The reasons for this may be that for some of the methods, multiplicities across both markers and transcripts are not accounted for while for other methods, information common across transcripts and markers is not utilized. These issues are addressed by the MOM approach to eQTL mapping.

11.4.1 Mixture Over Markers (MOM) Model

Kendziorski et al. [21] developed an approach designed to account for multiplicities across both markers and transcripts while controlling an overall expected posterior FDR. The model assumes a transcript j maps nowhere with probability p_0 or maps to marker m with probability p_m, such that $\sum_{m=0}^{M} p_m = 1$. The marginal distribution of expression measurements $\mathbf{y}_j = \{y_{j1}, y_{j2}, \ldots, y_{jn}\}$ is then given by

$$p_0 f_0(\mathbf{y}_j) + \sum_{m=1}^{M} p_m f_m(\mathbf{y}_j), \qquad (11.3)$$

where f_m is the predictive density of the data if transcript j maps to marker m; f_0 is the predictive density when the transcript maps nowhere. Specifically, suppose transcript abundance measurements y_{ji} arise independently from some observation distribution $f_{\text{obs}}(\cdot | \mu_{j,\cdot}, \theta)$. The dependence among the underlying means $\mu_{j,\cdot}$ is captured by a distribution $\pi(\mu)$. Within this setting, $f_0(\mathbf{y}_j) = \int \left(\prod_{i=1}^{n} f_{\text{obs}}(y_{ji} | \mu) \right) \pi(\mu) \, d\mu$. For a transcript that maps to marker m, the underlying expression means defined by the marker genotype groups are not equal ($\mu_{j,0} \neq \mu_{j,1}$), but both are assumed to come from $\pi(\mu)$. The governing distribution is then

$$f_m(\mathbf{y}_j) = f_0\left(\mathbf{y}_j^0\right) \, f_0\left(\mathbf{y}_j^1\right), \qquad (11.4)$$

where $y_j^{0(1)}$ denotes the set of transcript j values for animals with genotype $0(1)$.

Model fit proceeds via the EM algorithm. Once the parameter estimates are obtained, posterior probabilities of mapping nowhere or to any of the M locations can be calculated via Bayes rule. For instance, the posterior probability that transcript j maps to location $l, l = 0, \ldots, M$, is given by

$$\frac{p_l f_l(\mathbf{y}_j)}{p_0 f_0(\mathbf{y}_j) + \sum_{m=1}^{M} p_m f_m(\mathbf{y}_j)} . \qquad (11.5)$$

With the MOM approach, a transcript is identified to be differentially expressed (DE) if the posterior probability of DE exceeds some threshold. The threshold is the smallest posterior probability such that the average posterior probability of all transcripts exceeding the threshold is larger than $1 - \alpha$. In order to make a transcript-specific call, highest posterior density (HPD) regions are constructed. A main advantage of this approach is that the operating characteristics are well understood. When model assumptions hold, the transcript-specific posterior expected FDR is controlled at $\alpha \cdot 100\%$. This is shown theoretically [32] and in simulation studies [21]. A second advantage is that the magnitude of the posterior probabilities can be used as evidence either in favor of or against a particular transcript mapping. Furthermore, these probabilities are comparable across transcripts. This type of information is not obtained using p-value-based methods.

The main disadvantage of MOM is that the genomic regions identified are limited by their size, which may be large as analysis is conducted at genotyped markers only. When dense maps are not available [21, 37], this limitation can be a serious one. The biological techniques currently available to search for genes in large genomic regions (e.g., candidate gene approach, congenic lines) can take years and, as a result, additional statistical methods capable of narrowing down regions are necessary. In the next section, we propose a method for interval mapping of eQTL.

11.5 MOM Interval Mapping

Consider a set of L locations spanning the entire genome. As in MOM, we imagine that the transcript may map nowhere with probability p_0 or to any of the L locations with probability $p_l, l = 1, 2, \ldots, L$. We stress that a location l need not be a genotyped marker. As in Section 11.4.1, transcript j is mapped to location l if $\mu_{j,l}^0 \neq \mu_{j,l}^1$, where $\mu_{j,l}^{0(1)}$ denotes the latent mean level of expression for transcript j for the population of individuals with genotype $0(1)$ at location l. Let z_j^l be an indicator of whether transcript j maps to location l. If l is at a marker, the predictive density under the alternative hypothesis is as before $f_l(\mathbf{y}_j) = f_0(\mathbf{y}_j^0) f_0(\mathbf{y}_j^1)$, where the grouping is determined by the marker's genotype. However, when l is between markers, the decomposition is no longer valid. Instead, we have the following

$$f_l(\mathbf{y}_j) = \int f_l(\mathbf{y}_j | g^l) \, p(g^l | \mathcal{M}) \, dg^l,$$

where

$$f_l(\mathbf{y}_j | g^l) = \int\int \prod_{i \in \mathcal{G}_0^l} f_{\mathrm{obs}} \left(y_{ji} | \mu_j^0 \right) \prod_{i \in \mathcal{G}_1^l} f_{\mathrm{obs}} \left(y_{ji} | \mu_j^1 \right)$$

$$\times \pi \left(\mu_j^0 \right) \pi \left(\mu_j^1 \right) d \left(\mu_j^0 \right) d \left(\mu_j^1 \right).$$

Here, $g^l = (g_1^l, g_2^l, \ldots, g_n^l)$ denotes the unknown genotype vector at location l; $\mathcal{G}_{0(1)}^l$ denotes the individuals with genotype 0(1) at location l. Under the null hypothesis, the predictive density of the data, $f_0(\mathbf{y}_j)$ can be calculated as before since it does not rely on genotype groupings.

Theoretically, parameter estimates for mixing proportions and hyperparameters are obtained via the EM algorithm and, as before, the posterior probability for transcript j mapping to location l is given by

$$p \left(z_j^l = 1 | \mathbf{y}, \mathcal{M} \right) = \frac{p(z_j^l = 1) \int f_l(\mathbf{y}_j | g^l) p(g^l | \mathcal{M}) \, dg^l}{p(\mathbf{y}_j | \mathcal{M})}, \qquad (11.6)$$

where $p(z_j^l = 1)$ is the prior probability transcript j maps to location l; $\mathbf{y}$ and $\mathcal{M}$ denote the expression and marker data, respectively.

In practice, evaluation of this integral can be prohibitive. At a particular location l, the conditional distribution of the genotype vector given the expression and marker data, $p(g^l | \mathcal{M})$, depends on the two markers flanking l. Since g^l is a vector of length n, there are 2^n possible genotypes, and as a result, the integral in (11.6) is a very large mixture (when n is even moderately large). One option is to restrict to fewer possibilities since many genotype vectors have very small probabilities. However, as the number of individuals in the study gets large (> 200), this quickly becomes computationally infeasible even with the restriction.

11.5.1 Pseudomarker-MOM

To address the 2^n problem, we use importance sampling as was done in [38] for traditional QTL mapping. First, multiple versions of *pseudomarkers* are sampled from $p(g^l | \mathcal{M})$; equation (11.6) is then replaced by its Monte Carlo approximation. In simulating the pseudomarkers, one could use a simple Markov chain structure where the putative QTL genotype at a given location only depends on the two flanking markers. However, this does not work well when the marker data contains genotyping errors or noninformative markers. Instead, we consider a hidden Markov model (HMM) as was done in R/qtl [4] where the "true" marker genotypes follow a Markov chain, and the observed marker genotypes are characterized by distributions conditional on the underlying state process.

Suppose for each location l, Q genotype vectors are sampled from the proposal distribution $p(\mathbf{g}|\mathcal{M})$, where $\mathbf{g} = \{g^1, g^2, \ldots, g^L\}$, to yield $(g_1^l, g_2^l, \ldots, g_Q^l)$, for $l = 1, \ldots, L$. Then equation (11.6) can be approximated by

$$p\left(z_j^l = 1|\mathbf{y}, \mathcal{M}\right)$$

$$\approx \frac{p_j^l \sum_{q=1}^{Q} f_l\left(y_j|g_q^l\right)}{\left(1 - \sum_{l'=1}^{L} p_j^{l'}\right) \sum_{q=1}^{Q} f_0(y_j) + \sum_{l'=1}^{L} p_j^{l'} \sum_{q=1}^{Q} f_{l'}\left(y_j|g_q^{l'}\right)} , \quad (11.7)$$

where p_j^l is $p(z_j^l = 1)$. This approach is effectively an extension of the MOM model evaluated by averaging over pseudomarkers. We therefore refer to it as pseudomarker-MOM.

11.5.2 Two-Stage Approach

Pseudomarker-MOM can be applied to grids of varying sizes (i.e., varying L) to localize eQTL at and in between markers. However, as the computational burden increases with L, very fine searches can be prohibitive. Fortunately in many cases, eQTL regions can be identified using a first pass with a fairly sparse grid followed by pseudomarker-MOM in interesting regions. In particular, if each mapping transcript has only 1 eQTL, then under some mild conditions, the expected posterior probability of a transcript mapping to a particular marker is a nonincreasing function of the recombination frequency between that marker and the eQTL (for support, see appendix). As a result, the marker regions picked by the first scan are those regions nearest the eQTL. Once the regions are defined, pseudomarker-MOM can be used to localize the eQTL with greater accuracy. Simulation studies shown in the next section suggest that this two-stage approach works quite well, even under more general conditions.

11.5.3 Simulation Results

To assess the performance of the two-stage approach, we performed a small set of simulation studies. The simulations are in no way designed to capture the many complexities of eQTL data, but rather to provide some preliminary information on operating characteristics of the approach in simple settings. Twenty simulated data sets were generated. Each contained 5,000 transcripts

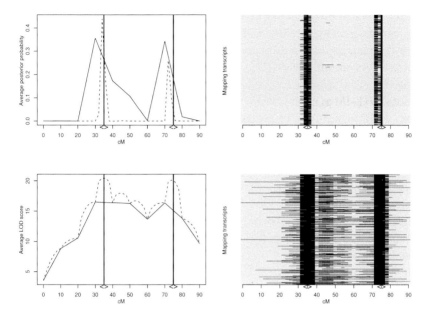

Fig. 11.1. The upper left panel shows the average posterior probabilities of linkage at every marker. The solid curve represents MOM, and the dashed one is from pseudomarker-MOM with pseudomarker spacing of 2 cM. The solid black vertical lines and the "<>" symbols on the x-axis indicate eQTL positions. The upper right panel shows the 96.8% HPD region (red) for the eQTL locations of the mapping transcripts. The lower left panel shows the average LOD scores at every marker. The solid curve is from marker regression and the dashed curve is from standard QTL-IM mapping every 2 cM. The lower right panel shows the 1-LOD drop interval (red) around the true eQTL locations.

and 100 individuals genotyped at 10 markers evenly spaced every 10 cM on a single chromosome. Intensity values were obtained as described in [21]. The proportion of DE transcripts was set to 10% and two eQTL were considered (at 35 cM and 75 cM).

The two-stage approach was applied to the simulated data. In the first stage, genome locations making up the 96.8% HPD region were selected from the average posterior probability profile obtained using MOM. Pseudomarker-MOM was then applied across a 2-cM grid spanning the locations, with 100 pseudomarker realizations ($Q = 100$). For comparison, we applied QTL-IM to each transcript and obtained genome-wide LOD score cutoffs based on the approximation given in [34].

Figure 11.1 (upper left panel) shows the posterior probability profile, averaged across the mapping transcripts for one simulation (results are representative of those observed in the other 19 simulations). The eQTL regions are identified both by MOM and pseudomarker-MOM. MOM picks up a wide peak over the true eQTL positions, but pseudomarker-MOM provides much greater accuracy. Figure 11.1 (upper right panel) shows the 96.8% HPD regions for *individual* mapping transcripts (96.8% is used to compare with the QTL-IM results below). As shown, the eQTL are identified correctly for most of the transcripts.

Traditional QTL-IM as implemented in R/qtl was considered for comparison (for details on R/qtl, see [4]). Figure 11.1 (lower left panel) shows the LOD profile averaged across mapping transcripts. The regions containing the eQTL have the highest average LODs, but the average LOD scores are overall very high for mapping transcripts and it is not clear what cutoff one should use in order to correctly identify the eQTL regions.

To compare with the HPD regions obtained using pseudomarker-MOM, 96.8% "confidence intervals" were constructed around each eQTL using a 1-LOD drop interval around peak LOD scores [30]. We use quotes here to stress that these intervals can be biased. In general, they have been shown to be too small and the bootstrap procedure has been recommended [41]. For a large number of transcripts in repeated simulations, obtaining bootstrap samples is computationally prohibitive. In addition, for our purposes of comparison, confidence intervals that are slightly too small biases the results in favor of QTL-IM as eQTL appear to be better localized. It is not always clear which peaks to construct confidence intervals around (see the lower left panel of Figure 11.1 which shows many peaks). To give QTL-IM the best possible result, we considered a 10-cM window around the first eQTL (35 cM) and defined the LOD peak as the highest LOD within that window. The 1-LOD drop interval was then constructed. This was repeated for the second eQTL. Of course, in practice, one does not have the luxury of knowing where to choose these peaks and only the largest peak would be identified. For these simulations, this method of identifying eQTL favors QTL-IM. Even so, the traditional approach provides less precise estimates of eQTL locations when compared with pseudomarker-MOM.

11.5.4 Diabetes Study Results

The favorable results observed in our simulation study are also observed in a case study investigating the genetic basis of diabetes. The details of the experiment are described in [21]. Briefly, an F_2 cross was generated from two parental strains differing in diabetes susceptibility. The cross contained 60 animals, each genotyped at 194 locations across the genome. Affymetrix MOE430 chips were used to obtain 45,265 phenotypes for 60 members of the F_2. Following some initial preprocessing, RMA values were considered for

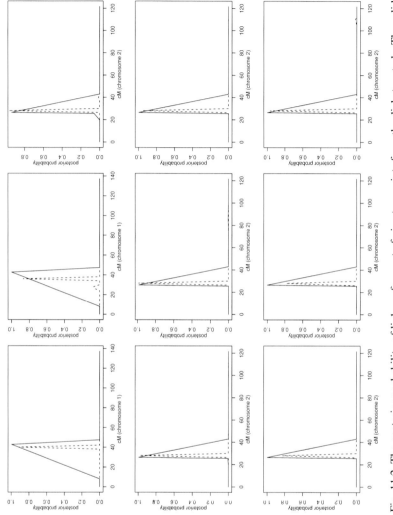

Fig. 11.2. The posterior probability of linkage for a set of nine transcripts from the diabetes study. The solid lines give results from MOM and the dashed lines are from pseudomarker-MOM every 2 cM.

40,738 transcripts. The 145 marker locations with over 90% of the individuals genotyped were selected from the full set of 194 markers.

The two-stage approach was applied to the data along with QTL-IM. For QTL-IM, LOD score thresholds were determined by transcript-specific permutations. Nine transcripts known to be involved in diabetes [24] are shown in Figure 11.2. These nine are among the transcripts identified by MOM if FDR is controlled at 5%. The LOD profiles for these same transcripts are shown in Figure 11.3. The solid lines represent MOM and marker regression in Figures 11.2 and 11.3, respectively. The dashed lines represent pseudomarker-MOM and QTL-IM in the corresponding figures. As in the simulation study, pseudomarker-MOM provides a more precise localization of eQTL regions. Furthermore, for five of the nine transcripts, the LOD score does not exceed the threshold for significance; these transcripts would have been missed by QTL-IM.

11.6 Discussion

The microarray has revolutionized traditional QTL mapping studies. Instead of considering at most a handful of traits, investigators now have the opportunity to map thousands. With this opportunity comes a number of challenges in both experimental design and analysis, most of which have not yet been addressed.

We have here considered the problem of identifying mapping transcripts and the genomic locations to which they map. Initial attempts to address this problem involved applying traditional QTL mapping methods to each trait in isolation, followed by adjustments for some multiplicities. This allows for eQTL identification at and in between markers. However, we note that caution should be used when interpreting any results derived from these approaches as the operating characteristics of QTL methods applied in the eQTL setting are not known. In particular, the power to identify eQTL could be low as information common across transcripts is not utilized. At the same time, FDR could be inflated as some multiplicities are accounted for while others are not.

Kendziorski et al. [21] proposed a Bayesian approach that combined data across both markers and transcripts, facilitating simultaneous localization of eQTL while controlling an overall expected posterior FDR. Their approach, the MOM model, allows for the identification and rank ordering of eQTL and hot spots. Section 11.5.1 proposed pseudomarker-MOM, an extension of MOM allowing for interval mapping. A main advantage of MOM and pseudomarker-MOM is that the operating characteristics are well understood in the context of the models. Of course, diagnostics must always be checked and biological

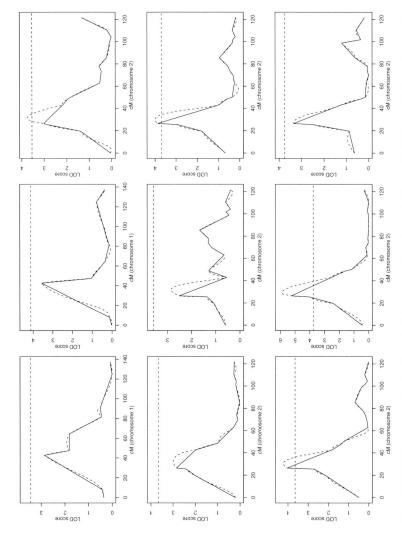

Fig. 11.3. LOD score profiles for the set of nine transcripts shown in Figure 11.2. The solid lines give results from marker regression and the dashed lines are from QTL-IM every 2 cM. The horizontal dashed line represents the 95th percentile of the maximum LOD score from 5,000 permutations.

results validated. To this end, our preliminary evaluation using both simulated and case study data is encouraging.

In summary, much more work is required before the analysis of eQTL data becomes routine. It seems that a clever application of methods designed to handle traditional quantitative traits is limited. It is certainly true that some very useful information has been derived using these approaches, much like the fold-change analysis provided information in early microarray studies. However, significant improvement can be gained by more carefully considering the relevant multiplicities, the hierarchical nature of the data, and the error rates of most interest in any particular study. Advances in addressing these issues will ensure that maximal information is derived from these powerful experiments.

Appendix

If (i) for each mapping transcript, there is only 1 eQTL and (ii) the prior probability of a transcript mapping to a marker is equal for all markers, then the posterior probability of DE will be highest at the marker nearest the eQTL. For our model, we make no prior assumptions regarding the location of mapping transcripts and thus the assumption of equality imposed in (ii) is not very restrictive.

Proof: For algebraic simplicity, consider a backcross.

We assume the lognormal-normal (LNN) model described in [22]. First assume the eQTL is located at a marker (so the genotypes are known). Let n_0 and n_1 denote the number of animals having genotype 0 and 1, respectively, at the eQTL. The log predictive density of mRNA expression for transcript j evaluated at the eQTL position can be written as

$$
\begin{aligned}
\log(f_1^*(y_j)) = {} & -\frac{n_0}{2}\log(2\pi) - \frac{n_0 - 1}{2}\log(\sigma^2) - \frac{1}{2}\log\left(\sigma^2 + n_0\tau_0^2\right) \\
& -\frac{\sum_{i \in G_0}\left(y_{ji}^0 - \mu_0\right)^2}{2\left(\sigma^2 + n_0\tau_0^2\right)} + \frac{\tau_0^2\left[\left(\sum y_{ji}^0\right)^2 - n_0\sum\left(y_{ji}^0\right)^2\right]}{2\sigma^2\left(\sigma^2 + n_0\tau_0^2\right)} \\
& -\frac{n_1}{2}\log(2\pi) - \frac{n_1 - 1}{2}\log(\sigma^2) - \frac{1}{2}\log\left(\sigma^2 + n_1\tau_0^2\right) \\
& -\frac{\sum_{i \in G_1}\left(y_{ji}^1 - \mu_0\right)^2}{2\left(\sigma^2 + n_1\tau_0^2\right)} + \frac{\tau_0^2\left[\left(\sum y_{ji}^1\right)^2 - n_1\sum\left(y_{ji}^1\right)^2\right]}{2\sigma^2\left(\sigma^2 + n_1\tau_0^2\right)}
\end{aligned}
$$

$$\text{(A.1)}$$

Since $n_0 + n_1$ is fixed for a given experiment, the quantity in A.1 that varies across different marker locations is

$$-\frac{1}{2}\log\left(\sigma^2 + n_0\tau_0^2\right) - \frac{1}{2}\log\left(\sigma^2 + n_1\tau_0^2\right)$$

$$+\frac{\tau_0^2\left(\sum y_{ji}^0 + \frac{\mu_0\sigma^2}{\tau_0^2}\right)^2}{2\sigma^2\left(\sigma^2 + n_0\tau_0^2\right)} + \frac{\tau_0^2\left(\sum y_{ji}^1 + \frac{\mu_0\sigma^2}{\tau_0^2}\right)^2}{2\sigma^2\left(\sigma^2 + n_1\tau_0^2\right)}. \qquad (A.2)$$

When an eQTL is located in between markers, at some location l having recombination frequency r with the eQTL, (A.2) evaluated at marker location l becomes

$$-\frac{1}{2}\log\left(\sigma^2 + (n_0(1-r) + n_1 r)\tau_0^2\right) - \frac{1}{2}\log\left(\sigma^2 + (n_1(1-r) + n_0 r)\tau_0^2\right)$$

$$+\frac{\tau_0^2\left(\sum y_{ji}^{'0} + \frac{\mu_0\sigma^2}{\tau_0^2}\right)^2}{2\sigma^2(\sigma^2 + (n_0(1-r) + n_1 r)\tau^2)} + \frac{\tau_0^2\left(\sum y_{ji}^{'1} + \frac{\mu_0\sigma^2}{\tau_0^2}\right)^2}{2\sigma^2(\sigma^2 + (n_1(1-r) + n_0 r)\tau^2)}, \qquad (A.3)$$

where the unknown eQTL genotypes for the AA and Aa groups are now incorporated in $y_{ji}^{'0}$ and $y_{ji}^{'1}$, respectively.

Using distribution theory, we have

$$\sum_i y_{ji}^{'0} + \frac{\mu_0\sigma^2}{\tau_0^2} \sim N\left(\mu_0(n_0(1-r) + n_1 r) + \frac{\mu_0\sigma^2}{\tau_0^2}, v_0^2\right).$$

$$\sum_i y_{ji}^{'1} + \frac{\mu_0\sigma^2}{\tau_0^2} \sim N\left(\mu_0(n_0(1-r) + n_1 r) + \frac{\mu_0\sigma^2}{\tau_0^2}, v_1^2\right),$$

where $v_0^2 = (\sigma^2 + \tau_0^2)(n_0(1-r) + n_1 r) + \tau_0^2(n_0(n_0 - 1)(1-r)^2 + n_1(n_1 - 1)r^2)$ and $v_1^2 = (\sigma^2 + \tau_0^2)(n_1(1-r) + n_0 r) + \tau_0^2(n_1(n_1 - 1)(1-r)^2 + n_0(n_0 - 1)r^2)$.

Furthermore,

$$\frac{\left(\sum_i v_{ji}^{'0} + \frac{\mu_0\sigma^2}{\tau_0^2}\right)^2}{v_0} \sim \chi_1^2(\delta).$$

with noncentral parameter $\delta = \dfrac{\left(\mu_0(n_0(1-r) + n_1 r) + \frac{\mu_0\sigma^2}{\tau_0^2}\right)^2}{v_0^2}$. Similarly, we can obtain

the distribution of $\dfrac{\left(\sum_i y_{ji}^{'1} + \frac{\mu_0\sigma^2}{\tau_0^2}\right)^2}{v_1}$.

With this, the expectation of (A.3) becomes

$$-\frac{1}{2}\log\left(\sigma^2 + (n_0(1-r) + n_1 r)\tau_0^2\right)$$

$$-\frac{1}{2}\log\left(\sigma^2 + (n_1(1-r) + n_0 r)\tau_0^2\right) + (I) + (II), \qquad (A.4)$$

where

$$(I) = \frac{\tau_0^2}{2\sigma^2} \frac{\left(\sigma^2 + \tau_0^2\right)(n_0(1-r) + n_1 r) + \tau_0^2(n_0(n_0-1)(1-r)^2 + n_1(n_1-1)r^2)}{\sigma^2 + \tau_0^2(n_0(1-r) + _1 r)}$$
$$+ \frac{\mu_0^2\left(\sigma^2 + \tau_0^2(n_0(1-r) + n_1 r)\right)}{2\sigma^2 \tau_0^2}.$$

$$(II) = \frac{\tau_0^2}{2\sigma^2} \frac{\left(\sigma^2 + \tau_0^2\right)(n_1(1-r) + n_0 r) + \tau_0^2(n_1(n_1-1)(1-r)^2 + n_0(n_0-1)r^2)}{\sigma^2 + \tau_0^2(n_1(1-r) + n_0 r)}$$
$$+ \frac{\mu_0^2\left(\sigma^2 + \tau_0^2(n_1(1-r) + n_0 r)\right)}{2\sigma^2 \tau_0^2}.$$

The derivative of (A.4) with respect to r is a little messy but can be shown to be negative for $0 \leq r \leq \frac{1}{2}$ and equal to 0 for $r = \frac{1}{2}$. Therefore, (A.3) is maximized when $r = 0$. In other words, the posterior probability of DE at the test location closest to the eQTL is maximized in expectation.

Bibliography

[1] D. Botstein, R.L. White, M.H. Skolnick, and R.W. David. Construction of a genetic linkage map in man using restriction fragment length polymorphisms. *American Journal of Human Genetics*, 32:314–331, 1980.

[2] R.B. Brem, G. Yvert, R. Clinton, and L. Kruglyak. Genetic dissection of transcriptional regulation in budding yeast. *Science*, 296:752–755, 2002.

[3] K.W. Broman. Mapping expression in randomized rodent genomes. *Nature Genetics*, 37(3):209–210, 2005.

[4] K.W. Broman, H. Wu, S. Sen, and G.A. Churchill. R/qtl: Qtl mapping in experimental crosses. *Bioinformatics*, 19(7):889–890, 2003.

[5] L. Bystrykh, E. Weersing, B. Dontje, S. Sutton, M.T. Pletcher, T. Wiltshire, A.I. Su, E. Vellenga, J. Wang, K.F. Manly, L. Lu, E.J. Chesler, R. Alberts, R.C. Jansen, R.W. Williams, M. P. Cooke, and G. de Haan. Uncovering regulatory pathways that affect hematopoietic stem cell function using "genetical genomics". *Nature Genetics*, 37:225–232, 2005.

[6] E.J. Chesler, L. Lu, S. Shou, Y. Qu, J. Gu, J. Wang, H.C. Hsu, J.D. Mountz, N.E. Baldwin, M.A. Langston, D.W. Threadgill, K.F. Manly, and R.W. Williams. Complex trait analysis of gene expression uncovers polygenetic and pleiotropic networks that modulate nervous system function. *Nature Genetics*, 27:233–242, 2005.

[7] G.A. Churchill and R.W. Doerge. Empirical threshold values for quantitative trait mapping. *Genetics*, 138:963–971, 1994.

[8] N.J. Cox. An expression of interest. *Nature*, 430:733–734, 2004.

[9] R.W. Doerge, Z.-B. Zeng, and B.S. Weir. Statistical issues in the search for genes affecting quantitative traits in experimental populations. *Statistical Science*, 12:195–219, 1997.

[10] P. Dumas, Y. Sun, G. Corbeil, S. Tremblay, Z. Pausova, V. Kren, D. Krenova, M. Pravenec, P. Hamet, and J. Tremblay. Mapping of quantitative trait

loci (qtl) of differential stress gene expression in rat recombinant inbred strains. *Journal of Hypertension*, 18(5):545–551, 2000.

[11] J. Dupuis, P.O. Brown, and D. Siegmund. Statistical methods for linkage analysis of complex traits from high resolution maps of identity by descent. *Genetics*, 140:843–856, 1995.

[12] J. Dupuis and D. Siegmund. Statistical methods for mapping quantitative trait loci from a dense set of markers. *Genetics*, 151:373–386, 1999.

[13] I.A. Eaves, L.S. Wicker, G. Ghandour, P.A. Lyons, L.B. Peterson, J.A. Todd, and R.J. Glynne. Combining mouse congenic strains and microarray gene expression analyses to study a complex trait: The nod model of type 1 diabetes. *Genome Research*, 12(2):232–243, 2002.

[14] E. Feingold, P.O. Brown, and D. Siegmund. Gaussian models for genetic linkage analysis using complete high resolution maps of identity-by-descent. *American Jornal of Human Genetics*, 53:234–251, 1993.

[15] N. Hubner, C.A. Wallace, H. Zimdahl, E. Petretto, H. Schulz, F. Maciver, M. Mueller, O. Hummel, J. Monti, V. Zidek, A. Musilova, V. Kren, H. Causton, L. Game, G. Born, S. Schmidt, A. Muller, S.A. Cook, T.W. Kurtz, J. Whittaker, M. Pravenec, and T.J. Aitman. Integrated transcriptional profiling and linkage analysis for identification of genes underlying disease. *Nature Genetics*, 37(3):243–253, 2005.

[16] R.A. Irizarry, B. Hobbs, F. Collin, Y.D. Beazer-Barclay, K.J. Antonellis, U. Scherf, and T.P. Speed. Exploration, normalization, and summaries of high density oligonucleotide array probe level data. *Biostatistics*, 4(2):249–264, 2003.

[17] R.C. Jansen. Studying complex biological systems using multifactorial perturbation. *Nature Reviews Genetics*, 4:145–151, 2003.

[18] R. Jansen and J.P. Nap. Genetical genomics: The added value from segregation. *Trends in Genetics*, 17:388–391, 2001.

[19] C. Jiang and Z-B. Zeng. Multiple trait analysis of genetic mapping of quantitative trait loci. *Genetics*, 140:1111–1127, 1995.

[20] C.L. Karp, A. Grupe, E. Schadt, S.L. Ewart, M. Keane-Moore, P.J. Cuomo, J. Kohl, L. Wahl, D. Kuperman, S. Germer, D. Aud, G. Peltz, and M. Wills-Karp. Identification of complement factor 5 as a susceptibility locus for experimental allergic asthma. *Nature Immunology*, 1:221–226, 2000.

[21] C.M. Kendziorski, M. Chen, M. Yuan, H. Lan, and A.D. Attie. Statistical methods for expression quantitative trait loci (eQTl) mapping. *Biometrics*, 62:19–27, 2006.

[22] C.M. Kendziorski, M.A. Newton, H. Lan, and M.N. Gould. On parametric empirical Bayes methods for comparing multiple groups using replicated gene expression profiles. *Statistics in Medicine*, 22:3899–3914, 2003.

[23] S.A. Knott and C.S. Haley. Multitrait least squares for quantitative trait loci detection. *Genetics*, 156:899–911, 2000.

[24] H. Lan, M. Chen, J.E. Byers, B.S. Yandell, D.S. Stapleton, C.M. Mata, E. Mui, M.T. Flowers, K.L. Schueler, K.F. Manly, R.W. Williams, C. Kendziorski, and A.D. Attie. Combined expression trait correlations and expression quantitative trait locus mapping. *PLoS Genetics*, 2(1):e6, 2006.

[25] E.S. Lander and D. Botstein. Mapping mendelian factors underlying quantitative traits using rflp linkage maps. *Genetics*, 121:185–199, 1989.

[26] C. Li and W.H. Wong. Model-based analysis of oligonucleotide arrays: Expression index computation and outlier detection. *Proceedings of the National Academy of Sciences USA*, 98:31–36, 2001.

[27] C. Li and W.H. Wong. Model-based analysis of oligonucleotide arrays: Model validation, design issues and standard error application. *Genome Biology*, 2:1–11, 2001.

[28] M.S. Lund, P. Sorenson, B. Guldbrandtsen, and D.A. Sorensen. Multitrait fine mapping of quantitative trait loci using combined linkage disequilibria and linkage analysis. *Genetics*, 163(1):405–410, 2003.

[29] M. Lynch and B. Walsh. *Genetics and Analysis of Quantitative Traits*. Sunderland: Sinauer, 1998.

[30] B. Mangin, B. Goffinet, and A. Rebai. Constructing confidence intervals for qtl location. *Genetics*, 138:1301–1308, 1994.

[31] M. Morley, C.M. Molony, T.M. Weber, J.L. Devlin, K.G. Ewens, R.S. Spielman, and V.G. Cheung. Genetic analysis of genome-wide variation in human gene expression. *Nature*, 430:743–747, 2004.

[32] M.A. Newton, A. Noueiry, D. Sarkar, and P. Ahlquist. Detecting differential gene expression with a semiparametric hierarchical mixture method. *Biostatistics*, 5:155–176, 2004.

[33] D.V. Nguyen, A.B. Arpat, N. Wang, and R.J. Carroll. DNA microarray experiments: Biological and technological aspects. *Biometrics*, 58:701–717, 2002.

[34] A. Rebai, B. Goffinet, and B. Mangin. Approximate thresholds for interval mapping test for qtl detection. *Genetics*, 138:235–240, 1994.

[35] A. Rebai, B. Goffinet, and B. Mangin. Comparing power of different methods of qtl detection. *Biometrics*, 51:87–99, 1995.

[36] K. Sax. The association of size differences with seed-coat pattern and pigmentation in *phaseolusvulgaris*. *Genetics*, 8:552–560, 1923.

[37] E.E. Schadt, S. Monks, T.A. Drake, A.J. Lusis, N. Che, V. Collnayo, T.G. Ruff, S.B. Milligan, J.R. Lamb, G. Cavet, P.S. Linsley, M. Mao, R.B. Stoughton, and S.H. Friend. Genetics of gene expression surveyed in maize, mouse and man. *Nature*, 422:297–302, 2003.

[38] S. Sen and G.A. Churchill. A statistical framework for quantitative trait mapping. *Genetics*, 159:371–387, 2001.

[39] J.D. Storey. The positive false discovery rate: A Bayesian interpretation and the q-value. *Annals of Statistics*, 31:2013–2035, 2003.

[40] J.D. Storey and R. Tibshirani. Statistical significance for genomewide studies. *Proceedings of the National Academy of Sciences USA*, 100(16):9440–9445, 2003.

[41] P.M. Visscher, R. Thompson, and C.S. Haley. Confidence intervals in qtl mapping by bootstrapping. *Genetics*, 143:1013–1020, 1996.

[42] M.L. Wayne and L.M. McIntyre. Combining mapping and arraying: An approach to candidate gene identification. *Proceedings of the National Academy of Sciences USA*, 99(23):14903–14906, 2002.

[43] Y.H. Yang, S. Dudoit, P. Luu, D.M. Lin, V. Peng, J. Ngai, and T.P. Speed. Normalization for cDNA microarray data: A robust composite method addressing single and multiple slide systematic variation. *Nucleic Acids Research*, 30(4):e15, 2002.

[44] G. Yvert, R.B. Brem, J. Whittle, J.M. Akey, E. Foss, E.N. Smith, R. Mackelprang, and L. Kruglyak. Transacting regulatory variation in *Saccharomyces cerevisiae* and the role of transcription factors. *Nature Genetics*, 35(1):57–64, 2003.

[45] L. Zhang, M.F. Miles, and K.D. Aldape. A model of molecular interactions on short oligonucleotide microarrays. *Nature Biotechnology*, 21:818–821, 2003.

12

Bayesian Mixture Models for Gene Expression and Protein Profiles

MICHELE GUINDANI, KIM-ANH DO, PETER MÜLLER,
AND JEFFREY S. MORRIS

The University of Texas M.D. Anderson Cancer Center

Abstract

We review the use of semiparametric mixture models for Bayesian inference in high-throughput genomic data. We discuss three specific approaches for microarray data, for protein mass spectrometry experiments, and for serial analysis of gene expression (SAGE) data. For the microarray data and the protein mass spectrometry we assume group comparison experiments, that is, experiments that seek to identify genes and proteins that are differentially expressed across two biologic conditions of interest. For the SAGE data example we consider inference for a single biologic sample. For all three applications we use flexible mixture models to implement inference. For the microarray data we define a Dirichlet process mixture of normal model. For the mass spectrometry data we introduce a mixture of Beta model. The proposed inference for SAGE data is based on a semiparametric mixture of Poisson distributions.

12.1 Introduction

We discuss semiparametric Bayesian data analysis for high-throughput genomic data. We introduce suitable semiparametric mixture models to implement inference for microarray data, mass spectrometry data, and SAGE data. The proposed models include a Dirichlet process mixture of normals for microarray data, a mixture of Beta distributions with a random number of terms for mass spectrometry data, and a Dirichlet process mixture of Poisson model for SAGE data. For the microarray data and the protein mass spectrometry data we consider experiments that compare two biologic conditions of interest. We assume that the aim of the experiment is to find genes and proteins, respectively, that are differentially expressed under the two conditions. For the SAGE example, we propose data analysis for a single biologic sample.

Several aspects of data analysis for microarray and other high-throughput gene and protein expression experiments give rise to mixture models. One important application of mixture models is THE flexible modeling of sampling distributions. This is attractive, for example, when the number of genes on a microarray is the relevant sample size, thus allowing flexible semiparametric representations. Such approaches are discussed, among others, in Broet et al. (2002), Dahl (2003), and Tadesse et al. (2005). The latter exploit the clustering implicitly defined by the mixture model to identify biologically interesting subclasses. Also, see Dahl (2006) and Tadesse et al. (2006) in this volume. In this chapter we review three approaches that are typical examples of this literature. In Section 12.2 we discuss the use of Dirichlet process mixtures for model-based inference about differential gene expression. In Section 12.3 we describe a mixture of Beta model for the mass/charge spectrum in MALDI-TOF mass spectrometry experiments. In Section 12.4 we introduce a semiparametric mixture of Poisson model for SAGE data.

Another important class of applications for mixture models in data analysis for high-throughput gene expression data is finite mixtures, with each term in the mixture corresponding to a different condition of interest. A typical example is the model used in Parmigiani et al. (2002) who construct a sampling model for observed gene expression in microarray experiments as a mixture of three terms corresponding to normal, under-, and overexpression. Newton et al. (2001) define a Gamma/Gamma hierarchical model with a mixture induced by an indicator for ties between two biologic conditions of interest. Kendziorski et al. (in press) use mixtures for expression QTL mapping. See also Chen and Kendziorski (2006) in this volume. Kendziorski et al. (2003) use finite mixtures to identify patterns of differential expression across multiple biologic conditions.

Naturally, the distinction between the two types of mixtures, that is, flexible mixtures for an unknown sampling model versus mixtures of submodels with a biologically meaningful interpretation, is not strict. A typical example is the use of semiparametric mixtures to define a probability model for clustering of genes or samples. Inference about clusters can often be interpreted as inference on biologically meaningful groups of genes or subpopulations corresponding to biologically distinct subtypes of a disease. From a modeling perspective, the intention of our distinction is to focus on semiparametric mixture models with a random and, at least in spirit, unconstrained size mixture.

Also, approaches that use hierarchical models to define flexible sampling models could alternatively be considered as mixture models. Collapsing the hierarchical model by marginalizing with respect to some intermediate level

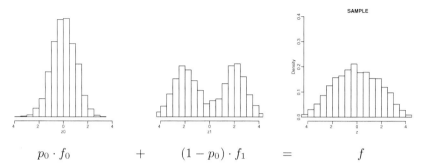

$$p_0 \cdot f_0 \qquad + \qquad (1 - p_0) \cdot f_1 \qquad = \qquad f$$

Fig. 12.1. Hypothetical distribution of difference scores for nondifferentially expressed (left, f_0) and differentially expressed genes (center, f_1), and the observed mixture (right, f). (See color plate 12.1.)

parameters one can often rewrite the hierarchical model as a mixture. See, for example, Hein et al. (2005) or the chapter by Hein et al. (2006) in this volume.

In this chapter we only focus on the use of semiparametric mixtures to represent an unknown sampling model, that is, applications of infinite size mixtures, and will not discuss the other types of mixture models.

12.2 A Nonparametric Bayesian Model for Differential Gene Expression

We consider inference for microarray group comparison experiments. Assume that the data has been summarized as a set of difference scores, $z_i, i = 1, \ldots, n$, for n genes. The difference score z_i could be, for example, a two-sample t-statistic for observed fluorescence intensities for gene i in samples under two biologic conditions of interest. See Efron et al. (2001) for a discussion of appropriate data preprocessing and Baggerly et al. (2006), in this volume, for an explanation of the experimental setup and important issues in data analysis for such experiments. We assume that the set $i = 1, \ldots, n$ of genes is partitioned into a subset of differentially expressed genes and nondifferentially expressed genes. Inference proceeds by assuming that for differentially expressed genes, the difference scores z_i arise by independent sampling from some unknown distribution f_1; for nondifferentially expressed genes, z_i are independent samples from an unknown distribution f_0. For a reasonable choice of difference scores, the distribution f_0 should be a unimodal distribution centered at zero. The distribution f_1 should be a bimodal distribution with symmetric modes to the left and right of zero corresponding to over- and underexpressed genes. Figure 12.1 shows possible histograms for observed difference scores generated from f_0 and f_1. Of course, the partition into differentially and nondifferentially expressed genes is unknown. Thus, instead of samples from f_0 and f_1, we can only work with the sample z_i, $i = 1, \ldots, n$, generated from a mixture of f_0 and f_1. Let p_0 denote the unknown proportion of nondifferentially expressed genes. We assume

$$z_i \overset{iid}{\sim} f(z) = p_0 \, f_0(z) + (1 - p_0) \, f_1(z), \quad i = 1, \ldots, n. \tag{12.1}$$

The main goal of inference in the two-group comparison microarray experiment can be formally described as the deconvolution of (12.1). We introduce a latent indicator variable $r_i \in \{0, 1\}$ to rewrite (12.1) equivalently as a hierarchical model

$$p(z_i \mid r_i = j) = f_j(z_i)$$
$$Pr(r_i = 0) = p_0. \tag{12.2}$$

The latent variable r_i can be interpreted as indicator for gene i being differentially expressed. Efron et al. (2001) propose cleverly chosen point estimates for p_0, f_0, and f_1 and report the implied inference for r_i. To develop the point estimate they introduce an additional set of difference scores, $z_i, i = n + 1, \ldots, 2n$. The additional difference scores are generated using the same original data, but deliberately computing difference scores for samples under the same biologic conditions. Thus,

$$z_i \sim f_0(z_i), \quad i = n + 1, \ldots, 2n,$$

for this additional null sample.

In Do et al. (2005) we propose a model-based semiparametric Bayesian approach to inference in this problem. We recognize f_0, f_1, and p_0 as unknown quantities and proceed by defining a suitable prior probability model. Probability models for unknown functions, including distributions such as f_0 and f_1 in this problem, are known as nonparametric Bayesian models. See, for example, Müller and Quintana (2004) for a recent review of non-parametric Bayesian inference. The term "non-parametric" is a misnomer, as the random functions are infinite dimensional parameters. However, the name is traditionally used because implied posterior inference closely resembles inference under classical non-parametric methods.

In choosing a prior probability model for f_0 and f_1 we face two competing aims. On one hand we wish to generalize traditional parametric models, like a normal sampling model. On the other hand we want to retain as much computational simplicity as possible. This leads us to use a mixture of normal model, with a nonparametric prior on the mixing measure. Inference under this model is almost as straightforward as under a simple normal model, yet, subject to some technical constraints, the mixture of normal model can approximate arbitrary sampling distributions. As probability model for the mixing measure we use a Dirichlet process (DP) prior (Ferguson, 1973; Antoniak, 1974). For reasons of computational simplicity and ease of interpretation, the DP prior is one of the most widely used nonparametric Bayes models. The DP model has two parameters, a base measure and a total mass parameter. We write $G \sim DP(G^*, M)$ to indicate that G has a DP prior with a base measure G^* and total mass M. The base measure has the interpretation as mean measure, in fact $E(G) = G^*$. The total mass parameter can be interpreted as a precision parameter. The larger the M, the closer the random G will be to G^*. Another important implication of the total mass parameter is mentioned below.

In summary, we assume the following model. Let $N(z; m, s)$ denote a normal distribution for the random variable z, with moments (m, s). We define a probability model for the random distributions f_0 and f_1 as

$$f_j(z) = \int N(z; \mu, \sigma) \, dG_j(\mu) \quad G_j \sim DP(G_j^*, M). \qquad (12.3)$$

One of the critical properties of the DP prior is that a DP-generated random measure is almost surely discrete. Thus the integral in (12.3) is simply a sum over all point masses in G_j. The total mass parameter M determines the distribution of the weights attached to these point masses. Mixture models with respect to a mixing measure with DP prior, such as (12.3), are known as mixture of DP (MDP) models and are widely used in nonparametric Bayesian inference. See, for example, MacEachern and Müller (2000) for a review of such models.

We complete the model given by the likelihood (12.2) and prior (12.3) with a hyperprior on the base measures G_j^*. We assume $G_0^* = N(0, \tau^2)$ with a conjugate inverse Gamma hyperprior on τ^2, and $G_1^* = \frac{1}{2}N(-b, \tau^2) + \frac{1}{2}N(b, \tau^2)$ with a conjugate normal hyperprior on b. Finally, we assume a Beta prior for p_0, $p_0 \sim Be(\alpha, \beta)$. The hyperparameters α, β, and M are fixed.

Inference in the proposed model is implemented by Markov chain Monte Carlo (MCMC) simulation. See Do et al. (2005) for a detailed description of the posterior MCMC algorithm. A direct implication of the models (12.2) and (12.3) is that the marginal posterior probability of differential expression, $Pr(r_i = 1 \mid \text{data})$, is the same for all genes with equal difference score z_i. Thus posterior inference can be summarized as a function $Pr(r_i = 1 \mid z_i = z, \text{data})$. Starting with model (12.2), a straightforward use of Bayes theorem shows

$$Pr(r_i = 0 \mid z_i = z, f_0, f_1, p_0) = p_0 \, f_0(z) / \underbrace{[p_0 \, f_0(z) + (1 - p_0) \, f_1(z)]}_{f(z)}.$$

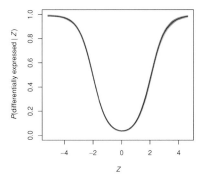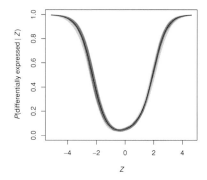

Fig. 12.2. $\bar{P}_1(z)$: posterior mean probability of differential expression as a function of the observed difference score z (solid black line). The left figure conditions on the full data, z_i, $i = 1, \ldots, 2n$, including the null data. The right figure does not make use of the null data, conditioning only on z_i, $i = 1, \ldots, n$. The dark gray shaded band shows the central 50% posterior density interval. Light gray shows a 75% posterior interval. The dark and light gray shaded areas are very narrow and can hardly be distinguished from the posterior mean curve.

Let $P_1 = p_0\, f_0/f$. Then the posterior expectation $\bar{P}_1 = E(P_1 \mid \text{data})$ is exactly the desired marginal posterior probability of differential expression, $\bar{P}_1 = Pr(r_i = 1 \mid z_i = z, \text{data})$. Figure 12.2 shows posterior inference for a simulation experiment. The figure shows the simulation truth, the reported posterior mean curve $\bar{P}_1(z)$, and pointwise posterior credible intervals for $P_1(z)$. The curve $\bar{P}_1(z)$ allows one to readily read off the marginal posterior probability of differential expression for each gene. In contrast to reasonable but ad hoc point estimates, the reported probabilities are interpreted as marginal probabilities in one coherent encompassing probability model. This leads to a straightforward definition, evaluation, and control of false discovery rates. See Newton et al. (2004) or Do et al. (2005) for a discussion.

12.3 A Mixture of Beta Model for MALDI-TOF Data

Matrix-assisted laser desorption – time of flight (MALDI-TOF) experiments allow the investigator to simultaneously measure abundance for a large number of proteins. Details of the experimental setup are described, for example, in Baggerly et al. (2003) and also in the chapter by Baggerly et al. (2006) in this volume. Briefly, the biological sample for which we wish to determine protein abundance is fixed in a matrix. A laser beam is used to break free and ionize individual protein molecules. The experiment is arranged such that ionized proteins are exposed to an electric field that accelerates molecules along a flight tube. On the other end of the flight tube, molecules hit a detector that records a

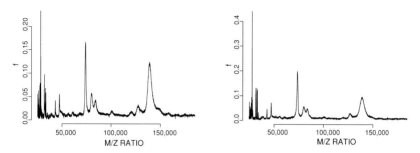

Fig. 12.3. Spectra for a normal samples (left) and a tumor samples (right), on grid of size $I = 60,000$.

histogram of number of molecules that hit over time. Assuming that all ionized molecules carry a unit charge, the time of flight is deterministically related to the molecule mass. The histogram of detector events over time can therefore be changed to a histogram of detector events over protein masses. Allowing for multiple charges, the mass scale is replaced by a scale of mass/charge ratios. The histogram of detector events is known as mass/charge spectrum. Figure 12.3 shows typical spectra.

Ideally, each protein that is present in the original probe should correspond to a peak in the spectrum. Because of the random initial velocities, when proteins are ionized by the laser impact we would expect to see peaks rather than sharp lines even in an idealized experiment. Many additional artifacts of the experiment add to the idealized description, leading to an additional baseline that adds to the protein peaks. See the data shown in Figure 12.3.

Assume we observe spectra for experiments $k = 1, \ldots, K$. Let $y_k(m_i)$ denote the recorded count for sample k at mass/charge grid point m_i, and let $f_k(m_i)$ denote the assumed underlying cleaned spectra corresponding to detected proteins only. The desired inference about the unknown protein abundance in the original probes can be formalized as (i) removing noise and baseline from the observed spectra y_{ki} to impute f_k; (ii) finding peaks in f_k; and (iii) reporting the relative sizes of these peaks. The relative size of the peaks corresponds to the relative abundance of the corresponding protein in the probe. If samples are collected under different biologic conditions, we need additional inference about different versus equal abundance of different proteins.

In Müller et al. (2006) we develop a nonparametric Bayes model to allow such inference. Based on the above stylized description of the experiment, we consider y_k as the empirical histogram of detector events. We represent it as a mixture of a baseline B_k corresponding to detector noise, protein fragments, etc., and a cleaned spectrum f_k:

$$p_k(m) = p_{0k} \, B_k(m) + (1 - p_{0k}) \, f_k(m).$$

The spectrum f_k is a sum of peaks, with each detected protein contributing a peak centered at its mass/charge value. The experimental arrangement implies a finite support for f_k. Motivated by nonparametric models for random distributions on a finite support developed in Petrone (1999) and Robert and Rousseau (2002), we use a mixture of Beta distributions to define the random distribution f_k. The location for each Beta kernel is interpreted as the mass/charge ratio of the protein giving rise to this peak. To facilitate later interpretation, we use a nonstandard parameterization of the Beta distribution. We write $Be(x; \, \epsilon, \alpha)$ for a Beta kernel for the random variable x, with mean and standard deviation ϵ and α (with appropriate constraints on α).

Let x denote the biologic condition of sample k. We assume a two-group comparison, that is, $x \in \{0, 1\}$. Then

$$f_k(m) = \sum_{j=1}^{J} w_{xj} \, \text{Beta}(m; \, \epsilon_j, \alpha_j). \tag{12.4}$$

In words, the kth spectrum is a mixture of Beta kernels, corresponding to J distinct proteins with mass/charge values ϵ_j. The relative weight w_{xj}, that is, relative abundance of protein j, is assumed the same for all samples under the same biologic condition. For reasons of technical convenience we chose a similar mixture of Beta prior for the baseline B_k. Different hyperparameters reflect the fact that the baseline is much smoother than f_k and we expect fewer terms in the mixture. $B_k(m) = \sum_{j=1}^{J_k} v_{kj} \, \text{Beta}(m; \, \eta_{kj}, \beta_{kj})$. The sizes of the mixtures are random. We use truncated Poisson priors for J and J_k, $k = 1, \ldots, K$. Baseline B_k and mean spectrum f_k are combined to define the distribution of mass/charge ratios $p_k = p_{0k} \, B_k + (1 - p_{0k}) \, f_k$. Following the idealized description of the experimental setup, the sampling model is random sampling from p_k. Let $y_k = (y_{ki}, \, i = 1, \ldots, I)$ denote the empirical spectrum for the kth sample over the grid of mass/charge values. Typically I is large, say 60,000, defining a very fine grid. Let $\theta = (J, J_k, w_{xj}, v_{kj}, \epsilon_j, \alpha_j, \eta_i, \beta_i, \, x = 0, 1, \, j = 1, \ldots, J, \, k = 1, \ldots, K, \, i = 1, \ldots, J_k)$ denote the parameter vector. The likelihood is

$$\log p(y_k \mid \theta) = \sum_{i=1}^{I} y_{ki} \log p_k(m_i). \tag{12.5}$$

Instead of the random sampling model (12.5) many authors use a regression likelihood, assuming normal residuals, $y_{ki} \sim N(p_k(m_i), \sigma^2)$. Little changes in the following discussion if we were to replace (12.5) by this regression likelihood.

The model is completed with a prior for the Beta parameters and the weights. For the weights w_{xj} we use a hierarchical prior with indicators λ_j for ties

$$\lambda_j = I(w_{0j} = w_{1j}).$$

Posterior inference on the λ_j and the locations ϵ_j summarizes the desired inference on proteins that are differentially expressed across the two groups of samples.

Implementation of posterior inference requires MCMC over a varying dimension parameter space, as the dimension of the parameter space depends on the sizes J and J_k of the mixtures. We use reversible jump MCMC (RJMCMC) as proposed in Green (1995) and, specifically for mixture models, in Richardson and Green (1997). See Müller et al. (2006) for a detailed description of the MCMC algorithm.

A minor complication arises in reporting and summarizing posterior inference about distinct proteins and their mass/charge ratios. The mixture f_k only includes exchangeable indices j, leading to the complication that the Beta kernel corresponding to a specific protein might have different indices at different iterations of the posterior MCMC simulation. In other words, the protein identity is not part of the probability model. To report posterior inference on the mean abundance of a given protein requires additional postprocessing to match Beta kernels that correspond to the same protein across iterations. We use a reasonable ad hoc rule. Any two peaks j and h with a difference in masses below a certain threshold are counted as arising from the same protein. Specifically, we use the condition $|\epsilon_j - \epsilon_h| < 0.5\alpha_j$ to match peaks. Here j indexes the peak that was imputed in an earlier MCMC iteration than the peak h. The problem of reporting inference related to the terms in a mixture is known as the label switching problem (Holmes, et al. 2005).

Figure 12.4 summarizes estimated masses and abundance of detected proteins. Assuming that the main inference goal is to identify proteins with differential expression across the two biologic conditions, we focus on inference about the indicator for differential expression, $1 - \lambda_j$. The figure indicates all protein masses with $Pr(\lambda_j = 0 \mid data, \ldots) > 50\%$, that is, with posterior probability greater than 50% for differential expression. The probability is evaluated conditional on the protein being present in the probe (therefore the "..." in the conditioning set). Also, only proteins are reported in the figure that have posterior probability greater than 5% of being present, that is, a peak being identified at the corresponding mass. In a data analysis, the list of reported protein masses

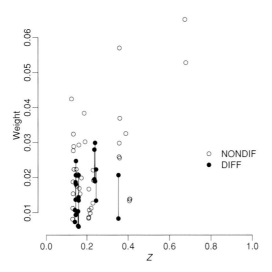

Fig. 12.4. Posterior mean abundance of detected proteins. All peaks with posterior probability of differential expression greater than 50% are marked as solid dots, with a line combining $\overline{w}_{0j} = E(w_{0j} \mid \text{data})$ and $\overline{w}_{1j}$. Mass/charge ratios on the horizontal axis are rescaled to the unit interval.

would now be compared against a list of known protein masses to match the discovered peaks with specific proteins.

12.4 A Semiparametric Mixture Model for SAGE Data

Consider data from a SAGE (Serial Analysis of Gene Expression) experiment. See Baggerly et al. (2006) for a description of the experimental setup, and the nature of the data. We consider inference for data from one biologic sample. Let y_i, $i = 1, \ldots, k$, denote observed tag frequencies for k distinct transcripts. Let $n = \sum y_i$ denote the total number of recorded transcripts, and let π_i denote the unknown true abundance of the ith transcript in the probe. For large y_i, the empirical frequency $\hat{\pi}_i = y_i / n$ is an appropriate point estimate for π_i. The associated uncertainty, formalized as variance of the maximum likelihood estimator or as posterior standard deviation in a suitable model, is negligible. However, for scarce tags with small π_i, more elaborate estimates are required. The empirical frequency for scarce tags includes considerable sampling variability. Also, when the data includes samples across different biologic conditions, the inference goal might not be restricted to estimating the transcript frequencies. For discrimination and classification, additional inference about differences in transcript frequencies, and related probability statements are required. In addition to inference on π_i for a specific tag i, one might be interested in the distribution of tag frequencies across different transcripts. This can be achieved by model-based posterior inference.

Morris et al. (2003) introduce an approach that is based on a hierarchical model with a mixture of two Dirichlet distributions as population distribution prior for the π_i. See Morris et al. (2006) in this volume for a review of this approach. Building on this model, we introduce a semiparametric Bayesian mixture model, replacing the two-component mixture of Dirichlet distributions by an unknown random measure, with a nonparametric Bayesian prior model.

For the following model construction it is convenient not to condition on n. In other words, instead of assuming that the set of observed counts arise as a multinomial sample with cell frequencies π_i, we assume that, conditional on hyperparameters, the counts y_i arise as independent samples from some distribution. Specifically, we assume that the counts y_i are sampled from a mixture of Poisson model. Let $Poi(x;\ \lambda)$ denote a Poisson distribution for the random variable x with parameter λ. We assume

$$y_i \sim \int Poi(y_i;\ \lambda)\, dG(\lambda),$$

$i = 1, \ldots, n$, independently conditional on G. We specify a prior distribution for the mixture model by assuming a nonparametric prior on the mixing measure, choosing a DP prior as in (12.3),

$$G \sim DP(G^*, M). \tag{12.6}$$

The mixture model can alternatively be written as a hierarchical model

$$y_i \mid \lambda_i \sim Poi(\lambda_i) \text{ with } \lambda_i \sim G. \tag{12.7}$$

The discrete nature of the DP random measure G implies a positive probability for ties among the λ_i. We denote with L the number of distinct values.

A minor complication arises from the fact that $y_i = 0$ is not observed; it is censored. Let k_0 denote the number of tags with nonzero count, that is the number of tags recorded in a SAGE library as shown in Baggerly et al. (2006). One could augment the model to include inference on k, $k \geq k_0$. Alternatively, we follow Stollberg et al. (2000), and fix k by imputing a point estimate for the unknown number of unobserved tags, that is, tags with $y_i = 0$.

Models (12.6) and (12.7) define a DP mixture of Poisson distributions. Such models are popular choices for nonparametric Bayesian data analysis. See, for example, MacEachern and Müller (2000) for a review of such models, including implementation of posterior inference by MCMC simulation. Choosing the base measure G^* to be conjugate with the Poisson distribution we define a conjugate

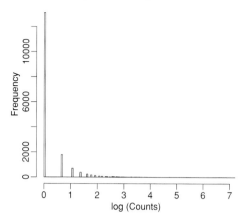

Fig. 12.5. Observed tag counts y_i. The highly skewed nature is typical of for SAGE data.

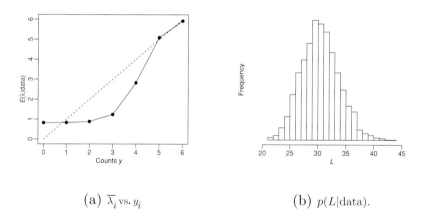

(a) $\overline{\lambda}_i$ vs. y_i.   (b) $p(L|\text{data})$.

Fig. 12.6. Posterior means $\overline{\lambda}_i = E(\lambda_i \mid \text{data})$ versus observed counts y_i (panel a). Note the strong shrinkage for small counts. For large counts, $y_i > 6$, posterior shrinkage quickly becomes negligible. Posterior distribution for the number of clusters L (panel b).

DP mixture, greatly facilitating the MCMC implementation. Let Ga(x; α, β) denote a Gamma distribution with mean α/β. We use

$$G^*(\lambda) = \text{Ga}(x; \ \alpha, \ \beta),$$

with fixed hyperparameters α and β.

To illustrate the model we implemented posterior inference for a SAGE library reported in Zhang et al. (1997). The same data was used in Morris et al. (2003), and is available at http://www.sagenet.org/SAGEData/NC1.htm. It records counts for $k_0 = 17,703$ distinct transcripts, with a total number of

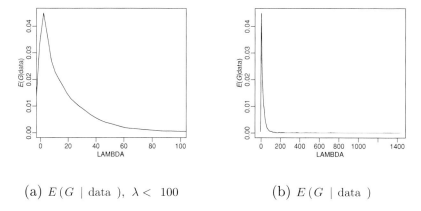

(a) $E(G \mid \text{data})$, $\lambda < 100$ (b) $E(G \mid \text{data})$

Fig. 12.7. Estimated mixing measure G. The left panel zooms in on the lower end, $\lambda < 100$. The highly skewed nature of $G^* = E(G \mid \text{data})$ reflects the same feature in the recorded data y_i.

$n = \sum y_i = 49,610$ recorded tags. We use the estimate from Stollberg et al. (2000), and set $k = 25,336$, with $y_i = 0$ for $i = k_0 + 1, \ldots, k$, that is, we estimate the number of tags with censored counts $y_i = 0$, as $\sum I(y_i = 0) = 8,072$. Figure 12.5a shows a histogram of observed counts y_i in the data. Figure 12.6 summarizes posterior inference for the transcript abundances. The figure plots posterior mean estimates $E(\lambda_i \mid \text{data})$ versus observed counts y_i. The nature of the shrinkage follows patterns reported in Morris et al. (2003). For censored tags, with $y_i = 0$, the posterior mean estimate inflates the maximum likelihood estimate and reports $E(\lambda_i \mid \text{data}) \approx 0.9$. For rare tags with nonzero counts, posterior inference shrinks the maximum likelihood estimate. For abundant posterior tags, posterior inference is driven only by the observed counts. And $E(\lambda_i \mid \text{data}) \approx y_i$. Figure 12.7 shows the estimated distribution of tag abundances λ_i.

12.5 Summary

We have illustrated the use of mixture models for Bayesian inference with gene expression and proteomics data. We focused on the use of mixtures as a flexible class of distributions to parameterize random distributions. Another important use of mixtures arises in models where the submodels in the mixture correspond to different biologic conditions. Such models are extensively reviewed in other chapters in this volume.

   We introduced DP mixtures of normals models to model microarray gene expression data, DP mixtures of Poissons to model tag counts in SAGE data, and location/scale mixtures of Beta kernels to represent mass/charge spectra in protein mass spectrometry experiments. The underlying theme in all three applications is the use of model-based inference, with a probability model on the random distribution (or mass/charge spectrum). This is in contrast to traditional, and very reasonable, multistep methods. The power of the model-based methods lies in the full probabilistic description of all related uncertainties. Many important inference problems go beyond point estimates. For example, consider the decision problem of flagging genes for differential expression, or the problem of identifying a set of proteins that can serve as biomarker panel, or sample size choice for a microarray experiment. A decision theoretic answer to these question relies on a description of all uncertainties in one coherent probability model.

Acknowledgments

Kim-Anh Do was partially supported by NIH University of Texas SPORE in Prostate Cancer grant CA90270. Jeff Morris was supported by NCI grant CA107304. Michele Guindani and Peter Müller were supported by NCI grant CA75981.

Bibliography

Antoniak, C. E. (1974), "Mixtures of Dirichlet processes with applications to Bayesian nonparametric problems," *The Annals of Statistics*, 2, 1152–1174.

Baggerly, K. A., Coombes, K. R., and Morris, J. S. (2006), "An introduction to high-throughput bioinformatics data," in *Bayesian Inference for Gene Expression and Proteomics,* Do, K.-A., Müller, P., and Vannucci, M., New York: Cambridge University Press, pp. 1–39.
Bayesian Mixture Models for Gene Expression and Protein Profiles

Baggerly, K. A., Morris, J. S., Wang, J., Gold, D., Xiao, L. C., and Coombes, K. R. (2003), "A comprehensive approach to analysis of MALDI-TOF proteomics spectra from serum samples," *Proteomics*, 3, 1667–1672.

Broet, P., Richardson, S., and Radvanyi, F. (2002), "Bayesian hierarchical model for identifying changes in gene expression from microarray experiments," *Journal of Computational Biology*, 9, 671–683.

Chen, M. and Kendziorski, C. (2006), "Interval mapping for expression quantitative trait loci," in *Bayesian Inference for Gene Expression and Proteomics,* Do, K.-A., Müller, P., and Vannucci, M., New York: Cambridge University Press, pp. 219–237.

Dahl, D. (2003), "Modeling differential gene expression using a Dirichlet process mixture model," in *2003 Proceedings of the American Statistical Association, Bayesian Statistical Sciences Section*, Alexandria, VA: American Statistical Association.

Dahl, D. (2006), "Model-based clustering for expression data via a Dirichlet process mixture model," in *Bayesian Inference for Gene Expression and Proteomics,* Do, K.-A., Müller, P., and Vannucci, M., New York: Cambridge University Press, pp. 201–218.

Do, K.-A., Müller, P., and Tang, F. (2005), "A Bayesian mixture model for differential gene expression," *Journal of the Royal Statistical Society C*, 54, 627–644.

Efron, B., Tibshirani, R., Storey, J. D., and Tusher, V. (2001), "Empirical Bayes analysis of a microarray experiment," *Journal of the American Statistical Association*, 96, 1151–1160.

Ferguson, T. S. (1973), "A Bayesian analysis of some nonparametric problems," *The Annals of Statistics*, 1, 209–230.

Green, P. J. (1995), "Reversible jump Markov chain Monte Carlo computation and Bayesian model determination," *Biometrika*, 82, 711–732.

Hein, A., Richardson, S., Causton, H., Ambler, G., and Green, P. (2005), "BGX: A fully Bayesian integrated approach to the analysis of Affymetrix GeneChip data," *Biostatistics*, 6, 349–373.

Hein, A.-M. K., Lewin, A., and Richardson, S. (2006), "Bayesian hierarchical models for inference in microarray data," in *Bayesian Inference for Gene Expression and Proteomics,* Do, K.-A., Müller, P., and Vannucci, M., New York: Cambridge University Press, pp. 53–74.

Holmes, C. C., Jasra, A., and Stephens, D. A. (2005), "Markov chain Monte Carlo methods and the label Switching problem in Bayesian mixture modeling," *Statistical Science*, 20, 50–67.

Kendziorski, C. M., Chen, M., Yuan, M., Lan, H., and Attie, A. (in press), "Statistical methods for expression trait loci (eQTL) mapping," *Biometrics*.

Kendziorski, C. M., Newton, M., Lan, H., and Gould, M. (2003), "On parametric empirical Bayes methods for comparing multiple groups using replicated gene expression profiles," *Statistics in Medicine*, 22, 3899–3914.

MacEachern, S. N. and Müller, P. (2000), "Efficient MCMC schemes for robust model extensions using encompassing Dirichlet process mixture models," in *Robust Bayesian Analysis*, eds. Ruggeri, F. and Ríos-Insua, D., New York: Springer-Verlag, pp. 295–316.

Morris, J. S., Baggerly, K. A., and Coombes, K. R. (2003), "Bayesian shrinkage estimation of the relative abundance of MRNA transcripts using SAGE," *Biometrics*, 59, 476–486.

Morris, J. S., Baggerly, K. A., and Coombes, K. R. (2006), "Shrinkage estimation for SAGE data using a mixture Dirichlet prior," in *Bayesian Inference for Gene Expression and Proteomics,* Do, K.-A., Müller, P., and Vannucci, M., New York: Cambridge University Press, pp. 254–268.

Müller, P., Do, K.-A., Bandyopadhyay, R., and Baggerly, K. (2006), "A Bayesian mixture model for protein biomarker discovery," Technical Report, M.D. Anderson Cancer Center.

Müller, P. and Quintana, F. A. (2004), "Nonparametric Bayesian data analysis," *Statistical Science*, 19, 95–110.

Newton, M., Noueriry, A., Sarkar, D., and Ahlquist, P. (2004), "Detecting differential gene expression with a semiparametric hierarchical mixture model," *Biostatistics*, 5, 155–176.

Newton, M. A., Kendziorski, C. M., Richmond, C. S., Blattner, F. R., and Tsui, K. W. (2001), "On differential variability of expression ratios: Improving statistical inference about gene expression changes from microarray data," *Journal Computational Biology*, 8, 37–52.

Parmigiani, G., Garrett, E. S., Anbazhagan, R., and Gabrielson, E. (2002), "A statistical framework for expression-based molecular classification in cancer," *Journal of the Royal Statistical Society B*, 64, 717–736.

Petrone, S. (1999), "Bayesian density estimation using Bernstein polynomials," *Canadian Journal of Statistics*, 27, 105–126.

Richardson, S. and Green, P. J. (1997), "On Bayesian analysis of mixtures with an unknown number of components," *Journal of the Royal Statistical Society B*, 59, 731–792.

Robert, C. and Rousseau, J. (2002), "A mixture approach to Bayesian goodness of fit," Technical Report, CEREMADE.

Stollberg, J., Urschitz, J., Urban, Z., and Boyd, C. (2000), "A quantitative evaluation of SAGE," *Genome Research*, 10, 1241–1248.

Tadesse, M., Sha, N., Kim, S., and Vannucci, M. (2006), "Identification of biomarkers in classification and clustering of high-throughput data," in *Bayesian Inference for Gene Expression and Proteomics,* Do, K.-A., Müller, P., and Vannucci, M., New York: Cambridge University Press, pp. 97–115.

Tadesse, M., Sha, N., and Vannucci, M. (2005), "Bayesian variable selection in clustering high-dimensional data," *Journal of the American Statistical Association*, 100, 602–617.

Zhang, L., Zhou, W., Velculescu, V., Kern, S., Hruban, R., Hamilton, S., Vogelstein, B., and Kinzler, K. (1997), "Gene expression profiles in normal and cancer cells," *Science*, 276, 1268–1272.

13

Shrinkage Estimation for SAGE Data Using a Mixture Dirichlet Prior

JEFFREY S. MORRIS, KEITH A. BAGGERLY,
AND KEVIN R. COOMBES

The University of Texas M.D. Anderson Cancer Center

Abstract

Serial analysis of gene expression (SAGE) is a technique for estimating the gene expression profile of a biological sample. Any efficient inference in SAGE must be based upon efficient estimates of these gene expression profiles, which consist of the estimated relative abundances for each mRNA species present in the sample. The data from SAGE experiments are counts for each observed mRNA species, and can be modeled using a multinomial distribution with two characteristics: skewness in the distribution of relative abundances and small sample size relative to the dimension. As a result of these characteristics, a given SAGE sample will fail to capture a large number of expressed mRNA species present in the tissue. Standard empirical estimates of the relative abundances effectively ignore these missing, unobserved species, and consequently tend to also overestimate the abundance of the scarce observed species comprising a vast majority of the total. In this chapter, we review a new Bayesian procedure that yields improved estimates for the missing and scarce species without trading off much efficiency for the abundant species. The key to the procedure is the mixture Dirichlet prior, which stochastically partitions the mRNA species into abundant and scarce strata, with each stratum modeled with its own multivariate prior, a scalar multiple of a symmetric Dirichlet. Simulation studies demonstrate that the resulting shrinkage estimators have efficiency advantages over the maximum likelihood estimator for SAGE scenarios simulated.

13.1 Introduction

Serial analysis of gene expression (SAGE) is a method for estimating the gene expression profile of a biological sample of interest. In this chapter, we review a method introduced in Morris, Baggerly, and Coombes (2003) for obtaining Bayesian shrinkage estimates of these profiles using a fully specified probability model. Bayesian inference using this method is straightforward since the estimators arise from a coherent probability model. An outline of the chapter is as follows.

In Section 13.2, we provide an overview of SAGE and motivate the use of the multinomial likelihood to model the resulting data, and then in Section 13.3 we describe some standard methods for estimating multinomial relative frequencies. After explaining why we believe these standard approaches are inadequate for SAGE data, we review a method based on the mixture Dirichlet prior. Section 13.4 describes the prior and Section 13.5 provides implementation details for obtaining posterior mean estimates for the mRNA species' relative abundances. In Section 13.6, we present the results of a simulation study demonstrating the benefit of shrinkage estimation based on the mixture Dirichlet prior, and Section 13.7 contains some conclusions.

13.2 Overview of SAGE

13.2.1 Measuring Gene Expression

The central dogma in genetics is that DNA is used as a template to make mRNA molecules, which then assemble the proteins that perform the biological tasks of a living organism. The "expression level" of a gene refers to the amount of its corresponding mRNA present in a cell, which is taken to be a rough surrogate for how active that gene is in coding its protein. Levels of gene expression are important to study in cancer research, as well as other biological applications. It is often of interest to compare the gene expression profiles of different biological samples, for example to identify genes differentially expressed across biological conditions (e.g., cancer/normal) or clinical outcomes (e.g., response to chemotherapy/no response).

The most common method for measuring gene expression is cDNA hybridization using microarrays, which can simultaneously measure the expression levels of the genes represented on the array, typically numbering in the thousands. In this method, sequences of DNA from the genes of interest are arranged on an array, either by spotting or direct synthesis. The sample of interest is then labeled and hybridized with the targets on the array. The amount of material hybridized to each target is estimated by measuring the corresponding staining intensity. After normalization, these intensities are used as an estimate of the expression levels of the target genes. Note that microarrays are a "closed system," since they only provide information on the prespecified genes that have been placed on the array.

An alternative method for measuring gene expression is serial analysis of gene expression (SAGE), introduced by Velculescu et al. (1999). Unlike microarrays, SAGE is an "open system," since one need not prespecify the genes of interest. It is possible to obtain expression level estimates for any gene expressed in the sample. First, a sample of n mRNA transcripts are selected from the biological sample and complementary cDNA strands are constructed. Commonly, the number of transcripts sampled is between $n = 10,000$ and $100,000$. For each selected transcript, a 10-base region at a specific location within its sequence is isolated, sequenced, and recorded. This sequence is called a tag. Ideally, these tags uniquely identify the source mRNA, and in practice this is roughly true. Thus, the relative expression level of a gene, measured by the relative quantity of the corresponding mRNA species, is approximated by the relative frequency of its corresponding SAGE tag. The data from a SAGE experiment consists of the counts for each unique tag observed in the sample. The collection of these counts for a biological sample is called a "SAGE library."

13.2.2 Characterizing SAGE Data

Suppose that from a SAGE sample consisting of n transcripts, we obtain a library containing k^* unique tags, with the counts for each unique tag represented by X_i, $i = 1, \ldots, k^*$, with $\sum_{i=1}^{k^*} X_i = n$. In a typical library, the number of unique tags observed is between $k^* = 3,000$ and $30,000$. By the nature of the sampling, it is very likely that the SAGE sample has failed to capture a number of mRNA species present in the biological sample. Let k_0 be the number of these "missing species," and $k = k^* + k_0$ the true number of expressed transcripts in the sample. If we knew k_0 or at least had an estimate of it, we could append our data set with $X_i = 0$, for $i = k^* + 1, \ldots, k$, to include the zero counts for the missing species.

Assuming the sampling of mRNA proceeds in a roughly independent fashion, the vector $\underline{X} = (X_1, \ldots, X_k)'$ can be modeled as a random draw from a multinomial distribution with parameters n and $\underline{\pi} = (\pi_1, \ldots, \pi_k)'$, with $\sum_{i=1}^{k} \pi_i = 1$. The vector $\underline{\pi}$ characterizes the relative expression profile of the biological sample, with π_i representing the true relative abundance of the mRNA species corresponding to unique tag i. These are the main parameters of interest in SAGE, and efficient inference depends on efficient estimation of these parameters. It is estimated that a typical cell contains roughly 300,000 mRNA transcripts, so frequently the π_i are reported as fractions over 300,000 to represent "mean copies of the transcript per cell."

Table 13.1 summarizes the distribution of relative frequencies across tags estimated by pooling together a series of large colon cancer SAGE libraries

Table 13.1. *Skewness in SAGE Data*

Copies/cell	% of Tags	% of Mass
≤ 5	89.9	23
5–50	9.2	30
50–500	0.8	27
500–5,000	0.1	20

Source: (Velculescu et al. 1999).

(Velculescu et al. 1999). Note that a vast majority of the observed tags have relative expression levels of no more than 5 per cell, that is, $\pi_i \leq 5/300,000$. Although containing almost 90% of all unique tags, this group only accounts for 23% of the total probability mass; the π_i for the unique tags in this group sum to 0.23. There are progressively fewer genes with larger relative frequencies. Only 1/1,000 of genes are present at rates of over 500 per cell, but these few abundant genes account for almost as much probability mass as the scarcest ones. The 1% most abundant tags account for almost 50% of the total probability mass of the sample.

Thus, we see that there are a small number of "abundant" genes, and a large number of "scarce" genes. This is an inherent characteristic of SAGE data, and gene expression in general. We could say from this that the distribution of the π_i is very strongly skewed right. Note that this skewness, along with the fact that n is not large relative to k, contributes to the fact that a large number of mRNA species are missing from any given SAGE sample.

13.3 Methods for Estimating Relative Abundances

13.3.1 Maximum Likelihood Estimation

It is typical to estimate the relative abundances for mRNA species π_i by the standard empirical estimators $\widehat{\pi}_{i,\mathrm{MLE}} = X_i/n$. These are trivial to compute and are maximum likelihood estimators (MLEs), so are asymptotically efficient. Thus, for large enough samples, they can be shown to outperform all other estimators. However, since $n \approx k$ and the distribution of π_i is strongly skewed, a SAGE library is essentially a small sample, even with values of n that seem "large." In this setting, the MLE performs well for the relatively few abundant species, but has undesirable properties for the scarce species comprising the vast majority of the total number of unique tags. For a given SAGE sample, it underestimates the relative frequency for all missing tags, and as a result, tends to overestimate the relative frequencies of the scarce observed tags.

The estimator for each missing tag is zero, which we know is less than the true value. As a result of the relative frequency constraint that the π_i's must sum to 1, this implies that the MLE tends to, on average, overestimate the relative frequencies for the nonmissing tags, that is, $\sum_{i:\,X_i>0} \widehat{\pi}_{i,\text{MLE}} > \sum_{i:\,X_i>0} \pi_i$. The genes with small but nonzero counts will be the ones most likely to be overestimated. Thus, for a given data set, the MLE will underestimate π_i for any species with zero counts, and tend to overestimate π_i for genes with small nonzero counts.

To further illustrate this point, consider the following toy example. Suppose we have a biological sample with 51 expressed genes. One is abundant with relative frequency $\pi_i = 0.50$, and the other 50 are scarce with $\pi_i = 0.01$. Suppose we sample 20 transcripts and record the counts for each. On average, 40 of the 50 scarce tags will be missing, with the other 10 occurring once. Thus, our estimate for a scarce tag will either be much smaller (0) or much larger (≥ 0.05) than the true value. In this effectively small sample setting, these estimators are limited as to how well they can estimate the relative abundances of the scarce tags.

We would like to find an estimator that improves on the MLE. We would like for it to give positive estimates when $X_i = 0$, which would require shrinking the estimates for the genes with counts greater than zero in order to honor the relative frequency contstraint $\sum_{i=1}^{k} \pi_i = 1$. This can be accomplished by specifying a prior distribution for $\underline{\pi}$ and using a Bayesian estimator.

13.3.2 Bayesian Estimation with a Symmetric Dirichlet Prior

The Dirichlet distribution is commonly used as a prior distribution with the multinomial likelihood, since it is conjugate. When there is no prior knowledge on which of the multinomial categories are more likely than the others, it is common practice to set all Dirichlet parameters to be the same a priori, which we refer to as a *symmetric Dirichlet* with parameter θ, or SymmDir(θ). A common choice for this hyperparameter is $\theta = 1$, described by Jeffreys (1961, Section 3.23), and corresponding to a k-variate generalization of the Uniform distribution.

In that case, the posterior distribution of $\underline{\pi}$ is Dirichlet with parameters $\theta + X_i$ for $i = 1, \ldots, k$. The posterior mean for π_i is $\widehat{\pi}_{i,\text{DIR}} = \frac{X_i + \theta}{n + k\theta}$, which can also be written as $(\frac{n}{n+k\theta}) * X_i/n + (\frac{k\theta}{n+k\theta}) * 1/k$. Thus, we see that the posterior mean is a weighted average of the MLE and the prior mean, with the weight determined largely by the sample size. As n gets very large, the estimator is approximately X_i/n, the MLE. When n is smaller, there is more weight given to the prior mean, $1/k$.

Now, consider our toy example again, this time using the posterior mean estimator with this Dirichlet prior, assuming $\theta = 1$. When $X_i = 0$, $\widehat{\pi}_{i,\text{DIR}} = 1/71 = 0.014$, and when $X_i = 1$, $\widehat{\pi}_{i,\text{DIR}} = 2/71 = 0.028$. These are both closer to the true value of 0.01 than the MLE. In fact, it can be shown that, for the scarce genes in this toy example, the Bayesian estimators are always closer to the truth than the MLEs, no matter when X_i is! However, this estimator performs abysmally for the abundant gene. When $X = 10$, we see the posterior mean estimate is 0.15, versus the MLE of 0.50. Recall the true value was 0.50. We see in our example that the Bayesian method with Dirichlet prior results in improved estimation for the scarce species relative to the MLE, but induces a severe bias that results in horrible estimates for the abundant species. This is not just true in this contrived example, but these results would also hold for real SAGE data.

13.3.3 Robin Hood and Nonlinear Shrinkage

Following is an analogy to illustrate the heuristics behind this problem. We know that the MLEs yield zero relative frequency estimates for all species not seen in our SAGE sample. Since we know that there are a large number of true mRNA species out there with positive relative frequencies that were simply missed by our random sampling procedure, we would like to have some positive probability mass for these species. Because of the relative frequency constraint, this means we need to decrease the estimators for some of the observed classes. There is no free lunch; in order to "pay" the zero count classes, we need to "steal" some probability mass from the other classes.

A Bayesian estimator will do this. Because the Bayesian posterior mean takes a weighted average of the prior mean and empirical estimator, it will result in a positive relative frequency estimate for the zero counts, and will shrink the estimates for tags with empirical estimates greater than the prior mean. The form of the prior determines how this shrinkage is done; that is, who do we "steal from" to "pay the zeroes."

The simple symmetric Dirichlet performs linear shrinkage, so steals the most mass from the "richest" or most abundant classes. This prior could be called a "Robin Hood" prior, since it steals from the rich to pay the poor. This is reasonable when we truly believe the multinomial classes are exchangeable, since then it is likely that any very large count is an aberration, and so should be shrunken the most. However, in settings like SAGE where we know there is a great deal of heterogeneity in the relative frequencies, this type of shrinkage is undesirable and, as we see from our simulation studies, leads to very poor estimators.

In SAGE, we would like a prior that is the opposite of a Robin Hood prior. It would be best to "steal" from the most "poor" classes, those with low counts, and leave the "rich" alone, since the sampling properties of the problem suggest that the poorest classes are the ones whose empirical probability estimates are holding on to the mass rightfully belonging to the zero classes. In other words, we would like an estimator that shrinks the MLEs in a nonlinear fashion, where classes with large counts are left largely unaffected, but those with small counts are shrunken.

This idea of nonlinear shrinkage has been implemented in other statistical settings. For example, in wavelet regression, noise is removed from a functional signal by shrinking wavelet coefficients toward zero in such a way that the smallest wavelet coefficients, likely to consist mostly of noise, are shrunken the most, while the large coefficients, likely to consist of signal, are left largely unaffected. In that setting, this shrinkage is achieved by using a prior that is a mixture of a Normal and point mass at zero (Vidakovic 1998), or alternatively a mixture of two Normals, one with a small and the other with a large variance (Chipman, Kolaczyk, and McCulloch, 1997). Here we accomplish nonlinear shrinkage via a mixture Dirichlet prior, which we now describe.

13.4 Mixture Dirichlet Distribution

One reason the symmetric Dirichlet prior fails in this context is that it inaccurately represents the population of relative frequencies in SAGE. It assumes that all k classes are a priori exchangeable, with relative frequencies of $1/k$, while in reality they are very heterogeneous. As previously mentioned, the characteristics of gene expression suggest that there should be a small number of very abundant tags, and a very large number of scarce tags. However, we typically do not know a priori which tags will be abundant. We quantify this prior knowledge through the following mixture Dirichlet prior, introduced by Morris, Baggerly, and Coombes (2003). This distribution stochastically partitions the tags into scarce and abundant strata, each of which has its own multivariate distribution, a scalar multiple of a symmetric Dirichlet.

13.4.1 Prior Specification

In order to specify this prior, we first introduce a new set of parameters $\{\lambda, \pi^*, \underline{q}\}$. Each unique tag is assumed to belong to one of two classes, either "abundant" or "scarce." The parameter $\lambda_i = 1$ indicates that unique tag i belongs to the abundant class. We assume a priori that $\lambda_i \sim \text{Bernoulli}(P)$, where P represents the prior proportion of unique tags belonging to the abundant class. Let the indices of tags belonging to the scarce and abundant classes be represented by $\mathcal{S} = \{i: \lambda_i = 0\}$ and $\mathcal{A} = \{i: \lambda_i = 1\}$, which are of length $k_S = \sum_{i=1}^{k}(1 - \lambda_i)$ and $k_A = \sum_{i=1}^{k} \lambda_i$, respectively. The parameter $\pi^* = \sum_{i=1}^{k} \lambda_i X_i$ represents the "abundant mass," and is given a Beta($\alpha_{\pi^*}, \beta_{\pi^*}$).

The vector $\underline{q} = (q_1, \ldots, q_k)'$ contains the relative frequencies for each unique tag *within its class*. Given $\underline{\lambda}$, $\underline{q}$ is partitioned into $\underline{q}_S = \underline{\pi}_S/(1 - \pi^*)$ and $\underline{q}_A = \underline{\pi}_A/\pi^*$. If $\lambda_i = 1$, then the q_i represents the relative proportion of abundant mass attributable to tag i, while if $\lambda_i = 0$, q_i represents the relative proportion of scarce mass attributable to tag i. The vectors $\underline{q}_A$ and $\underline{q}_S$ are assumed to each follow symmetric Dirichlet distributions of dimension k_A and k_S and parameters θ_A and θ_S, respectively. This construct allows the scarce and abundant tags to have their own prior distributions, yet honors the relative frequency constraint $\sum_{i=1}^{k} \pi_i = 1$. If k_0 is unknown, we give it an improper prior $f(k_0) \propto k_0^{-1}$, which was suggested by Jim Berger as a good reference prior in this context (personal communication, 2002).

Following is a summary of our mixture Dirichlet prior structure.

$$\underline{q}_A|\underline{\lambda} = \text{Symmetric Dirichlet}(\theta_A),$$
$$\underline{q}_S|\underline{\lambda} = \text{Symmetric Dirichlet}(\theta_S),$$
$$\lambda_i \sim \text{Bernoulli}(P),$$
$$\pi^* = \text{Beta}(\alpha_{\pi^*}, \beta_{\pi^*}),$$
$$f(k_0) \propto k_0^{-1}.$$

The relative frequencies for the individual multinomial classes are constructed using these quantities as follows: $\pi_i = \{q_i \pi^*\}^{\lambda_i} \{q_i(1 - \pi^*)\}^{(1-\lambda_i)}$.

This prior yields a nonlinear shrinkage profile, whereby the scarce species are shrunken strongly toward zero while the abundant species are more or less left alone, leaving positive mass for the missing species we know are there. Figure 13.1 contains shrinkage curves for a SAGE sample of size $n = 10,000$ for the MLE and Bayesian estimators with symmetric Dirichlet prior with $\theta = 1$ and a mixture Dirichlet prior with $\theta_A = 1$, $\theta_S = 0.5$, and $P = 0.005$. Note the linear and nonlinear shrinkage profiles that characterize the symmetric and mixture Dirichlet priors, respectively.

13.4.2 Selection of Prior Hyperparameters

The hyperparameters θ_A, θ_S, and P largely determine the shape of the shrinkage curve. In general, larger values of θ_A and θ_S lead to stronger shrinkage toward the prior means within the abundant and scarce classes, respectively. Because

Shrinkage Curves
***n* = 10,000**

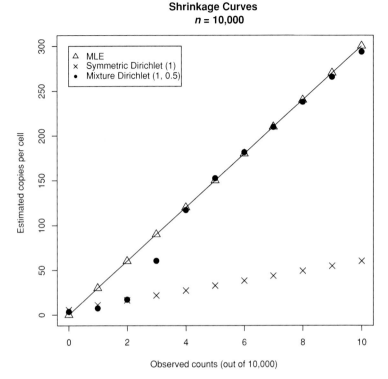

Fig. 13.1. Shrinkage curves for Bayesian estimators using symmetric and mixture Dirichlet priors for SAGE data with $n = 10,000$ and $k = 44,984$. The shrinkage plots plot the Bayesian posterior mean estimates versus the observed counts to demonstrate their shrinkage profiles relative to the MLE, given by the line. The hyperparameters of the mixture Dirichlet are $\theta_S = 0.5$ and $\theta_A = 1.0$, with $P = 0.005$ and a Uniform prior for π^*. The hyperparameter for the symmetric Dirichlet is $\theta = 1.0$. This plot only gives the shrinkage plot for observed counts from 0 to 10. If it were extended to include larger counts, the mixture Dirichlet would remain relatively close to the MLE line, while the symmetric Dirichlet would continue on its linear course, moving further away from the MLE.

we would like more shrinkage for scarce tags, we recommend making $\theta_S > \theta_A$. However, making θ_A too small will have the side effect of making the boundary between scarce and abundant species too sharp, which can hinder the efficiency of the shrinkage estimator. We have found that $\theta_S = 1$ and $\theta_A = 0.5$ have worked well in the examples we have tried. The hyperparameter P has a strong influence on the location of the boundary between scarcity and abundance. We have found that values of P between 0.005 and 0.03 seem to work well in practice, with P larger as n is larger.

13.5 Implementation Details

With the mixture Dirichlet prior, there is no closed form expression for the posterior distribution of $\underline{\pi}$ that would allow efficient random variate generation. The following Markov chain Monte Carlo (MCMC) procedure can be used to obtain posterior samples from this distribution.

(i) For $i = 1, \ldots, k$, sample λ_i from Bernoulli(α_i), with $\alpha_i = Pr(\lambda_i = 1 | \lambda_{(-i)}, \underline{X}, P)$, and $\lambda_{(-i)}$ is the set of all λ_j, $j = 1, \ldots, k$, except for the ith one. The formula for α_i is given below. Based on this sample, redefine the sets of indices $\mathcal{A} = \{i \colon \lambda_i = 1\}$ and $\mathcal{S} = \{i \colon \lambda_i = 0\}$.

(ii) Sample π^* from its complete conditional distribution, which is Beta($\alpha_{\pi^*} + n_A, \beta_{\pi^*} + n_S$).

(iii) Sample $\underline{q}_A$ and $\underline{q}_S$ from their complete conditional distributions, which are symmetric Dirichlets of dimension k_A and k_S and parameters $\{X_i + \theta_A, i \in \mathcal{A}\}$ and $\{X_i + \theta_S, i \in \mathcal{S}\}$, respectively.

(iv) If one wishes to update k_0, the number of "missing species," then sample k_0 from $f(k_0 | \underline{X}^*, \underline{\lambda}, \theta_S, P)$ using a Metropolis step, where $\underline{X}^*$ is the vector containing all $X_i > 0$ from our sample. Details for this step are given below.

Given these posterior samples, then, posterior samples of π_i are constructed by $\pi_i = \{q_i \pi^*\}^{\lambda_i} \{q_i(1 - \pi^*)\}^{(1-\lambda_i)}$.

In step (i), the probability $\alpha_i = O_i/(O_i + 1)$, where O_i is the conditional posterior odds that tag i is abundant, which is the product of the prior odds $P/(1 - P)$ and the conditional Bayes Factor BF_i, given by

$$BF_i = \left\{ \frac{\Gamma(n_{A(-i)} + \alpha_{\pi^*} + X_i)\Gamma(n_{S(-i)} + \beta_{\pi^*})}{\Gamma(n_{A(-i)} + \alpha_{\pi^*})\Gamma(n_{S(-i)} + \beta_{\pi^*} + X_i)} \right\} \tag{13.1}$$

$$\times \left\{ \frac{\Gamma(n_{A(-i)} + k_{A(-i)}\theta_A)\Gamma(n_{S(-i)} + k_{S(-i)}\theta_S + X_i + \theta_S)}{\Gamma(n_{A(-i)} + k_{A(-i)}\theta_A + X_i + \theta_A)\Gamma(n_{S(-i)} + k_{S(-i)}\theta_S)} \right\}$$

$$\times \left\{ \frac{\Gamma(k_{A(-i)}\theta_A + \theta_A)\Gamma(k_{S(-i)}\theta_S)}{\Gamma(k_{A(-i)}\theta_A)\Gamma(k_{S(-i)}\theta_S + \theta_S)} \right\} \left\{ \frac{\Gamma(\theta_A + X_i)\Gamma(\theta_S)}{\Gamma(\theta_A)\Gamma(\theta_S + X_i)} \right\}.$$

$\Gamma(x) = \int_0^\infty \exp(-u)u^{x-1} \, du$ is the Gamma function, $k_{A(-i)} = \sum_{j \neq i} \lambda_i$ and $k_{S(-i)} = \sum_{j \neq i}(1 - \lambda_i)$ are the number of abundant and scarce tags, leaving out species i, and $n_{A(-i)} = \sum_{j \neq i} X_i \lambda_i$ and $n_{S(-i)} = \sum_{j \neq i} X_i(1 - \lambda_i)$ are the total abundant and scarce counts, again leaving out species i. The first and second factors (in curly braces) arise from two Dirichlet multinomial distributions for the observed tag counts in $\mathcal{A}$ and $\mathcal{S}$. The third and fourth factors arise from a Beta-binomial distribution for k_A and k_S. Note that this expression differs from the expression (3) in Morris, Baggerly, and Coombes (2003), which contains typographical errors.

In step (iv), to update k_0, we generate a proposal value $k'_0 \sim N(k_0, \sigma_{k_0})$ for some chosen proposal standard deviation σ_{k_0}. We accept this new proposal with probability $\min(1, \gamma)$, given by

$$\gamma = \frac{\Gamma\{(k_S^* + k'_0)\theta_S\}\Gamma\{n_S + (k_S^* + k'_0)\theta_S\}}{\Gamma\{(k_S^* + k_0)\theta_S\}\Gamma\{n_S + (k_S^* + k_0)\theta_S\}\}} \tag{13.2}$$

$$\times \frac{\Gamma(k_S^* + k'_0 + 1)\Gamma(k'_0 + 1)k'_0}{\Gamma(k_S^* + k_0 + 1)\Gamma(k_0 + 1)k_0} (1 - P)^{k'_0 - k_0},$$

where $k_S^* = \sum_{i=1}^{k^*}(1 - \lambda_i)$. The first two terms on the second line come from the fact that the generalized multinomial distribution must be used when the number of zero-class categories are unknown, which includes an extra combinatoric term into the likelihood (see Boender and Kan 1987). In updating k_0, we assume that all missing species are scarce, that is, $\lambda_i = 0$ for all i: $X_i = 0$.

13.6 Simulation Study

In Morris, Baggerly, and Coombes (2003), a simulation study was performed to compare the relative performance of four estimators in estimating the relative frequencies of mRNA transcripts in SAGE: the MLE, a Bayesian estimator with symmetric Dirichlet prior, a Bayesian estimator with the mixture Dirichlet prior, and an alternative empirical Bayes-based shrinkage estimator from Good (1953).

13.6.1 Description of Simulation

The simulation was based on a true set of relative frequencies π obtained by pooling together the observed counts from six SAGE libraries from breast cancer tissue in a study at M.D. Anderson Cancer Center. All totaled, these data consist of 495,947 sequenced tags, with $k = 44,984$ unique tags, assumed to represent different mRNA species. There were 684 (1.5%) of the tags with relative frequencies greater than 50 copies per cell, accounting for 41% of the total mRNA mass. With such a large number of sequenced tags, our hope is that the set of observed relative frequencies from this pooled sample is a reasonable approximation for the distribution of true relative frequencies of mRNA transcripts in a biological tissue sample.

Simulations were performed with SAGE sample sizes of $n = 10,000$ and $n = 50,000$ transcripts. For each, 100 samples of size n were randomly generated from a multinomial population with relative frequencies $\underline{\pi}$. For each sample, $\underline{\pi}$ was estimated using various estimators: (1) maximum likelihood and Bayesian posterior means using the (2) symmetric Dirichlet prior with $\theta = 1$, and (3) the mixture Dirichlet prior with $\theta_S = 0.5$ and $\theta_A = 1.0$, and (4) a shrinkage estimator described by Good (1953), and attributed to Turing. This estimator is empirical Bayes and involves substituting a smoothed histogram of the observed counts for the histogram of true counts. For the mixture Dirichlet, $P = 0.005$ was used for the $n = 10,000$ simulation, and $P = 0.01$ was used for the $n = 50,000$ simulations. The total number of mRNA transcripts k was assumed known at 44,984, and π^* was given a Uniform prior. The estimates were based on 2,000 MCMC iterations obtained after a burn-in of 100.

The squared error loss for each of the three estimators was computed for each of the $k = 44,984$ species in each data set. The squared error loss for species i in data set j, SE_{ij}, is given by $(\widehat{\pi}_{ij} - \pi_i)^2$. From this, the mean square error for each species i was computed as $MSE_i = 100^{-1} \sum_{j=1}^{100} SE_{ij}$. These measures compared the performance for each individual species over repeated sampling. Overall performance averaging over species was assessed using integrated mean square error, $IMSE = \sum_{i=1}^{k} MSE_i$. In order to compare estimators for each given data set, the integrated square error for each sample j was computed as $ISE_j = \sum_{i=1}^{k} SE_{ij}$. All these summary measures were rescaled by a factor of 10^7 for readability.

13.6.2 Results

Figure 13.2 summarizes the simulation results for the $n = 10,000$ and $n = 50,000$ simulations. For each simulation, the relative efficiency of the three estimators to the MLE for each species is plotted against the true relative abundance. The relative efficiency for species i for estimator l is given by $RE_{il} = MSE_{i,\text{MLE}}/MSE_{il}$. To make the plot more readable, the relative efficiencies for species with similar true abundances were averaged together and plotted as a single circle, with the size of the circle made proportional to the log of the number of species averaged at that abundance.

First, consider the performance of the symmetric Dirichlet. For both sample sizes, the estimator was more efficient than the MLE for scarce tags, but performed increasingly poorly for more abundant tags, with the relative efficiency close to zero for the most abundant ones. The IMSE for $n = 10,000$ and $n = 50,000$ were 4,489 and 1,546, respectively, versus 995 and 201 for the MLE. This was what we expected based on our discussion in Section 13.3.2.

For $n = 10,000$, the mixture Dirichlet estimator showed efficiency improvements of more than 35% over the MLE based on IMSE (IMSE = 995 for MLE

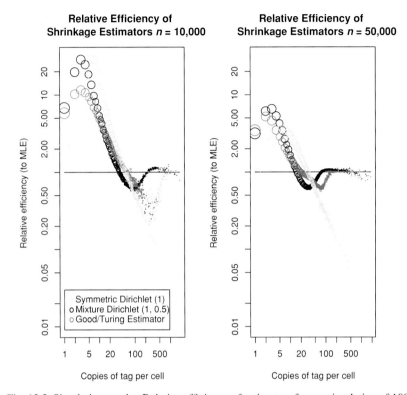

Fig. 13.2. Simulation results. Relative efficiency of estimators from a simulation of 100 multinomial samples of size 10,000 and 50,000 taken from a SAGE-like population. The horizontal axis consists of true relative frequencies multiplied by 300,000 to represent number of copies per cell containing 300,000 total mRNA transcripts. To aid presentation, the results for unique tags with like true relative frequencies have been combined, and the size of each plotted circle made proportional to the log(number of unique tags) with that true relative frequency.

vs. 643 for mixture Dirichlet). Efficiency gains of this order were seen for every one of the 100 simulated data sets, as measured by ISE. For the scarce tags (0–50 copies per cell), the mixture method was more efficient with RE of up to 25. These scarce tags account for 98.4% of the total number of unique tags. In the region of 200–1,000 copies per cell (0.37% of total tags), its performance was essentially equivalent to the MLE. For an intermediate range (50–200 copies per cell, 1.2% of tags) and for the most abundant tags (>1,000 copies per cell, 0.03% of tags), the mixture method was outperformed by the MLE, with minimum RE near 0.60. Turing's estimator had identical IMSE to the mixture Dirichlet (643), with slightly extended regions of improved efficiency

(0–60 copies per cell) and reduced efficiency (60–500 copies per cell) within the parameter space.

For $n = 50,000$, the mixture Dirichlet again had smaller IMSE than the MLE (166 vs. 201), outperforming the MLE for scarce tags (0–15 copies per cell, 93.5% of total), with RE of up to 6, with less efficiency than the MLE for an intermediate range (15–50 copies per cell, 4.9% of total), and equivalent for the abundant tags. The magnitude of improvement for scarce tags was again larger than the efficiency loss in the intermediate range (RE > 0.50). Turing's estimator had a slightly smaller IMSE (160) than the mixture Dirichlet, and again had extended regions of improved efficiency (0–20 copies per cell) and reduced efficiency (20–150 copies per cell) within the parameter space.

13.7 Conclusion

We have introduced a new method for estimating the relative abundance profiles of SAGE tags that explicitly takes into account the skewed nature of the data and as a result can have efficiency advantages over the MLE. Its key benefit is that the nonlinear shrinkage profile imposed by our prior helps correct for some of the sampling limitations in the data. Other methods could be constructed that yield nonlinear shrinkage profiles, and would likely experience similar types of efficiency gains (and tradeoffs) as our method.

Turing's estimator cited in Good (1953) had similar performance to ours, although it is not model-based. Blades et al. (in press) propose a mixture model for SAGE data that partitions the data into scarce and abundant tags based on whether they belong to the linear or noise portions of a log(number of tags) vs. log(frequency of tags) plot. The nonlinear shrinkage profile inherent in their method results in more shrinkage for intermediate and abundant tags than ours, with shrinkage for tags with observed counts into the 10's and 100's.

The fact that our method flows naturally from a fully specified coherent probability model gives it several inferential advantages over other more ad hoc methods. First, we obtain posterior samples from the joint distribution of all tags' expression levels, from which any inference, univariate or multivariate, can be obtained. For example, estimates, posterior intervals, density estimates, and Bayesian hypothesis tests are available for any quantities derivable from the relative frequencies for any set of tags, including fold-change differences. The efficiency advantages seen in estimation should translate to inferential procedures with better properties. For example, fold-change assessments involving species with very small counts in one group should be more accurate using inferential procedures based on the shrinkage estimator introduced here.

Another advantage of this method is that it can give an estimate of k_0, the number of missing species, and thus can estimate k, the total number of unique mRNA transcripts expressed in the biological sample. In that case, it is important to first apply a method to correct likely sequencing errors before applying the procedure described in this chapter, for example the procedures described by Colinge and Feger (2001) or Blades, Parmigiani, and Velculescu (in press). We believe these estimates of k should be taken with a grain of salt, however, since they are still based on a severely oversimplified model for the distribution of the π_i across species, consisting of a mixture of 2 symmetric Dirichlets. It would be interesting to consider other more flexible prior distributions for $\underline{\pi}$ that do an even better job of accommodating the heterogeneity seen in these expression data. This would likely lead to even better shrinkage estimators for $\underline{\pi}$ as well as improved estimates of the number of mRNA species present in the sample, k.

Acknowledgment

This work was partially supported by a grant from the National Cancer Institute (CA-107304).

Bibliography

Blades N., Kern, S., Jones, J., and Parmigiani, G. (2003). Denoising SAGE libraries: A mixture model approach.

Blades, N., Parmigiani, G., and Velculescu, V. (2003). Error estimation in SAGE libraries.

Boender, C. G. E. and Kan, A. H. G. R. (1987). A multinomial Bayesian approach to the estimation of population and vocabulary size. *Biometrika* **74**, 849–856.

Chipman, H. A., Kolaczyk, E. D., and McCulloch, R. E. (1997). Adaptive Bayesian wavelet shrinkage. *Journal of the American Statistical Association*, **92**, 1413–1421.

Colinge, J. and Feger, G. (2001). Detecting the impact of sequencing errors on SAGE data. *Bioinformatics* **17**(9), 840–842.

Good, I. J. (1953). The population frequencies of species and the estimation of population parameters. *Biometrika* **40**, 237–264.

Jeffreys, H. (1961). *Theory of Probability*, 3rd ed. Oxford: Clarendon Press.

Morris, J. S., Baggerly, K. A., and Coombes, K. R. (2003). Bayesian shrinkage estimators of the relative abundance of mRNA transcripts using SAGE. *Biometrics* **59**, 476–486.

Velculescu, V. E., et al. (1999). Analysis of human transcriptomes. *Nature Genetics* **23**, 387–388.

Vidakovic, B. (1998). Nonlinear wavelet shrinkage with Bayes rules and Bayes factors. *Journal of the American Statistical Association* **93**, 173–179.

14

Analysis of Mass Spectrometry Data Using Bayesian Wavelet-Based Functional Mixed Models

JEFFREY S. MORRIS

The University of Texas M.D. Anderson Cancer Center

PHILIP J. BROWN

University of Kent

KEITH A. BAGGERLY AND KEVIN R. COOMBES

The University of Texas M.D. Anderson Cancer Center

Abstract

In this chapter, we demonstrate how to analyze MALDI-TOF/SELDI-TOF mass spectrometry data using the wavelet-based functional mixed model introduced by J. S. Morris and R. J. Carroll (wavelet-based functional mixed models. *Journal of the Royal Statistical Society, Series B*, in 2006, which generalizes the linear mixed model to the case of functional data. This approach models each spectrum as a function, and is very general, accommodating a broad class of experimental designs and allowing one to model nonparametric functional effects for various factors, which can be conditions of interest (e.g., cancer/normal) or experimental factors (blocking factors). Inference on these functional effects allows us to identify protein peaks related to various outcomes of interest, including dichotomous outcomes, categorical outcomes, continuous outcomes, and any interactions among factors. Functional random effects make it possible to account for correlation between spectra from the same individual or block in a flexible manner. After fitting this model using Markov chain Monte Carlo, the output can be used to perform peak detection and identify the peaks that are related to factors of interest, while automatically adjusting for nonlinear block effects that are characteristic of these data. We apply this method to mass spectrometry data from a University of Texas M.D. Anderson Cancer Center experiment studying the serum proteome of mice injected with one of two cell lines in one of two organs. This methodology appears promising for the analysis of mass spectrometry proteomics data, and may have application for other types of proteomics data as well.

14.1 Introduction

MALDI-TOF is a mass-spectrometry-based proteomics method that yields spiky functional data, with peaks corresponding to proteins present in the biological sample. SELDI-TOF is a type of MALDI-TOF instrument in which the surface of the chips is specially coated to bind only certain types of proteins. An introduction to these technologies can be found in Chapter 1. In this chapter, we apply a new Bayesian method for modeling spiky functional data (Morris and Carroll in 2006) to analyze these data. This chapter reviews the material in Morris et al. (2006). This method yields posterior samples of fixed effect functions, which can be used to identify differentially expressed peaks while adjusting for potentially nonlinear block effects that are typical in these data.

In Section 14.2, we introduce our example data set and describe important preprocessing methods and standard analysis approaches in the existing litera- ture. In Section 14.3, we describe the functional mixed model upon which our method is based. We introduce wavelets and describe a Bayesian, wavelet-based method for fitting the functional mixed model in Section 14.4. We describe how to apply this method to MALDI-TOF data to detect peaks, identify differen- tially expressed peaks, and adjust for block effects, and we provide concluding discussions in Sections 14.5 and 14.6.

14.2 Overview of MALDI-TOF

14.2.1 Example

At the University of Texas M.D. Anderson Cancer Center, we conducted a SELDI-TOF experiment to study proteins in the serum of mice implanted with cancer tumors. The study included 16 nude mice. A tumor from one of two cancer cell lines was implanted into one of two organs (brain or lung) within each mouse. The cell lines were A375P, a human melanoma cancer cell line with low metastatic potential, and PC3MM2, a highly metastatic human prostate cancer cell line.

After a period of time, a blood sample was taken, from which the serum was extracted and then placed on a SELDI chip. This chip was run on the SELDI- TOF instrument twice, once using a low laser intensity and the other using a high laser intensity, yielding two spectra per mouse. The low laser intensity spectrum tends to measure the low molecular weight proteins more efficiently, while the higher laser intensity yields more precise measurements for proteins with higher molecular weights. This resulted in a total of 32 spectra, two per mouse. Since the measurements for the very low mass regions are unreliable, for this analysis we kept only the part of the spectrum between 2,000 and 14,000 Da, a range which contains roughly 24,000 observations per spectrum.

Our primary goals were to assess whether differential protein expression is more tightly coupled to the host organ site or to the donor cell line type, and to identify any protein peaks differentially expressed by organ site, by cell line, and/or their interaction. Typically, spectra from different laser intensities are analyzed separately. This is inefficient since spectra from both laser intensities contain information on the same proteins. We wanted to perform these analyses combining information across the two laser intensities, which required us to adjust for the systematic laser intensity effect and account for correlation between spectra obtained from the same mouse.

14.2.2 *Preprocessing MALDI-TOF/SELDI-TOF Data*

A number of preprocessing steps must be performed before modeling MALDI-TOF or SELDI-TOF data. It has been shown that inadequate or ineffective preprocessing can make it difficult to extract meaningful biological information from the data (Baggerly et al. 2003, 2004; Sorace and Zhan 2003). These steps include baseline correction, normalization, and denoising. The baseline, which is frequently seen in spectra, is a smooth underlying function that is thought to be largely due to a large cloud of particles striking the detector in the early part of the experiment and signal saturation (Malyarenko et al. 2005). This is an artifact that must be removed. Normalization refers to a constant multiplicative factor that is used to adjust for spectrum-specific variability, for example to adjust for different amounts of protein ionized and desorbed from the sample. Denoising is done to remove white noise from the spectrum that is largely due to electronic noise from the detector. In recent years, various methods have been proposed to deal with these issues. In the analysis presented in this chapter, we used the methods described by Coombes et al. (2005b). The first two columns of Figure 14.1 contain the raw spectrum and corresponding preprocessed spectrum for low- and high-intensity laser scans from one mouse, and demonstrate the effects of preprocessing. A more thorough discussion of these issues can be found in Chapter 1.

We used linear interpolation to downsample the observations within each spectrum to a 2,000-unit grid, equally spaced on the time scale. The third column in Figure 14.1 contains the interpolated spectra corresponding to the preprocessed spectra in the second column. Visual inspection of the raw and interpolated spectra revealed virtually no differences. The interpolation was performed for computational convenience. Further optimization of our code for fitting the functional mixed model described in this chapter will allow us to

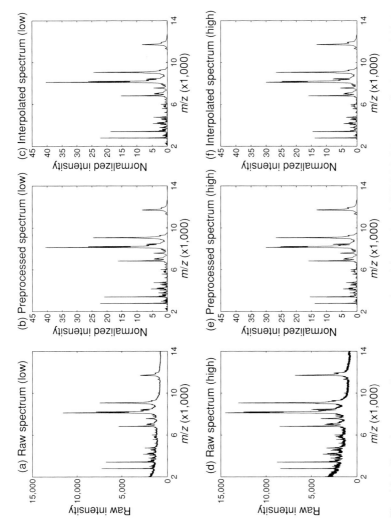

Fig. 14.1. Sample spectra. Raw, preprocessed, and interpolated SELDI-TOF spectra for low- and high-intensity laser scans for one mouse. Note that these spectra are characterized by many peaks corresponding to proteins present in the sample.

model the entire spectrum without downsampling. All analyses were performed on the interpolated, preprocessed spectra.

Some recent case studies (Baggerly et al. 2003, 2004; Conrads and Veenstra 2005; Coombes et al. 2005a; Hu et al. 2005; Sorace and Zhan 2003; Villanueva et al. 2005) have demonstrated that the MALDI-TOF instrument can be very sensitive to experimental conditions. Spectra can vary substantially for samples collected at different locations or stored under different conditions. Also, spectra obtained on different days can appear different from one another. These differences can be manifest in changes in both the intensities and locations of the peaks (i.e., both the y and x axes; see Figure 14.7). They are sometimes so large in magnitude that they swamp the biological differences that are of primary interest (Coombes et al. 2005a). Thus, it is important to take care in the experimental design phase to ensure that these factors are not counfounded with factors of interest, thus introducing systematic biases between the spectra from different treatment groups. Even when not confounded, it is still important to account for these block effects when modeling the spectra.

14.2.3 Peak Detection vs. Functional Modeling

It is common to use a two-step approach to analyze mass spectrometry data (Baggerly et al. 2003; Coombes et al. 2003, 2005b; Morris et al. 2005; Yasui et al. 2003). First, some type of feature detection algorithm is applied to identify peaks in the spectra, and then a quantification for each peak is obtained for each spectrum, for example, by taking the intensity at a local maximum or computing the area under the peak. Assuming there are p peaks and N spectra, this results in a $p \times N$ matrix of *protein expression levels* that is somewhat analogous to the matrix of mRNA expression levels obtained after preprocessing microarray data. Second, this matrix is analyzed using methods similar to those used for microarrays to identify peaks differentially expressed across experimental conditions.

This two-step approach is (i) intuitive since it focuses on the peaks, the most scientifically relevant features of the spectra, and (ii) convenient, since it can borrow from a wide array of available methods developed for microarrays. However, it also has disadvantages. First, since group comparisons are done only after peak detection, using this approach could result in not detecting important differences in low-intensity peaks if the peak detection algorithm is not sensitive enough. Important information can be lost in the reduction from the full spectrum to the set of detected peaks. Second, using this approach may not provide a natural way to account for block effects that affect the spectra in both the x and y axes.

Mass spectra can also be viewed as functional data. Let $y_i(x)$ denote the ith spectrum after preprocessing, but before peak detection. The observation $y_i(x)$ contains an intensity measurement from spectrum i associated with mass per unit charge value x. These functions are irregular, characterized by many peaks corresponding to proteins present in the tissue sample. An alternative to the two-step approach described above is to model the spectra as functions, in the spirit of functional data analysis (Ramsay and Silverman 1997). This is the approach we take in this chapter. Specifically, we describe a Bayesian functional modeling approach based on the functional mixed model, generalizing the linear mixed model equation for potentially irregular functional data. Since it involves modeling the entire spectrum, this method may detect significant group differences for very low abundance peaks that might be missed by peak detection algorithms. Further, by allowing a very flexible nonparametric representation of the fixed and random effects, this method can simultaneously model the functional effects of a number of factors, such as experimental factors of interest and nuisance factors related to the experimental design. These nonparametrically modeled effects can account for differences on both the x and y axes. In the subsequent sections, we introduce the functional mixed model, describe our method for fitting it, and demonstrate how to apply it to MALDI-TOF data.

14.3 Functional Mixed Models

Suppose we observe n functional profiles $Y_i(t)$, $i = 1, \ldots, n$, all defined on the compact set $\mathcal{T} \in \Re^1$. A functional mixed model for these profiles is given by

$$Y_i(t) = \sum_{j=1}^{p} X_{ij} B_j(t) + \sum_{k=1}^{m} Z_{ik} U_k(t) + E_i(t), \tag{14.1}$$

where X_{ij} are covariates, $B_j(t)$ are functional fixed effects, Z_{ik} are elements of the design matrix for functional random effects $U_k(t)$, and $E_i(t)$ are residual error processes. Here, we assume that $U_k(t)$ are independent and identically distributed (iid) mean-zero Gaussian processes with covariance surface $Q(t_1, t_2)$, and $E_i(t)$ are iid mean-zero Gaussian processes with covariance surface $S(t_1, t_2)$, with $U_k(t)$ and $E_i(t)$ assumed to be independent. The matrix Q is the covariance function for the random effect functions $k = 1, \ldots, m$, and S is the covariance function for the residual error processes for the n curves, after conditioning on the fixed and random effects. This model is a special case of the one discussed by Morris and Carroll (2006), and is also equivalent to the functional mixed model discussed by Guo (2002).

Suppose all observed profiles are sampled on the same equally spaced grid $\mathbf{t} = (t_h; h = 1, \ldots, T)$ of length T. Let Y be the $n \times T$ matrix containing the observed profiles on the grid, with each row containing one observed profile on the grid $\mathbf{t}$. A discrete, matrix-based version of this mixed model can be written as

$$Y = XB + ZU + E. \tag{14.2}$$

The matrix X is an $n \times p$ design matrix of covariates; B is a $p \times T$ matrix whose rows contain the corresponding *fixed effect functions* on the grid $\mathbf{t}$. B_{jh} denotes the effect of the covariate in column j of X on the response at time t_h. The matrix U is an $m \times T$ matrix whose rows contain *random effect functions* on the grid $\mathbf{t}$, and Z is the corresponding $n \times m$ design matrix. Each row of the $n \times T$ matrix E contains the residual error process for the corresponding observed profile. We assume that the rows of U are iid MVN($\mathbf{0}, Q$) and the rows of E are iid MVN($\mathbf{0}, S$), independent of U, with Q and S being $T \times T$ covariance matrices that are discrete evaluations of the covariance surfaces in (14.1) on the grid.

This model is very flexible and can be used to represent a wide range of functional data. The fixed effect functions may be group mean functions, interaction functions, or functional linear effects for continuous covariates, depending on the structure of the design matrix. The random effect functions provide a convenient mechanism for modeling between-function correlation, for example when multiple profiles are obtained from the same individual. The model places no restrictions on the form of the fixed or random effect functions. Since the forms of the covariance matrices Q and S are also left unspecified, it is necessary to place some type of structure on these matrices before fitting this model.

Guo (2002) introduced frequentist methodology for fitting this model, whereby the functions are represented as smoothing splines and the matrices Q and S are assumed to follow a particular fixed covariance structure based on the reproducing kernel for the spline. By using smoothing splines, one implicitly makes certain assumptions about the smoothness of the underlying functions that are not appropriate for the irregular, spiky functions encountered in MALDI-TOF. Also, the structures assumed for the Q and S matrices in that paper, while appropriate for very smooth data, are not flexible enough to accommodate the complex types of curve-to-curve deviations encountered for irregular spiky functional data like MALDI-TOF data. Morris and Carroll (2006) introduced a Bayesian wavelet-based method for fitting this model which uses wavelet shrinkage for regularization and allows more flexible structures for Q and S, and thus is better suited for the spiky functions encountered in MALDI-TOF data.

14.4 Wavelet-Based Functional Mixed Models

We give a brief overview of wavelets and wavelet regression, then describe the Bayesian wavelet-based approach for fitting the functional mixed model introduced by Morris and Carroll (2006), which extended the work of Morris et al. (2003). This method is described in detail by Morris and Carroll (in press), and applied to accelerometer data with an extension to partially missing functional data in the paper by Morris et al. (in press).

14.4.1 Wavelets and Wavelet Regression

Wavelets are families of basis functions that can be used to represent other functions, often very parsimoniously. A wavelet series approximation for a function $y(t)$ is given by

$$y(t) = \sum_k c_{J,k}\phi_{J,k}(t) + \sum_{j=1}^{J}\sum_k d_{j,k}\psi_{j,k}(t), \qquad (14.3)$$

where J is the number of scales, and k ranges from 1 to K_j, the number of coefficients at scale j. We define the scale index j such that higher j refers to a coarser level of detail. The functions $\phi_{J,k}(t)$ and $\psi_{j,k}(t)$ are father and mother wavelet basis functions that are dilations and translations of a father and mother wavelet function, $\phi(t)$ and $\psi(t)$, respectively, with $\phi_{j,k}(t) = 2^{-j/2}\phi(2^{-j}t - k)$ and $\psi_{j,k}(t) = 2^{-j/2}\psi(2^{-j}t - k)$. These wavelet coefficients comprise a location-scale decomposition of the curve, with j indexing the scales and k indexing the locations within each scale. The coefficients $c_{J,k}, d_{J,k}, \ldots, d_{1,k}$ are the *wavelet coefficients*. The $c_{J,k}$ are called the *smooth* coefficients, and represent smooth behavior of the function at coarse scale J, and the $d_{j,k}$ are called the *detail* coefficients, representing deviations of the function at scale j, where a smaller j corresponds to a finer scale. The wavelet coefficients at scale j essentially correspond to the differences of averages of 2^{j-1} time units, spaced 2^j units apart. In addition, by examining the phase properties of the wavelet bases, we can associate each wavelet coefficient on each scale with a specific set of time points.

Theoretically, each coefficient can be computed by taking the inner product of the function and the corresponding wavelet basis function, although in practice more efficient approaches are used. If the function is sampled on an equally spaced grid of length T, then the coefficients may be computed using a pyramid-based algorithm implementing the discrete wavelet transform (DWT) in just $O(T)$ operations. Applying the DWT to a row vector of observations $\mathbf{y}$ produces a row vector of wavelet coefficients $\mathbf{d} = (c_{J,1}, \ldots, c_{J,K_J}, d_{J,1}, \ldots, d_{J,K_J}, d_{J-1,1}, \ldots, d_{1,K_1})$. This transformation is a linear projection, so it may also be represented by matrix multiplication, $\mathbf{d} = \mathbf{y}W'$, with W' being the DWT projection matrix. Similarly, the inverse discrete wavelet transform (IDWT) may be used to project wavelet coefficients back into the data space, and can also be represented by matrix multiplication by the IDWT projection matrix W, the transpose of the DWT projection matrix. We use the method implemented in the Matlab Wavelet Toolbox (Misiti et al. 2000) for computing the DWT; other implementations can be used just as well.

Wavelets can be used to perform nonparametric regression using the following three-step procedure. Assume $y_i = f(t_i) + e_i$ for an equally spaced grid t_i. First, noisy data $\mathbf{y}$ are projected into the wavelet domain using the DWT, yielding empirical wavelet coefficients $\mathbf{d}$. The coefficients are then thresholded by setting to zero any coefficients smaller in magnitude than a specified threshold, and/or nonlinearly shrunken toward zero using one of a number of possible frequentist or Bayesian approaches. These result in estimates of the true wavelet coefficients, which would be the wavelet coefficients for the regression mean function f if there were no noise. Finally, these estimates are projected back to the original data domain using the IDWT, yielding a denoised nonparametric estimate of the true function. Since most signals may be represented by a small number of wavelet coefficients, yet white noise is distributed equally among all wavelet coefficients, this procedure yields denoised function estimates that tend to retain dominant local features of the function. We refer to this property as *adaptive regularization*, since the function is regularized (i.e., denoised or smoothed) in a way that adapts to the characteristics of the function. This property makes the procedure useful for modeling functions with many local features like peaks. References on wavelet regression can be found in the literature, in the work of Vidakovic (1999, Chapters 6 and 8), in Donoho and Johnstone (1995), Chipman, Kolaczyk, and McCulloch (1997), Vidakovic (1998), Abramovich, Sapatinas, and Silverman (1998), Clyde, Parmigiani, and Vidakovic (1998), and Clyde and George (2000).

14.4.2 Wavelet-Based Modeling of Functional Mixed Model

Morris and Carroll (2006) used a similar three-step procedure to fit the functional mixed model discussed in Section 14.3. First, the DWT is used to compute the wavelet coefficients for the N observed functions, effectively projecting these functions into the wavelet space. Second, a Markov chain Monte Carlo (MCMC) simulation is performed to obtain posterior samples of the model parameters in a wavelet-space version of the functional mixed model. Third, the IDWT is applied to the posterior samples, yielding posterior samples of the parameters in the data-space functional mixed model (14.2), which could be used to perform Bayesian inference. The wavelet-space modeling allows parsimonious yet flexible modeling of the covariance matrices Q and S, leading to computationally efficient code, and providing a natural mechanism for adaptively regularizing the random and fixed effect functions.

The projection in the first step is accomplished by applying the DWT to each row of Y, yielding a matrix of wavelet coefficients $D = YW'$, where W' is the DWT projection matrix. Row i of D contains the wavelet coefficients for profile i, with the columns corresponding to individual wavelet coefficients and double-indexed by scale j and location k. It is easy to show that the wavelet-space version of model (14.2) is

$$D = XB^* + ZU^* + E^*, \qquad (14.4)$$

where each row of $B^* = BW'$ contains the wavelet coefficients corresponding to one of the fixed effect functions, each row of $U^* = UW'$ contains the wavelet coefficients for a random effect function, and $E^* = EW'$ contains the wavelet-space residuals. The rows of U^* and E^* remain independent mean-zero Gaussian distributions, but with covariance matrices $Q^* = WQW'$ and $S^* = WSW'$.

Motivated by the whitening property of the wavelet transform, many wavelet regression methods in the single-function setting assume that the wavelet coefficients for a given function are mutually independent. In this context, this corresponds to making Q^* and S^* diagonal matrices. Allowing the variance components to differ across both wavelet scale j and location k yields $Q^* = \mathrm{diag}(q_{jk})$ and $S^* = \mathrm{diag}(s_{jk})$. This assumption reduces the dimensionality of Q and S from $T(T+1)/2$ to T, while still accommodating a reasonably wide range of nonstationary within-profile covariance structures for both the random effects and residual error processes. For example, it allows heteroscedasticity and differing degrees of smoothness for different regions of the curves, which are important characteristics of these matrices for MALDI-TOF spectra. Figure 1 in the paper by Morris and Carroll (2006) illustrates this point.

Next, an MCMC scheme is used to generate posterior samples for quantities of model (14.4). We use vague proper priors for the variance components and independent mixture priors for the elements of B^*. Specifically, the prior for B_{ijk}^*, the wavelet coefficient at scale j and location k for fixed effect function i, is a spike-slab prior given by $B_{ijk}^* = \gamma_{ijk}\mathrm{Normal}(0, \tau_{ij}) + (1 - \gamma_{ijk})\delta_0$, with

$\gamma_{ijk} \sim \text{Bernoulli}(\pi_{ij})$ and δ_0 being a point mass at zero. This prior is commonly used in Bayesian implementations of wavelet regression, including those by Clyde, Parmigiani, and Vidakovic (1998) and Abramovich, Sapatinas, and Silverman (1998). Use of this mixture prior causes the posterior mean estimates of the B_{ijk}^* to be nonlinearly shrunken toward zero, which results in adaptively regularized estimates of the fixed effect functions. The parameters τ_{ij} and π_{ij} are *regularization parameters* that determine the relative tradeoff of variance and bias in the nonparametric estimation. They may either be prespecified or estimated from the data using an empirical Bayes method; see the paper by Morris and Carroll (2006) for details.

There are three major steps in the MCMC scheme. Let Ω be the set of all covariance parameters indexing the matrices Q^* and S^*. The first step is a series of Gibbs steps to sample from the distribution of the fixed effect functions' wavelet coefficients conditional on the variance components and the data, $f(B^*|\Omega, D)$, which is a mixture of a point mass at zero and a Gaussian distribution. See the original paper (Morris and Carroll in press) for an expression for the mixing parameters, means, and variances of these distributions. The second step is to sample from the distribution of the variance components conditional on the fixed effects and data, $f(\Omega|B^*, D)$. We accomplish this using a series of random walk Metropolis-Hastings steps, one for every combination of (j, k). We estimate each proposal variance from the data by multiplying an estimate of the variance of the MLE by 1.5. An automatic procedure for selecting the proposal variances was necessary in order for our MCMC scheme to be automated and thus computationally feasible to implement in this very high-dimensional, highly parameterized setting. Note that we work with the marginalized likelihood with the random effects U^* integrated out when we update the fixed effects B^* and variance components Ω. This greatly improves the computational efficiency and convergence properties of the sampler over a simple Gibbs sampler that also conditions on the random effects. The stationary distribution for these first two steps is $f(B^*, \Omega|D)$. The third step is a series of Gibbs steps to update the random effects' wavelet coefficients from their complete conditional distribution, $f(U^*|B^*, \Omega, D)$, which is a Gaussian distribution. Note that this step is optional, and only necessary if one is specifically interested in estimating the random effect functions.

Posterior samples for each fixed effect function, $\{\mathbf{B}_i^{(g)}, g = 1, \ldots, G\}$, on the grid $\mathbf{t}$ are then obtained by applying the IDWT to the posterior samples of the corresponding complete set of wavelet coefficients $\mathbf{B}_i^{*(g)} = [B_{i11}^{*(g)}, \ldots, B_{iJK_J}^{*(g)}]$. This is similarly done for the random effect functions $\mathbf{U}_i$. If desired, posterior samples for the covariance matrices Q and S may also be computed using matrix multiplication $Q^{(g)} = W Q^{*(g)} W'$ and $S^{(g)} = W S^{*(g)} W'$, respectively.

Since $Q^{*(g)}$ and $S^{*(g)}$ are diagonal, this may be accomplished in an equivalent but more efficient manner by applying the two-dimensional version of the IDWT (2d-IDWT) to $Q^{*(g)}$ and $S^{*(g)}$ (Vannucci and Corradi 1999). These posterior samples of the quantities in model (14.2) may subsequently be used to perform any desired Bayesian inference. Code to fit the wavelet-based functional mixed model can be found online at the following URL: `http://biostatistics.mdanderson.org/Morris`.

14.5 Analyzing Mass Spectrometry Data Using Wavelet-Based Functional Mixed Models

In this section, we apply the Bayesian wavelet-based functional mixed model to analyze our example SELDI-TOF data set. Recall that this data set consisted of $N = 32$ spectra, $Y_i(t)$, $i = 1, \ldots, 32$, one low-intensity laser scan, and one high-intensity laser scan for each of 16 mice. Each mouse had one of two cancer cell lines (A375P or PC3MM2) injected in one of two organ sites (lung or brain). We were interested in identifying protein peaks differentially expressed between organs, between cell lines, and with significant interactions between any organ and cell line.

The functional mixed model we used to fit these spectra is given by

$$Y_i(t) = \sum_{j=0}^{4} X_{ij} B_j(t) + \sum_{k=1}^{16} Z_{ik} U_k(t) + E_i(t), \qquad (14.5)$$

where $X_{i0} = 1$ and corresponds to the overall mean spectrum $\beta_0(t)$, $X_{i1} = 1$ if the mouse was injected with the A375P cell line, -1 if PC3MM2, and corresponds to the cell line main effect function $\beta_1(t)$. Also, $X_{i2} = 1$ if the injection site was the lung and -1 if the injection site was the brain, and corresponds to the organ main effect function $\beta_2(t)$, while $X_{i3} = X_{i1} * X_{i2}$ and corresponds to the organ-by-cell line interaction function $\beta_3(t)$. Finally, we included a fixed effect function $\beta_4(t)$ to model the laser intensity effect, with corresponding covariate $X_{i4} = 1$ or -1 if the spectrum came from low- or high-intensity scans, respectively. We included random effects functions $U_i(t)$ for each mouse, $i = 1, \ldots, 16$, to model the correlation between spectra obtained from the same mouse, so $Z_{ik} = 1$ if and only if spectrum i came from mouse k.

We modeled the spectra on the time scale t because they were equally spaced on that scale, but plotted our results on the mass-per-unit-charge scale $(m/z, x)$, since that scale is biologically meaningful. In our wavelet-space modeling, we chose the Daubechies wavelet with vanishing 4th moments and performed the

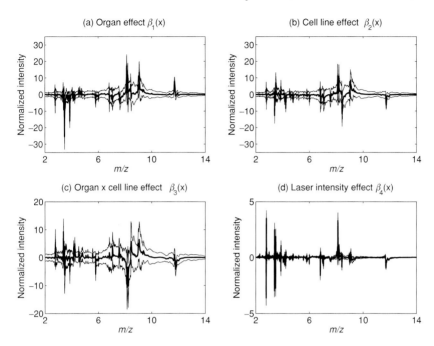

Fig. 14.2. Fixed effect curves. Posterior mean and 95% pointwise posterior credible bands for (a) organ main effect function, (b) cell line main effect function, (c) organ-by-cell-line interaction function, and (d) laser intensity effect function.

DWT down to $J = 11$ levels. We used a modified empirical Bayes procedure to estimate the shrinkage hyperparameters π_{ij} and τ_{ij}, $i = 1, \ldots, 5$, $j = 1, \ldots 10$, constraining $\tau \geq 10$ so there would be less bias in the estimation of peak heights, which we believed to be important in this context. We did almost no shrinkage ($\pi \approx 1$, $\tau = 1,000$) for wavelet level 11 or the scaling coefficients. After a burn-in of 1,000 iterations, we ran our MCMC scheme for a total of 20,000 iterations, keeping every 10th. The entire model fitting took 7 hours, 53 minutes in Matlab on a Windows 2000 Pentium IV 2.8 GHz machine with 2 GB RAM. Using random walk Metropolis transition probabilities, the acceptance probabilities for the roughly 2,000 sets of covariance parameters were all between 0.041 and 0.532, with median of 0.294, and 10th and 90th quantiles of 0.20 and 0.50.

Figure 14.2 contains the posterior means and 95% posterior credible bands for the organ and cell line main effect functions, the interaction function, and the laser intensity effect function. The interpretation of the organ main effect function $\beta_1(x)$, for example, is the difference between the mean spectra for lung- and brain-injected animals at m/z value x, after adjusting for the

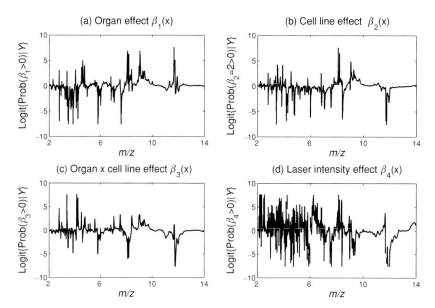

Fig. 14.3. Posterior probabilities. Logit transformed pointwise posterior probabilities of being greater than zero for (a) organ main effect function, (b) cell line main effect function, (c) organ-by-cell-line interaction function, and (d) laser intensity effect function.

functional effects of cell line, cell-line-by-organ interaction, and laser intensity. The spiky nature of these fixed effect functions indicates that differences in spectra between treatment groups are localized, and highlights the importance of using adaptive regularization methods with these data. Although difficult to see in these plots, there are a number of locations within the curves at which there is strong evidence of significant effects. These are evident in Figure 14.3, which contains the pointwise posterior probabilities of each fixed effect curve being greater than zero, $\mathrm{Prob}(\beta_j(x) > 0|\mathbf{Y})$. These significant regions are also evident if one zooms in on certain regions of the plots (e.g., see Figures 14.5 and 14.6).

14.5.1 Peak Detection

While it is not necessary to perform peak detection when using this functional analysis approach, it still may be useful to perform a peak-level analysis since the peaks are the biologically most relevant features of the spectra, and by restricting attention to the peaks, we can reduce the multiplicity problems inherent to performing pointwise inference on these curves. Morris et al. (2005) demonstrated that for MALDI-TOF data, it was possible to obtain more

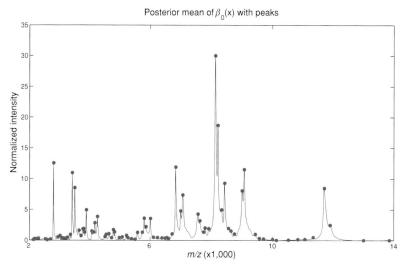

Fig. 14.4. Peak detection. Posterior mean for the overall mean spectrum, $\beta_0(t)$, with detected peaks indicated by the dots. A peak is defined to be a location for which its first difference and the first difference immediately preceding it are positive, and the first differences for the two locations immediately following it are negative. (See color plate. 14.4.)

sensitive and specific peak detection by performing the peak detection on the mean spectrum rather than on the individual spectra. In the present context, we can perform peak detection using the posterior mean estimate of the overall mean spectrum $\beta_0(t)$ and expect to see similar advantages. The adaptive regularization inherent to our estimation approach results in a natural denoising of this curve, reducing the number of spurious peaks detected.

In order to perform this peak detection, we applied the first difference operator $\triangledown$ to our regularized estimate of the mean spectrum $\Gamma_0(t) = \triangledown\beta_0(t) = \beta_0(t+1) - \beta_0(t)$. We considered a location t to be a *peak* if its first difference and the first difference immediately preceding it were positive ($\Gamma_0(t-1) > 0$ and $\Gamma_0(t) > 0$), and the first differences for the two locations immediately following it were negative ($\Gamma_0(t+1) < 0$ and $\Gamma_0(t+2) < 0$). This condition assured that this location was a local maximum, and the left and right slopes of the peak were monotone for at least two adjacent points.

Using this procedure, we found a total of 82 peaks out of the 2,000 observations within the spectrum. Figure 14.4 contains the posterior mean overall mean curve with peak locations indicated by dots. Based on visual inspection, this procedure appears to have done a reasonable job of identifying the peaks.

14.5.2 Identifying Peaks of Interest

We further investigated each fixed effect function at the m/z values corresponding to detected peaks. For each of the $j = 1, \ldots, 82$ peaks with locations t_j, and $i = 1, \ldots, 3$ comparisons of interest (organ main effect, cell line main effect, organ-by-cell-line interaction), we computed the minimum posterior probability for each fixed effect function to be greater than or less than zero, that is, $p_{ij} = \min[\Pr\{\beta_i(t_j) > 0 | D\}, \Pr\{\beta_i(t_j) < 0 | D\}]$. We determined a threshold ϕ below which a comparison was considered interesting and worthy of further investigation. To obtain ϕ, we first specified a small positive number α and sorted the p_{ij} from smallest to largest, $p_{(1)}, \ldots, p_{(246)}$. We defined ϕ to be $p_{(\delta)}$, where δ was the largest integer for which $\sum_{k=1}^{\delta}\{2p_{(k)} + (2G)^{-1}\} < \alpha$. Let G be the number of MCMC samples used to compute the posterior probabilities. The factor of 2 is included to adjust for the two-sided nature of the analysis, and the factor involving G adjusts for the limitation in precision for estimating p_{ij} that is due to the number of MCMC samples run. This approach provides a somewhat ad hoc procedure for multiplicity adjustment. More formal approaches will be investigated in future research. Note that for our example, the peaks flagged as significant are very strongly significant, so would likely be flagged by other procedures for adjusting for multiplicities.

We applied this procedure to our data using $\alpha = 0.01$, and found that $\phi = 0.0033$, and $\delta = 18$ of the p_{ij} were flagged as interesting. These 18 p_{ij} were from a total of 12 peaks. Table 14.1 lists the m/z values for these peaks, along with the p_{ij} values and a description of the interesting effect. Whenever an interaction effect was found to be interesting, the main effects for that peak were not considered. Out of these 12 peaks, we found 4 with organ main effects, 3 with cell-line main effects, 1 with both organ and cell-line main effects, and 4 associated with the organ-by-cell-line interaction effects.

We attempted to find information about the possible identity of the flagged peaks by running the estimated m/z values of the corresponding peaks through TagIdent, a searchable database (available at `http://us.exp asy.org/tools/tagident.html`) that contains the molecular masses and pH for proteins observed in various species. We searched for proteins emanating from both the source (human) and the host (mouse) whose molecular masses were within the estimated mass accuracy (0.3%) of the SELDI instrument from the peak found. This only gives an educated guess at what the protein identity of the peak could be; it would be necessary to perform an additional MS/MS experiment in order to definitively identify the peak. For illustration, we plotted posterior means and posterior pointwise credible intervals for the interesting effect functions in the neighborhood of the peaks at 3886.3, 5805.3, 7628.1,

Table 14.1. *Flagged Peaks from Proteomics Example*

Peak location	Effect type	p	Comment
3412.6	Interaction	<0.0005	PC3MM2>A375P for brain-injected only
3496.6	Organ	<0.0005	Only expressed in brain-injected mice
3886.3	Organ	<0.0005	Only expressed in brain-injected mice
4168.2	Interaction	0.0005	PC3MM2>A375P in brain-injected only
4252.1	Interaction	<0.0005	PC3MM2>A375P in brain-injected only
4814.2	Cell line	0.0030	PC3MM2>A375P
5805.3	Interaction	<0.0005	Brain>lung only for mice with A375P cell line
6015.2	Cell line	<0.0005	PC3MM2>A375P
7628.1	Organ	0.0015	Only expressed in brain-injected mice
8438.1	Cell line	0.0015	PC3MM2>A375P
9074	Organ	0.0020	Lung>brain
11721.0	Organ	<0.0005	Lung>brain
11721.0	Cell line	<0.0005	PC3MM2>A375P

Note: Location of peak (in Daltons per coulomb) is given, along with which effect was deemed significant, the associated posterior probability p, and a description of the effect.

and 11721.0 (Figures 14.5 and 14.6). In Figure 14.5(a), we see that the peak at 3886.3 is expressed more highly in brain-injected mice than in lung-injected mice. In fact, our observation of the posterior mean curves for the 4 organ-by-cell-line group mean curves ($\beta_0(x) + \beta_1(x) + \beta_2(x) + \beta_3(x)$, $\beta_0(x) + \beta_1(x) - \beta_2(x) - \beta_3(x)$, $\beta_0(x) - \beta_1(x) + \beta_2(x) - \beta_3(x)$, and $\beta_0(x) - \beta_1(x) - \beta_2(x) + \beta_3(x)$)) indicates that this peak does not even appear to be present in the serum proteomic profile of lung-injected mice; it is only in brain-injected mice. Using TagIdent, we found that this peak closely matched calcitonin gene-related peptide II precursor (CGRP-II, 3882.34 Da, pH 5.41). This peptide is in the mouse proteome, dilates blood vessels in the brain, and has been observed to be abundant in the central nervous system. This result may represent an important host response to the implanted tumor.

Figures 14.5(c) and (d) contain the posterior mean interaction main effect curve $\beta_3(x)$ and group mean functions, respectively, in the neighborhood of the peak at 5805.3 Da. The measurement corresponding to this protein is higher in brain-injected mice than in lung-injected mice only for those mice given cell line A375P. There is a protein in the human proteome, KiSS-16, with molecular weight of 5794.7 Da that is known to be highly expressed in metastasis-suppressed chromosome 6 melanoma hybrids.

Figures 14.6(a) and (b) contain the posterior mean organ main effect curve $\beta_1(x)$ and group mean functions, respectively, in the neighborhood of the peak

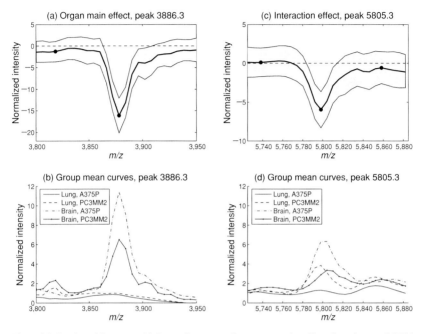

Fig. 14.5. Peaks of Interest. (a) Posterior mean for organ main effect function and 95% pointwise posterior credible bands for the peak near 3886.3. (b) Posterior mean for mean functions for each organ-by-cell-line group near the peak at 3886.3. (c) Posterior mean organ-by-cell-line interaction effect function and 95% pointwise posterior credible bands near the peak at 5805.3. (d) Posterior mean for mean functions for each organ-by-cell-line group near the peak at 5805.3.

at 7628.1 Da. This protein is only present in spectra from brain-injected mice. The protein neurogranin in the human proteome, with a molecular weight of 7618.47 Da, is active in synaptic development and remodeling in the brain.

Figures 14.6(c) and 14.6(d) contain the posterior mean and 95% posterior pointwise credible intervals for the organ and cell line main effects curves $\beta_1(x)$ and $\beta_2(x)$ in a neighborhood around the peak at 11721.0 Da, and Figure 14.6(e) contains the corresponding group mean curves. This protein has higher expression in the metastatic cell line PC3MM2 than the nonmetastatic cell line A375P, and in lung-injected mice than in brain-injected mice. There is a protein MTS1 in the mouse proteome with molecular mass 11721.4 Da that is known to be specifically expressed in different metastatic cells (Tulchinsky et al. 1990). A similar protein with a molecular mass of 11728.5 Da is present in the human proteome.

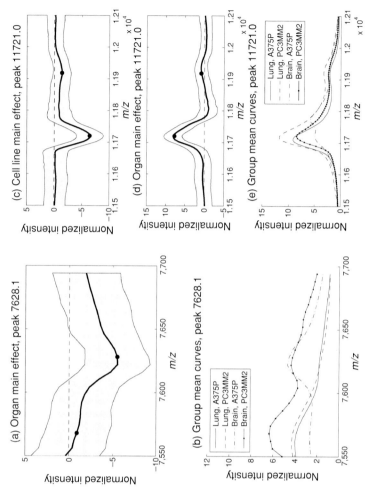

Fig. 14.6. Peaks of Interest. (a) Posterior mean for organ main effect function and 95% pointwise posterior credible bands for the peak near 7628.1. (b) Posterior mean for mean functions for each organ-by-cell-line group near the peak at 7628.1. (c) and (d) Posterior mean cell line and organ main effect functions, respectively, and 95% pointwise posterior credible bands near the peak at 11721.0. (e) Posterior mean for mean functions for each organ-by-cell-line group near the peak at 11721.0.

287

14.5.3 Nonparametric Modeling of Block Effects

The analysis described above identified a number of interesting peaks. Our ability to detect these differences was aided by the fact that we were able to combine information from both the low- and high-intensity laser spectra to perform our analysis, giving us greater power to detect differences. Recall that it is typical to analyze spectra with different laser intensities separately because there are systematic differences between the spectra, but this is inefficient since spectra from both laser intensities contain information about the same protein peaks.

Our inclusion of a nonparametric functional laser intensity effect $\beta_4(x)$ in the modeling allowed us to combine these in a common model. The interpretation of this effect is the difference between the mean spectrum from the two laser intensities, after adjusting for the other functional effects in the model. The flexibility of the nonparametric modeling allows this factor to adjust for systematic differences in both the x and y axes. Figure 14.7 illustrates this point. Figure 14.7(a) contains the posterior mean laser effect function $\beta_4(x)$ and 95% posterior bounds in the region of two peaks at 3412.6 and 3496.6, while Figure 14.7(b) contains the posterior mean for the overall mean spectrum $\beta_0(x)$ in the same region. The pulse-like characteristics in the laser effect curve near the peak location demonstrate that the inclusion of this effect in the model adjusts for a slight misalignment in the peaks across the different laser intensity blocks, that is, differences in the x-axis. The mean curves for low-intensity laser $\beta_0(x) + \beta_4(x)$ and high-intensity laser $\beta_0(x) - \beta_4(x)$ (Figure 14.7(b)) demonstrate that the peak at 3412.6 in the overall mean curve is at a slightly higher m/z value for the low-intensity spectra and slightly lower m/z value for the high-intensity spectra. Figures 14.7(c) and 14.7(d) contain $\beta_4(x)$ and $\beta_0(x)$ in the neighborhood of the peak at 11721.0, and demonstrate that the nonparametric laser effect can also adjust for an additive offset in the mean peak intensity across blocks, that is, the y-axis.

This same strategy can be used in other MALDI-TOF data sets to adjust for systematic effects when spectra are run in batches, at different laboratories, and when samples are obtained from different locations, as long as these factors are not completely confounded with one of the other covariates of interest. This is important, since MALDI-TOF instruments are quite sensitive to these factors, and it is necessary to deal successfully with them in order to obtain reproducible results.

14.6 Conclusion

We have demonstrated how to use the newly developed Bayesian wavelet-based functional mixed model to model MALDI-TOF proteomics data. This method

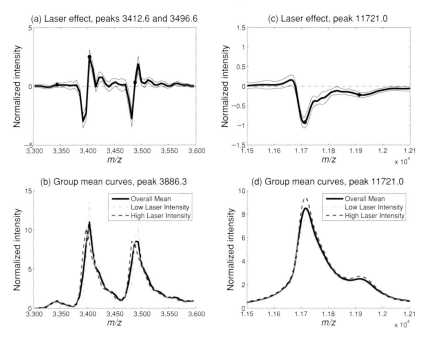

Fig. 14.7. Laser intensity effect. Posterior mean laser intensity effect near peaks of interest at (a) 3412.6 and 3496.6 and (c) 11721, along with 95% pointwise posterior credible bands. The red dots indicate the locations of peaks detected in the fitted mean spectrum. Panels (b) and (d) contain the corresponding fitted posterior mean curves for the overall mean and the laser intensity-specific mean spectra in the same two regions. Note that the nonparametrically estimated laser intensity effects are able to adjust for both shifts in location (x-axis, see (a) and (b)), and shifts in intensity (y-axis, see (c) and (d)). (See color plate 14.7.)

appears well suited to this context, for several reasons: the functional mixed model is very flexible; it is able to simultaneously model nonparametric functional effects of many covariates simultaneously, both factors of interest and nuisance factors such as block effects. Further, the random effect functions can be used to model correlation structure among spectra that might be induced by the experimental design. The wavelet-based modeling approach works well for modeling functional data with many local features like MALDI-TOF peaks since it results in adaptive regularization of the fixed effect functions, avoids attenuation of the effects at the peaks, and is reasonably flexible in modeling the between-curve covariance structures, accomodating autocovariance structures induced by peaks and heteroscedasticity allowing different between-spectrum variances for different peaks. Given the posterior samples produced by this method, we were able to perform peak detection and flag a number of peaks as interesting and worthy of future investigation. The efficiency of our analysis was increased because the random effect functions and a nonparametric laser-intensity-effect function allowed us to combine information across spectra obtained from different laser intensities. This strategy has more general application for calibrating spectra so data can be combined across different laboratories or batches. Our approach may also be useful for analyzing data from other proteomic platforms that generate functional data, and may be extended to model functional data on two-dimensional domains, including data from two-dimensional gel electrophoresis and liquid chromatography mass spectrometry.

Acknowledgment

This work was partially supported by a grant from the National Cancer Institute (CA-107304).

References

Abramovich, F., Sapatinas, T., and Silverman, B. W. (1998). Wavelet thresholding via a Bayesian approach. *Journal of the Royal Statistical Society, Series B*, 60, 725–749.

Baggerly, K. A., Morris, J. S., and Coombes, K. R. (2004). Reproducibility of SELDI Mass Spectrometry Patterns in Serum: Comparing Proteomic Data Sets from Different Experiments. *Bioinformatics*, 20(5): 777–785.

Baggerly, K. A., Morris, J. S., Wang, J., Gold, D., Xiao, L. C., and Coombes, K. R. (2003). A comprehensive approach to the analysis of matrix-assisted laser desorption/ionization-time of flight proteomics spectra from serum samples. *Proteomics*, 3(9), 1667–1672.

Chipman, H. A., Kolaczyk, E. D., and McCulloch, R. E. (1997). Adaptive Bayesian wavelet shrinkage. *Journal of the American Statistical Association*, 92, 1413–1421.

Clyde, M. and George, E. I. (2000). Flexible empirical Bayes estimation for wavelets. *Journal of the Royal Statistical Society, Series B*, 60, 681–698.

Clyde, M., Parmigiani, G., and Vidakovic, B. (1998). Multiple shrinkage and subset selection in wavelets. *Biometrika*, 85, 391–401.

Conrads, T. P. and Veenstra, T. D. (2005). What have we learned from proteomic studies of serum? *Expert Review of Proteomics*, 2(3), 279–281.

Coombes, K. R., Fritsche, H. A., Jr., Clarke, C., Cheng, J. N., Baggerly, K. A., Morris, J. S., Xiao, L. C., Hung, M. C., and Kuerer, H. M. (2003). Quality control and peak finding for proteomics data collected from nipple aspirate fluid using surface enhanced laser desorption and ionization. *Clinical Chemistry*, 49(10), 1615–1623.

Coombes, K. R., Morris J. S., Hu J., Edmonson S. R., and Baggerly K. A. , (2005a). Serum proteomics profiling: A young technology begins to mature. *Nature Biotechnology*, 23(3), 291–292.

Coombes K. R., Tsavachidis S., Morris J. S., Baggerly K. A., and Kobayashi R., (2005b). Improved peak detection and quantification of mass spectrometry data acquired from surface-enhanced laser desorption and ionization by denoising spectra using the undecimated discrete wavelet transform. *Proteomics*, 5, 4107–4117.

Donoho, D. L. and Johnstone, I. M., (1995). Adapting to unknown smoothness via wavelet shrinkage. *Journal of the American Statistical Association*, 90, 1200–1224.

Guo, W. (2002) Functional mixed effects models. *Biometrics*, 58, 121–128.

Hu J., Coombes K. R., Morris J. S., and Baggerly K. A. (2005). The importance of experimental design in proteomic mass spectrometry experiments: Some cautionary tales. *Briefings in Genomics and Proteomics*, 3(4), 322–331.

Malyarenko D. I., Cooke W. E., Adam B. L., Gunjan M., Chen H., Tracy E. R., Trosset M. W., Sasinowski M., Semmes O. J., and Manos D. M. (2005). Enhancement of sensitivity and resolution of SELDI TOF-MS records for serum peptides using time series analysis techniques. *Clinical Chemistry*, 51(1), 65–74.

Misiti M., Misiti Y., Oppenheim G., and Poggi J. M. (2000). *Wavelet Toolbox for Use with Matlab: User's Guide*. Natick, MA: Mathworks, Inc.

Morris J. S., Arroyo C., Coull B., Ryan L. M., Herrick R., and Gortmaker S. L. (in press). Using wavelet-based functional mixed models to characterize population heterogeneity in accelerometer profiles: A case study. *Journal of the American Statistical Association*.

Morris J. S. and Carroll R. J. (2006). Wavelet-based functional mixed models. *Journal of the Royal Statistical Society, Series B*, 68(2), 179–199.

Morris J. S., Coombes K. R., Koomen J, Baggerly K. A., and Kobayashi R. (2005). Feature extraction and quantification for mass spectrometry data in biomedical applications using the mean spectrum. *Bioinformatics*, 21(9), 1764–1775.

Morris J. S., Vannucci M., Brown P. J., and Carroll R. J. (2003). Wavelet-based nonparametric modeling of hierarchical functions in colon carcinogenesis. *Journal of the American Statistical Association*, 98, 573–583.

Morris, J. S., Brown, P. J., Herrick, R. C., Baggerly, K. A., and Coombes, K. R. (2006). Bayesian Analysis of Mass Spectrometry Proteomics Data using Wavelet Based Functional Mixed Models. UT MD Anderson Cancer Center, Department of Biostatistics and Applied Mathematics, Working Papers Series, working paper 22. http://www.bepress.com/mdandersonbiostat/paper22.

Ramsay, J. O. and Silverman, B. W. (1997). *Functional Data Analysis*. New York: Springer.

Sorace JM and Zhan M (June 9, 2003). A data review and re-assessment of ovarian cancer serum proteomic profiling. *BMC Bioinformatics*, 4–24.

Tulchinsky, E. M., Grigorian, M. S., Ebralidze, A. K., Milshina, N. I., and Lukanidin, E. M. (1990). Structure of gene MTS1, transcribed in metastatic mouse tumor cells. *Gene*, 87(2), 219–223.

Vannucci, M. and Corradi, F. (1999). Covariance structure of wavelet coefficients: Theory and models in a Bayesian perspective. *Journal of the Royal Statistical Society, Series B*, 61, 971–986.

Vidakovic, B. (1998). Nonlinear wavelet shrinkage with Bayes rules and Bayes factors. *Journal of the American Statistical Association*, 93, 173–179.

Vidakovic, B. (1999). *Statistical Modeling by Wavelets*. New York: Wiley.

Villanueva, J., Philip, J., Chaparro, C. A., Li, Y., Toledo-Crow, R., DeNoyer, L., Fleisher, M., Robbins, R. J., and Tempst, P. (2005). Correcting common errors in identifying cancer-specific peptide signatures. *Journal of Proteome Research*, 4(4), 1060–1072.

Yasui, T., Pepe, M., Thompson, M. L., Adam, B. L., Wright, G. L., Jr., Qu, Y., Potter, J. D., Winget, M., Thornquist, M., and Feng, Z. (2003). A data-analytic strategy for protein biomarker discovery: Profiling of high-dimensional proteomic data for cancer detection. *Biostatistics*, 4(3), 449–463.

15

Nonparametric Models for Proteomic Peak Identification and Quantification

MERLISE A. CLYDE, LEANNA L. HOUSE,
AND ROBERT L. WOLPERT
Duke University

Abstract

We present model-based inference for proteomic peak identification and quantification from mass spectroscopy data, focusing on nonparametric Bayesian models. Using experimental data generated from MALDI-TOF mass spectroscopy (matrix-assisted laser desorption ionization time-of-flight) we model observed intensities in spectra with a hierarchical nonparametric model for expected intensity as a function of time-of-flight. We express the unknown intensity function as a sum of kernel functions, a natural choice of basis functions for modeling spectral peaks. We discuss how to place prior distributions on the unknown functions using Lévy random fields and describe posterior inference via a reversible jump Markov chain Monte Carlo algorithm.

15.1 Introduction

The advent of matrix-assisted laser desorption/ionization such time-of-flight (MALDI-TOF) mass spectroscopy and related SELDI-TOF (surface enhanced laser desorption/ionization) allows the simultaneous assay of thousands of proteins, and has transformed research in protein regulation underlying complex physiological processes. This technology provides the means to detect large proteins in a range of biological samples, from serum and urine to complex tissues, such as tumors and muscle. With appropriate statistical analysis, one may explore patterns of protein expression on a large scale in high-throughput studies without the need for prior knowledge of which proteins may be present (Baldwin et al., 2001; Diamandis, 2003; Martin and Nelson, 2001; Petricoin and Liotta, 2003; Petricoin et al., 2002). As such, it becomes a discovery tool, identifying proteins and pathways that are linked to a biological process. In

293

applications, tens to thousands of spectra may be collected, leading to massive volumes of data. Each spectrum contains on the order of tens of thousands of intensity measurements, with an unknown number of peaks representing proteins of specific mass-to-charge ratios.

The combined effects of heterogeneity in protein composition of samples and other complexities due to the biochemical/physical processes of the measurement procedures lead to many challenges in identifying proteins or biomarkers that differentiate subgroups. Several steps, involving low-level processing of the spectra, such as calibration, filtering of noise, baseline subtraction, normalization, and peak detection, are often carried out in separate stages in order to identify the location of peaks (representing proteins) and to quantify their abundance; inadequate or incorrect methods may introduce substantial biases or create more challenges for later stages of analysis, such as classification of subjects (Coombes et al., 2005). In this chapter, we describe nonparametric statistical models for spectra that permit simultaneous filtering of noise and removal of baseline trends in conjunction with peak identification, quantification, and, ultimately, classification.

15.2 Kernel Models for Spectra

We describe the model for a single spectrum, which may be either a raw spectrum or the average of spectra from several laser shots, individuals, etc. (Morris et al., 2005). The raw data consist of a time series of intensities of ions striking the detector at recorded time intervals (each clock tick is 4ns). The data in Figure 15.1 represent the average spectrum from 10 laser shots for a single serum sample. Typically, TOFs are calibrated using known samples to provide associated mass/charge values via a quadratic (or higher polynomial) transformation. Following Malyarenko et al. (2005), we prefer to develop the model for intensity as a function of TOF rather than with mass/charge. We denote the observed intensity measurement at observed TOF $t \in \mathbb{T} \equiv [t_o, t_n]$ as Y_t, with expected intensity $\mathsf{E}[Y_t]$ given by the function $f(t)$. Nonparametric models (such as wavelets) have been highly successful in representing the unknown expected intensity function $f(t)$ (Coombes et al., 2004; Morris et al., 2005), expressing it as a linear combination of basis functions. Rather than using basis functions generated from a wavelet, we express the mean intensity through a linear combination of kernel functions

$$f(t) = b(t) + \sum_{j=1}^{J} k(t; \tau_j, \omega_j)\gamma_j \qquad (15.1)$$

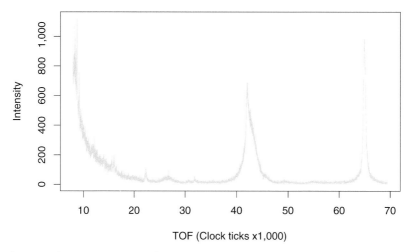

Fig. 15.1. The average spectrum from 10 laser shots for a single serum sample. The time axis denotes individual clock ticks with intensities recorded every 4 ns.

where $k(t; \tau_j, \omega_j)$ is proportional to a nonnegative density, such as a Gaussian or Cauchy kernel, and $b(t)$ represents the systematic background process.

The kernel model has several notable features that are attractive for modeling spectra. First, J, the number of terms in the expansion, is meaningful, representing the number of kernels (peaks) or proteins in the spectrum. As basis functions, the kernels also have an intuitive interpretation. Because of variations in their kinetic energy, ions of equivalent mass may reach the detector at different times, resulting in a spread or distribution of arrival times. In the case of single ion peaks, the literature suggests that peak shape should be symmetric with possibly Gaussian (Dass, 2001) or Cauchy (Kempka et al., 2004) forms. Kernels based on normalized densities, such as the Gaussian

$$ k(t; \tau_j, \omega_j) = \sqrt{\frac{\omega}{2\pi}} \; \exp\left(-\frac{\omega}{2}(t - \tau)^2\right) \qquad (15.2) $$

or Cauchy

$$ k(t; \tau_j, \omega_j) = \frac{\sqrt{\omega}}{\pi} \left(1 + \omega\,(t - \tau)^2\right)^{-1}, \qquad (15.3) $$

capture the spiky nature of peaks in the time domain and serve as natural choices for basis functions for expanding the mean function. In the parameterizations above, τ_j may be interpreted as the expected TOF for protein j. When normalized densities (that integrate to one) are used to construct the kernels, the coefficient γ_j corresponds to the area under the curve, which may be thought of as a measure of the concentration of protein j or of its abundance.

Finally, the parameter ω_j controls the width of peaks. Determining whether a given peak in the spectrum corresponds to a single protein or to two or more proteins is an issue of the resolving power of the mass spectrometer, which is characterized by its resolution. For a symmetric single ion peak with expected TOF τ_j, the resolution ρ_j at peak j is defined as

$$\rho_j = \frac{\tau_j}{\Delta \tau_j}, \tag{15.4}$$

where $\Delta \tau_j$ is the full peak width at 50% of the maximum height (FWHM) (Siuzdak, 2003) as illustrated in Figure 15.2. Solving for ω_j, we have

$$\omega_j = (2\rho_j/\tau_j)^2 \qquad \text{Cauchy kernel} \tag{15.5}$$
$$\omega_j = \log(4)(2\rho_j/\tau_j)^2 \qquad \text{Gaussian kernel} \tag{15.6}$$

or in general, for a symmetric kernel $k(t, \tau, \omega)$, $\omega = g_k(\tau, \rho)$ for g_k that satisfies (15.4).

Figure 15.3 illustrates how peak width increases as TOF increases (larger mass/charge). As the proteins in the figure have the same concentration (γ_j), the area under each curve is constant, but the height decreases inversely with the square of TOF. The two peaks at 3,000 and 3,015 clock ticks are too close to resolve as individual peaks by isolating the mode, but may be resolved through the model because the width is wider than expected for the particular TOF. Using the relationship in (15.4), available prior information about resolution can be translated into prior knowledge about ω_j, which will aid in resolving the number of proteins in a peak.

15.3 Prior Distributions

To make posterior inference about the unknown function f (which we will assume belongs to some separable Hilbert space $\mathbb{H}$), we must first propose a prior distribution for functions in $\mathbb{H}$. With the representation of $f(t)$ in (15.1), an intuitive construction begins by choosing any positive number $\nu^+ > 0$ and assigning J a Poisson distribution, $J \sim \mathsf{Poisson}(\nu^+)$ with mean ν^+. Conditionally on J, accord the $(\gamma_j, \tau_j, \omega_j)$ independent identical distributions, $(\gamma_j, \tau_j, \omega_j) \overset{\text{iid}}{\sim} \pi(d\gamma, d\tau, d\omega)$, where π is a probability distribution on $\mathbb{R}^+ \times \mathbb{T} \times \mathbb{R}^+$. This leads to the equivalent representation of $f(t)$ as a convolution of kernels of the form

$$f(t) = b(t) + \int_{\mathbb{T} \times \mathbb{R}^+} k(t; \tau, \omega)\, \mathbf{\Gamma}(d\tau, d\omega), \tag{15.7}$$

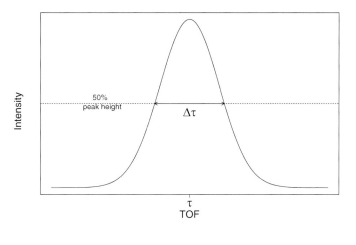

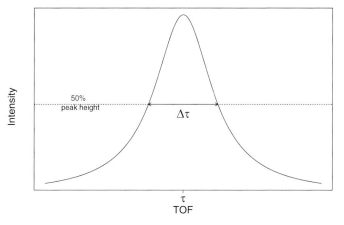

Fig. 15.2. Gaussian kernel with $\omega = 0.055$ (top) and Cauchy kernel (bottom) with $\omega = 0.04$ with expected TOF $\tau = 1{,}000$ ns. The resolution is the same in both cases $(\Delta\tau)/\tau = 100)$.

where

$$\Gamma(d\tau, d\omega) = \sum_{j=1}^{J} \gamma_j \delta_{\tau_j}(d\tau)\delta_{\omega_j}(d\omega)$$

is a discrete random Borel measure on $\mathbb{T} \times \mathbb{R}^+$ with a random number J jumps of random height γ_j at the random points (τ_j, ω_j).

More generally, the prior distribution $\pi(d\gamma, d\tau, d\omega)$ need not be proper (i.e., finite) for the random measure Γ (and the convolution) to be finite and well

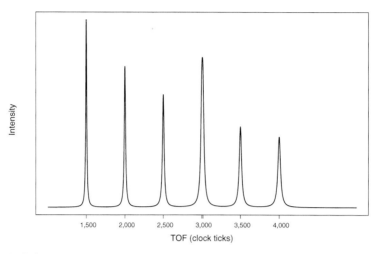

Fig. 15.3. Cauchy kernels with equal concentrations and constant resolution ($\rho = 100$). With equal concentrations, the heights are inversely related to the TOF, $2\rho/\tau_j$. The two peaks at 3,000 and 3,015 appear as a single peak, but the combined peak is wider than expected for the given resolution.

defined. In particular, a natural choice for modeling concentrations is with a Gamma random field prior, a special case of a Lévy random field prior, where we take

$$\Gamma \sim \mathsf{Lv}(\nu) \qquad (15.8)$$

with Lévy measure ν of the form

$$\nu(d\gamma, d\tau, d\omega) = \alpha\gamma^{-1} e^{-\beta\gamma} \mathbf{1}_{\{\gamma > 0\}} \, d\gamma \, \pi(d\tau, d\omega) \qquad (15.9)$$

for $\alpha > 0$ and $\beta > 0$ and for some finite measure $\pi(d\tau, d\omega)$ on $\mathbb{T} \times \mathbb{R}^+$. For disjoint sets $A_i \subset \mathbb{T} \times \mathbb{R}^+$, the random measure Γ assigns $\Gamma[A_i]$ independent Gamma distributions, $\Gamma[A_i] \sim \mathsf{Gamma}(\alpha\pi(A), \beta)$. For example, with $A_i = (t_i, t_{i+1}] \times \mathbb{R}^+$ and $\pi(d\tau, d\omega) = \mathbf{1}_{\tau \in \mathbb{T}} \, d\tau\pi(d\omega))$, the random variable $\Gamma[A_i]$ represents the total abundance of proteins with expected TOFs in the interval $(t_i, t_{i+1}]$. While other approaches may be used to construct a prior for $f(t)$, the Gamma random field, which is a stationary independent increment field, ensures that our prior beliefs are specified coherently across all possible partitions of TOF. Because the Gamma random field prior assigns probability 1 to nonnegative functions f, we are assured that the expected intensity will always be nonnegative.

Infinite Lévy measures ν, such as in the Gamma random field in (15.9), lead to a random measure Γ with an infinite number of support points J a priori, as the mean

$$\nu^+(\alpha, \beta) \equiv \nu(\mathbb{R}^+, \mathbb{T}, \mathbb{R}^+) = \int\int\int_{\mathbb{R}^+ \times \mathbb{T} \times \mathbb{R}^+} \nu(d\gamma, d\tau, d\omega) \qquad (15.10)$$

in the Poisson distribution is infinite. As the Lévy measure ν, however, satisfies the bound

$$\int\int\int_{\mathbb{R}^+ \times \mathbb{T} \times \mathbb{R}^+ \times K} (1 \wedge |\gamma|)\, \nu(d\gamma, d\tau, d\omega) < \infty, \qquad (15.11)$$

tractable computation may be obtained by the approximation

$$\nu_\epsilon(d\gamma, d\tau, d\omega) \equiv \nu(d\gamma, d\tau, d\omega)\mathbf{1}_{\gamma > \epsilon}, \qquad (15.12)$$

which will lead to finite

$$\nu_\epsilon^+(\alpha, \beta) \equiv \nu_\epsilon(\mathbb{R}^+, \mathbb{T}, \mathbb{R}^+) \qquad (15.13)$$

and hence finite J (almost surely). This approximation may be viewed as incorporating just the J largest intensities into the mean $f(t)$. Although we may expect on the order of $30-50$ proteins (Campa et al., 2003) and hence finite J, the total number of protein products may be much higher due to protein modifications, such as the addition of matrix adducts or addition/loss of other ions, or isotopic differences in protein composition. For $\epsilon > 0$, J corresponds to the number of peaks or proteins in the spectra with expected intensity greater than ϵ, thus the choice of ϵ may be guided by expected noise levels and overall resolution. For more details concerning Lévy random fields and approximations, see Cont and Tankov (2004); Jacod and Shiryaev (1987); Khinchine and Lévy (1936); Maruyama (1970); Sato (1999); Wolpert and Ickstadt (1998a,b); Wolpert and Taqqu (2005).

To complete the Gamma random field prior we must specify a joint distribution for τ_j and ω_j. Without prior information on the distribution of the mass/charge of expected proteins, a default choice is to take τ_j uniform over $\mathbb{T}$. Given existing databases of proteins and associated masses, one can construct a more informative prior for τ_j for a given proteomic application.

Because information is available regarding resolution, we develop priors for resolution, rather than directly placing a prior distribution on the parameter ω_j, which governs peak width. Because the resolution ρ_j depends on only characteristics of the mass spectrometer (laser and detector settings, experimental conditions) and not on the kernel representation, this provides a model independent method for assessing prior distributions for ω_j. Resolution may differ among peaks, primarily because of variation in ion kinetic energy. We develop a hierarchical prior distribution for peak resolution ρ_j, with $\rho_j|\varrho \overset{\text{iid}}{\sim} \pi(\rho_j \mid \varrho)$, which allows for variation in resolution from peak to peak, and place a prior distribution on the overall resolution ϱ to correspond to expected ranges. Because the width at 50% of the peak height is a function of the kernel parameters, the relationship between peak resolution ρ_j and τ_j given by equation (15.4) may be used to find the distribution of the peak width parameter ω_j given τ_j for any kernel parameterization. The hierarchical representation allows peak widths to vary slightly from protein to protein, but "borrows strength" from the ensemble of peaks and information regarding the overall resolution.

The prior may be restated in hierarchical fashion as

$$f(t) = \beta\{\beta_0 + k_b(t, \tau_0, \omega_0)\gamma_0 + \sum_{j=1}^{J} k(t, \tau_j, \omega_j)\gamma_j\}$$

$$\gamma_j \mid J, \epsilon \overset{\text{iid}}{\sim} \mathsf{Gamma}(0, 1; \epsilon) \qquad \text{for } j = 0, \ldots, J$$

$$\tau_j \mid J \overset{\text{iid}}{\sim} \mathsf{Uniform}(\mathbb{T}) \qquad \text{for } j = 1, \ldots, J$$

$$\rho_j \mid J \overset{\text{iid}}{\sim} \mathsf{LogNormal}(\varrho, 0.05) \qquad \text{for } j = 1, \ldots, J$$

$$\omega_j = g_k(\tau_j, \rho_j) \qquad \text{for } j = 1, \ldots, J$$

$$J \mid \alpha, \epsilon \sim \mathsf{Poisson}\left(v_\epsilon^+(\alpha, 1)\right)$$

where in the distribution for γ_j, $\mathsf{Gamma}(0, b; \epsilon)$ represents a truncated Gamma distribution with density proportional to $\gamma^{-1}\exp(-b\gamma)$ on $[\epsilon, \infty)$ and normalizing constant $\mathsf{E}_1(b\epsilon)$ ($\mathsf{E}_1(z)$ is the Exponential Integral function (Abramowitz and Stegun, 1970, Section 5.1)). In the above reformulation, the intensities $\{\gamma_j\}$ all have scale 1; however, the parameter β can be thought of as an overall spectrum-specific scale parameter used to adjust the intensities and background parameters. The function g_k used to transform ρ_j to ω_j is given in (15.5) and (15.6) for the Cauchy and Gaussian kernels, respectively. For MALDI data, we represent $b(t)$ as an overall constant plus a kernel fixed at the initial time $\tau_0 \equiv t_0$ (near 8000 clock ticks),

$$b(t) = \beta\{\beta_0 + k(t, \tau_0, \omega_0)\gamma_0\}, \qquad (15.14)$$

which effectively captures much of the high intensity measurements below 2,000 Da.

Prior distributions at higher stages of the hierarchy depend on prior knowledge about the anticipated number of proteins J_0 and the choice of ϵ and are taken to be weakly data-dependent. The prior on the overall scaling parameter

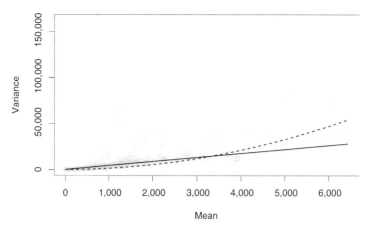

Fig. 15.4. Means and variances of intensities using a sliding window of 50 clock ticks. The solid line represents a robust fit of the model with the variance linear in the mean (Gamma model), while the dashed line represents the robust fit to a model for the variance that is quadratic in the mean (LogNormal model).

β depends on the data through the sum of the observed intensities, and is chosen so that the expected intensity at any point in time is roughly 0.01% of the total observed intensity. The prior on ρ leads to 95% of the resolution values being between roughly 80 and 125, based on our experience with similar data. Finally, the Gamma prior on the parameter α in the Lévy measure ν (15.9) leads to J having a negative binomial distribution marginally with expected value J_0 (the anticipated number of proteins), and provides robustness to a fixed choice of α.

15.4 Likelihood

Posterior inference about parameters in the model requires specification of an appropriate likelihood. Because intensity measurements are nonnegative, both Gamma and LogNormal distributions are reasonable candidates that allow the variance to depend on the mean. Under the Gamma model the variance is proportional to the mean, while with the LogNormal, the variance is proportional to the square of the mean. To explore which model is more appropriate, we took running windows of 50 clock ticks and computed the mean and variance of intensity (Y_t) in each window. We used a robust quantile regression (Koenker and D'Orey, 1994) to fit the linear and quadratic models for variance as function of the mean (Figure 15.4). Overall, the linear relationship between the mean and variance appears to be more appropriate over a larger range of the data.

Based on the exploratory analysis, we adopt the following Gamma model for intensities:

$$Y_t - \min(Y_t) + c \mid f(t), \phi \overset{iid}{\sim} \text{Gamma}\,(f(t)\phi, \phi) \qquad (15.15)$$

parameterized with mean $f(t)$ and variance $f(t)/\phi$ to accommodate the nonconstant variability present in spectra. To avoid problems with evaluating the likelihood at zero, we add a small constant c to the data (allowing c to be random and estimated from the data did not change inferences).

To complete our model specification, we need to choose a prior for ϕ. From experiments using blank chips, where there is no signal but just pure noise, we observe intensities ranging from 20 to 25, or for the average of 10 spectra, we would expect standard deviations around $1.1 - 1.3$. From the robust regression line in Figure 15.4, the slope estimate is 4.3, which provides another estimate of $1/\phi$, the variance inflation factor. We take the prior for ϕ to be Gamma(0.5, 1), which provides reasonable coverage of these values (roughly 30% of the mass is in the interval), but puts 50% of the mass on values of ϕ less than 1/4.3 allowing for greater prior uncertainty (lower precisions).

15.5 Posterior Inference

Given prior distributions on all unknowns, the number of proteins J, the locations τ_j, peak widths ω_j, peak resolutions ρ_j, and peak masses γ_j, as well as other parameters, α, β, etc., the posterior distribution of all unknowns is proportional to the likelihood of the data based on the Gamma model, multiplied by the prior distributions defined by the Gamma random field and other prior distributions at higher stages of the hierarchy. Marginal posterior distributions for most quantities of interest are not available analytically. The prior construction using Lévy random fields, however, permits tractable simulation of the posterior distribution via a reversible jump Markov chain Monte Carlo (RJ-MCMC) algorithm (Green, 1995). The RJ-MCMC algorithm proceeds by drawing computer simulations of the high-dimensional state vector $\{\alpha, \beta, \rho, J, \{\gamma_j, \tau_j, \omega_j\}_{j \leq J}\}$ and any other uncertain features. At each iteration, we randomly select to either increment J and add a new peak and associated parameters (Birth), decrement J and remove a peak (Death), or update peak or other parameters (Update); Birth/Death moves that allow a peak to be Split into two peaks or be Merged into a single peak are also included. Efficient computation is possible because updates to f based on adding/deleting or updating peaks bypass the need to invert large matrices that often arise in Gaussian approaches. Furthermore, because kernels are only computed as needed, memory requirements scale linearly with the sample size. For starting values, we have developed an EM algorithm (Dempster Laird and Rubin., 1977) to find modal estimates of the parameters in a single spectrum under an approximate Gaussian model, with positivity constraints. An R package for fitting these models is under development by the authors.

15.6 Illustration

To illustrate inference using the adaptive kernel model, we use the data from the average spectrum shown in Figure 15.1. We select hyperparameters in a Gamma prior distribution for α such that the prior mean number of peaks is $\mathsf{E}(J) = 30$, based on discussions with the researchers, who provided the data. The value of ϵ, which controls the minimum detectable peak mass, was set based on previous simulation experiments with similar levels of noise and overall total intensity. Using the Cauchy kernel, we ran the RJ-MCMC for 2 million iterations, thinning by 1,000, and kept the last 1,000 values for inference.

Figure 15.5 summarizes the marginal distribution of $1/\phi$ (the variance inflation factor) as well as joint draws of ρ_j and τ_j. The resolution ρ_j does not appear to vary systematically with TOF (or mass/charge), although the few areas with higher resolution suggest that the hierarchical model may be more appropriate than a model with one common resolution throughout. The figure also shows the cumulative distribution for relative concentration $\sum_{\tau_j \leq t} \gamma_j / \sum_{j=1}^{J} \gamma_j$ versus TOF t. Jumps in the cumulative distribution indicate locations of peaks in the spectrum.

At each iteration of the RJ-MCMC sampler, locations of the expected TOF (τ_j) are updated, with the number of peaks potentially changing. Point estimates of quantities of interest are computed from ergodic averages along the Markov chain or the maximum a posteriori (MAP) draw. Figure 15.6 illustrates the function estimates corresponding to the highest posterior probability draw (top) and to the posterior mean (model averaging).

The rug plot at the bottom of each plot indicates locations of peaks. A technical issue with using RJ-MCMC algorithms for peak identification involves summarizing a high-dimensional parameter vector of varying dimension. Under model averaging, we identify peaks or local modes by using the posterior distribution of the derivative process of the mean intensity function shown in Figure 15.7. Peak identification is carried out by finding where the derivative process crosses zero. This typically results in fewer peaks than the MAP draw, but identifies major peaks. Figure 15.7 illustrates that the model can capture features such as asymmetry and can differentiate between peaks composed of a single protein or multiple protein peaks. Despite the inherent flexibility

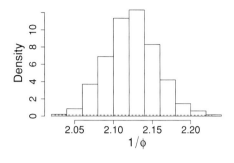

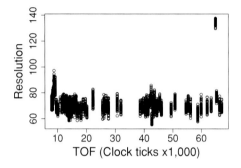

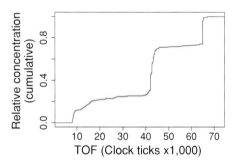

Fig. 15.5. Posterior distribution of $1/\phi$ with prior shown by the dashed curve (top), posterior draws of resolution ρ_j versus TOF τ_j (middle), and posterior draws of cumulative distribution of relative concentration $\sum_{\tau_j \leq t} \gamma_j / \sum_{j=1}^{J} \gamma_j$ as a function of TOF τ_j (bottom).

of nonparametric models, the prior information on resolution helps in resolving peaks, as peaks that are wider than expected will require multiple kernels (proteins) to fit well. The choice of the minimum peak size, ϵ, also prevents overfitting as extremely small coefficients that do not contribute much to the overall estimate are not included.

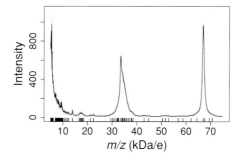

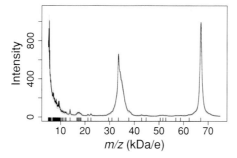

Fig. 15.6. Estimates of mean intensity from the highest posterior draw (top), and under model averaging (posterior mean) (bottom). The rug plot at the bottom indicates locations of peaks.

15.7 Summary

The use of kernels to generate basis functions in the nonparametric model for spectra provides the flexibility and adaptivity of wavelet methods, but additionally provides peak identification and protein quantification directly from model parameters τ_j and γ_j, respectively. The locations (τ_j) may be viewed as the expected TOF of protein j, with γ_j corresponding to its abundance. The parameters ω_j, which control kernel shape, are allowed to vary over time, providing adaptivity in both time and frequency, similar to wavelet regression models and signal processing representations using Gabor frames (Clyde and George, 2000; Clyde et al., 1998; Morris et al., 2005; Wolfe et al., 2004). Unlike these nonparametric regression models, the Gamma random field prior handles easily the nonnegativity constraints on parameters γ_j in the mean intensity function, but still achieves "sparse" local time-frequency representations. Tu et al. (2005) demonstrate that Lévy process priors for nonparametric regression provide excellent MSE (mean squared error) properties, outperforming translational invariant (nondecimated) wavelets in many cases.

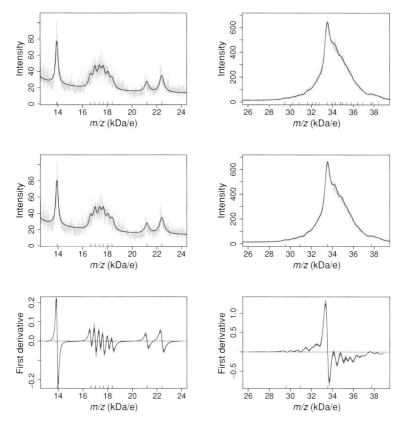

Fig. 15.7. Estimates of mean intensity from the highest posterior draw (top) and with model averaging (middle). The posterior distribution of the first derivative of the mean intensity is illustrated in the bottom row. The rug plot at the bottom of each graph indicates locations of peaks.

The single spectrum model may be extended to multiple spectra for classification problems or for discovering which proteins differentiate groups. In the case of multiple spectra, peak locations will not necessarily coincide, because of lack of alignment or sample-to-sample variability. Hierarchical models that allow expected TOF, τ_j, and relative abundances, γ_j, and other parameters to vary from spectrum to spectrum may be used to address alignment, normalization, calibration, and baseline adjustments. The hierarchical representation can easily accommodate replicate spectra from the same subject, day effects, or other aspects of the experimental design. For classification problems, such as identifying disease states (cancer, for example), separate hierarchical models may be fit within groups. For new subjects, one may find the probability of disease states given the new spectrum and observed data using estimates of the marginal predictive distributions under each group, and then finding the probability of cancer using Bayes Theorem. While these models do not identify directly proteins that are differentially expressed between the two (or more) groups, differences between the posterior distributions of the intensity function can be used to highlight regions with differential expression.

Acknowledgments

The authors would like to thank Ned Patz for providing the data used in this paper and Michael Fitzgerald for helpful discussions regarding MALDI-TOF and mass spectroscopy. This work was made possible by National Science Foundation grants DMS–0342172, DMS–0422400, and DMS–0406115.

Bibliography

Abramowitz, M. and Stegun, I. (1970) *Handbook of Mathematical Functions*. New York: Dover Publications, Inc.

Baldwin, M. A., Medzihradszky, K. F., Lock, C. M., Fisher, B., Settineri, T. A. and Burlingame, A. (2001) Matrix-assisted laser desorption/ionization coupled with quadrupole/orthogonal acceleration time-of-flight mass spectrometry for protein discovery, identification, and structural analysis. *Analytical Chemistry*, **73**, 1707–1720.

Campa, M. J., Fitzgerald, M. C. and Patz, E. F. (2003) Exploring the proteome with MALDI-TOF (editorial). *Proteomics*, **3**, 1659–1660.

Clyde, M. and George, E. I. (2000) Flexible empirical Bayes estimation for wavelets. *Journal of the Royal Statistical Society, Series B*, **62**, 681–698.

Clyde, M., Parmigiani, G. and Vidakovic, B. (1998) Multiple shrinkage and subset selection in wavelets. *Biometrika*, **85**, 391–401.

Cont, R. and Tankov, P. (2004) *Financial Modelling with Jump Processes*. London, UK: Chapman & Hall.

Coombes, K., Koomen, J., Baggerly, K., Morris, J. and Kobayashi, R. (2005) Understanding the characteristics of mass spectrometry data through the use of simulation. *Cancer Informatics*, **1**, 41–52.

Coombes, K., Tsavachidis, S., Morris, J., Baggerly, K., Hung, M. and Kuerer, H. (2005) Improved peak detection and quantification of mass spectrometry data acquired from surface-enhanced laser desorption and ionization by denoising spectra with the undecimated discrete wavelet transform. *Proteomics*, **5**, 4107–4117.

Dass, C. (2001) *Principles and Practice of Biological Mass Spectrometry*. New York: John Wiley & Sons.

Dempster, A. P., Laird, N. M. and Rubin, D. B. (1977) Maximumm likelihood from incomplete data via the EM algorithm. *J. Roy. Stat. Soc. B*, **39**(1), 1–38.

Diamandis, E. P. (2003) Point: Proteomic patterns in biological fluids: Do they represent the future of cancer diagnostics. *Clinical Chemistry*, **49**, 1272–1275.

Green, P. J. (1995) Reversible jump Markov chain Monte Carlo computation and Bayesian model determination. *Biometrika*, **82**, 711–732.

Jacod, J. and Shiryaev, A. N. (1987) *Limit Theorems for Stochastic Processes*, Vol. 288 of *Grundlehren der mathematischen Wissenschaften*. Berlin, DE: Springer-Verlag.

Kempka, M., Södahl, J., Björk, A. and Roeraade, J. (2004) Improved method for peak picking in matrix-assisted laser desorption/ionization time-of-flight mass spectrometry. *Rapid Communications in Mass Spectrometry*, **18**, 1208–1212.

Khinchine, A. Y. and Lévy, P. (1936) Sur les lois stables. *Comptes Rendus Hebdomadaires des Seances de l'Académie des Sciences. Académie des science (France), Serie* A. Paris, **202**, 374–376.

Koenker, R. W. and D'Orey, V. (1994) Computing regression quantiles. *Applied Statistics*, **43**, 410–414.

Malyarenko, D. I., Cooke, W. E., Adam, B.-L., Malik, G., Chen, H., Tracy, E. R., Trosset, M. W., Sasinowski, M., Semmes, O. J. and Manos, D. M. (2005) Enhancement of sensitivity and resolution of surface-enhanced laser desorption/ionization time-of-flight mass spectrometric records for serum peptides using time-series analysis techniques. *Clinical Chemistry*, **51**, 65–74.

Martin, D. B. and Nelson, P. S. (2001) From genomics to proteomics: Techniques and applications in cancer research. *Trends in Cell Biology*, **11**, 560–656.

Maruyama, G. (1970) Infinitely divisible processes. *Theory of Probabability and Its Applications*, **15**, 1–22.

Morris, J. S., Coombes, K. R., Koomen, J., Baggerly, K. A. and Kobayashi, R. (2005) Feature extraction and quantification for mass spectrometry in biomedical applications using the mean spectrum. *Bioinformatics*, **21**, 1764–1775.

Petricoin, E. I., Ardekani, A., Hitt, B., Levine, P., Fusaro, V., Steinberg, S., Mills, G., Simone, C., Fishman, D., Kohn, E. and Liotta, L. (2002) Use of proteomic patterns in serum to identify ovarian cancer. *The Lancet*, **359**, 572–577.

Petricoin, E. I. and Liotta, L. (2003) Mass spectrometry-based diagnostics: The upcoming revolution in disease detection. *Clinical Chemistry*, **49**, 533–534.

Sato, K.-I. (1999) *Lévy Processes and Infinitely Divisible Distributions*. Cambridge, UK: Cambridge University Press.

Siuzdak, G. (2003) *The Expanding Role of Mass Spectrometry in Biotechnology*. San Diego: MCC Press.

Tu, C., Clyde, M. A. and Wolpert, R. L. (2005) Lévy adaptive regression kernels. Technical Report, Institute of Statistics and Decision Sciences, Duke University.

Wolfe, P. J., Godsill, S. J. and Ng, W.-J. (2004) Bayesian variable selection and regularisation for time-frequency surface estimation. *Journal of the Royal Statistical Society, Series B*, **66**, 575–589.

Wolpert, R. L. and Ickstadt, K. (1998a) Poisson/gamma random field models for spatial statistics. *Biometrika*, **85**, 251–267.

Wolpert, R. L. and Ickstadt, K. (1998b) Simulation of Lévy random fields. In *Practical Nonparametric and Semiparametric Bayesian Statistics*, Vol. 133 of *Lecture Notes in Statistics* (eds. D. Dey, P. Müller and D. Sinha), pp. 227–242. New York: Springer Verlag.

Wolpert, R. L. and Taqqu, M. S. (2005) Fractional Ornstein-Uhlenbeck Lévy processes and the Telecom process: Upstairs and downstairs. *Signal Processing*, **85**, 1523–1545.

16

Bayesian Modeling and Inference for Sequence Motif Discovery

MAYETRI GUPTA
University of North Carolina at Chapel Hill

JUN S. LIU
Harvard University

Abstract

Motif discovery, which focuses on locating short sequence patterns associated with the regulation of genes in a species, leads to a class of statistical missing data problems. These problems are discussed first with reference to a hypothetical model, which serves as a point of departure for more realistic versions of the model. Some general results relating to modeling and inference through the Bayesian and/or frequentist perspectives are presented, and specific problems arising out of the underlying biology are discussed.

16.1 Introduction

The goal of motif discovery is to locate short repetitive patterns in DNA that are involved in the regulation of genes of interest. To fix ideas, let us consider the following paragraph modified from Bellhouse [4, Section 3, p. 5]:

Richard Bayes (1596–1675), a great-grandfather of Thomas Bayes, was a successful cutler in Sheffield. In 1643 Richard served in the rotating position of Master of the Company of Cutlers of Hallamshire. Richard was sufficiently well off that he sent one of his sons, Samuel Bayes (1635–1681) to Trinity College Cambridge during the Commonwealth period; Samuel obtained his degree in 1656. Another son, Joshua Bayes (1638–1703) followed in his father's footsteps in the cutlery industry, also serving as Master of the Company in 1679. Evidence of Joshua Bayes's wealth comes from the size of his house, the fact that he employed a servant and the size of the taxes that he paid. Joshua Bayes's influence may be taken from his activities in ...

Imagine that a person who has never seen the English language before looks at this paragraph and tries to make sense out of it (this is very much analogous to how we view the genome sequences of various species). Also imagine that

all the punctuation marks, capitalizations, and spaces have been taken away
from this paragraph so that available to him are collections of sequences like

> *richardbayes15961675agreatgrandfatherofthomasbayeswasas* ...
> *in1643richardbayesservedintherotatingpositionofmasterofthe* ...
> *richardwassufficientlywelloffthathesentoneofhissonssamuelbayes* ...
> ...

How should the non-English speaker proceed? The first natural question to
ask is, what might be an internal "linkage" of these sequences? This question
leads one to find the most commonly occurring "words" (or, rather, short subsequences of unknown length) that might characterize this paragraph. Indeed,
if one tries to list all the possible subsequences of length 5, the word "bayes"
pops up as the most frequent or "enriched" one. If one tries this on all segments
of length 10 or 11, "joshuabayes" tops the list. After these findings, you may
suggest to your collaborators (i.e., biologists) to investigate the properties of
"bayes" or "joshuabayes," which may ultimately lead to the discovery of the
great probabilist's name, although this paragraph per se mainly discusses a
few relatives of the probabilist. So, it appears that by looking for "significantly
enriched" words, one can indeed get some insight on a paragraph written in a
completely unknown language.

However, in order to make the above procedure statistically sound, one
needs (a) to model in what context a word is "significantly enriched" (thus,
a probabilistic structure for generating the observed text is needed); (b) a
strategy for determining the length(s) of the enriched word(s) to be discovered; and (c) an efficient computational strategy to find all enriched words. In
the genomic context, the problem is even more difficult because the "words"
used by the nature are never "exact," that is, certain "misspellings" can
be tolerated. Thus, one also needs (d) a probabilistic model to describe a
fuzzy word.

A simplified model leads to the following class of statistical problems.
Let X_{ij}, $j = 1, \ldots, L_i$, represent the ith observed genomic sequence (i.e.,
each X_{ij} takes four different values: A, C, G, and T, instead of the 26 letters in the English alphabet). Our first "null" statistical model is to assume
that each X_{ij} is the result of a toss of a four-sided die characterized by the
probability vector $\boldsymbol{\theta}_0 = (\theta_{0A}, \theta_{0C}, \theta_{0G}, \theta_{0T})$. The problem of interest is to infer
whether there exist subsequences corresponding to one or more enriched words.
That is, whether there are subsequences $\boldsymbol{Y}_{ia} = \{Y_{il} : l = a, \ldots, a + w - 1; 1 \leq
a \leq L_i - w + 1\}$ of $\{X_{ij} : 1 \leq j \leq L_i\}$ which are generated from a "run" of
tosses from w "special" dice, each characterized by the multinomial probability

vector $\boldsymbol{\theta}_m = (\theta_{m,A}, \ldots, \theta_{m,T})$. Thus, we now use a *product-multinomial* model, $[\boldsymbol{\theta}_1, \ldots, \boldsymbol{\theta}_w]$, to characterize a fuzzy word.

The values of $w, a, \boldsymbol{\theta}_0$, and $\boldsymbol{\theta}_m$ ($m = 1, \ldots, w$) are all unknown. The basic setup above constitutes a missing data problem which somewhat differs from standard missing data problems in two ways: (i) estimating the unknown locations a of the beginning of the "run" is generally considered to be of more interest than the values of the unknown parameters $\boldsymbol{\theta}$ and (ii) at an individual locus level, there exist experimental methods (even though expensive and potentially inaccurate) to verify the computational predictions.

The purpose of this chapter is to (i) explain in brief the biological background of the preceding problem in relation to gene regulatory binding site discovery, (ii) propose a Bayesian framework for its solution that serves as a point of departure for discussing more realistic versions of the problem, and (iii) describe some alternative models and methods designed to capture the complicating features arising in practice. We consider issues of model selection and robustness of the inference procedures that are especially relevant in the Bayesian context. Some of the problems have close connections in the rich literature on hidden Markov models (HMMs), to which relevant similarities will be discussed.

16.2 Biology of Transcription Regulation

With the completion of many genome sequencing projects, a challenge now facing biologists is to determine which parts of the genome encode for biological functions, and the mechanisms by which sequence information is "translated" into these functions. In *transcriptional* regulation, sequence signals upstream of each gene provide a target (the *promoter region*) for an enzyme complex called RNA polymerase (RNAP) to bind and initiate the transcription of the gene into *messenger* RNA (mRNA). Certain proteins called *transcription factors* (TFs) can bind to the promoter regions, either interfering with the action of RNAP and inhibiting gene expression, or enhancing gene expression. TFs recognize sequence sites that give a favorable binding energy, which often translates into a sequence-specific pattern ($\sim$8–20 base pairs long). Binding sites thus tend to be relatively well-conserved in composition – such a conserved pattern is termed as a "motif" (corresponding to the "key word" in the example of Section 16.1). For example, an important TF in *Escherichia coli*, the cyclic AMP receptor protein (CRP), recognizes a pattern of the form TGTGANNNNNNTCACA ("N" denotes that any one of the four nucleotides may be present) – but a substantial deviation from this pattern may sometimes be tolerated. It is estimated that $\sim$2,000 (out of a total of $\sim$30,000) genes in the human genome encode sequence-specific DNA-binding TFs [39]. For identifying and understanding the functional role of noncoding sequences in the human and other genomes, it would be valuable to identify all the sequence patterns that can be recognized by these proteins. Experimental detection of TF-binding sites (TFBSs) on a gene-by-gene and site-by-site basis is possible [8], but remains an extremely difficult and expensive task at a genomic level, especially as the amount of sequence to be analyzed increases. Computational methods that assume no prior knowledge of the pattern of the binding sites then become a necessary tool for aiding in their discovery.

16.3 Problem Formulation, Background, and General Strategies

One of the first motif-finding approaches was CONSENSUS, an information-theory-based progressive alignment procedure [35]. Assuming each sequence contains one motif site of width w, the objective was to find the set of sites maximizing "information content," that is, Kullback-Leibler entropy distance between the motif site composition and the background distribution: $\sum_{i=1}^{w} \sum_{j=1}^{J} f_{ij} \log_2 \left(\frac{f_{ij}}{f_{0j}} \right)$, where f_{ij} is the observed frequency of letter j in position i of the site, and f_{0j} denotes the corresponding background letter frequencies. CONSENSUS starts by examining all pairs of w-long subsequences (w-mers) in the first two sequences, and retains the top-scoring M (say, 50) motifs (each consisting of pairs of sites). Each of the M motifs is next aligned to all w-mers in the third sequence, again the top M motifs are retained, and the process is continued for all the sequences.

Other early statistical methods for finding motifs include an EM algorithm [9] based on a missing-data formulation [23], and a Gibbs sampling (GS) algorithm [22]. In both approaches, starting positions of true motif sites were treated as "missing" components of the observed sequence data. Under the assumption that there is exactly one motif site per sequence, an iterative procedure was used to alternately refine the motif description (parameters) and sample sites in the sequences that could represent instances of the motif. Later generalizations that allow for a variable number of motif sites per sequence were a Gibbs sampler [27, 31] and an EM algorithm for finite mixture models [2].

Another class of methods approach the motif discovery problem from a "segmentation" perspective. MobyDick [5] treats the motifs as "words" used by nature to construct the "sentences" of DNA and estimates word frequencies using a Newton–Raphson optimization procedure. The dictionary model was later extended to include "stochastic" words in order to account for variations in the motif sites [14] and a data augmentation (DA) [37] procedure introduced for finding such words.

Recent approaches to motif discovery have improved upon the previous methods in at least two primary ways: (i) improving and sensitizing the basic model to reflect realistic biological phenomena, such as multiple motif types in the same sequence, "gapped" motifs, and clustering of motif sites (cis-regulatory modules) [15, 29, 42], and (ii) using auxiliary data sources, such as gene expression microarrays, phylogenetic information, and the physical structure of DNA [7, 21]. Due to limitations of space, in this chapter we will mainly focus on (i) and indicate ways in which the Bayesian approach has facilitated making significant inroads into this field. We will primarily discuss de novo methods of discovering uncharacterized motifs in biological sequences, as opposed to scanning sequences with a previously (experimentally) determined motif representation to find probable matches.

16.3.1 Likelihood-Based Approaches to Motif Discovery

In Lawrence and Reilly [23], an EM algorithm was developed to estimate the motif pattern and infer the motif site locations. In their formulation, every sequence in the data set is assumed to contain one and only one motif site, and its start position is considered the "missing data" part of the model. In order to model multiple motif sites per sequence, Bailey and Elkan [2] present a simplified model (see Figure 16.1) in which the sequence data set is broken up conceptually into all overlapping subsequences of length w and each of these w-mers is assumed to be generated from one of the two classes: "motif" or "background." More precisely, denoting the set of all w-mers by $X = (X_1, X_2, \ldots, X_n)$, each w-mer $X_i = (x_{i1}, \ldots, x_{iw})$ is assumed to be generated from a two-component mixture model indexed by an unobserved group indicator Z_{ij}, where

$$Z_{ij} = \begin{cases} 1 & \text{if } X_i \text{ is a motif site of type } j \ (j = 1, 2), \\ 0 & \text{otherwise.} \end{cases}$$

A similar model is also presented in Liu et al. [27], where Z_{ij} is allowed to take on $J + 1$ possible values to accommodate J distinct motif types, and a GS strategy is proposed for the inference.

Let us write the set of parameters corresponding to the motif component and background as $\Theta_1 = (\theta_1, \ldots, \theta_w)$ and $\Theta_0 = (\theta_0, \ldots, \theta_0)$ (where $\theta_i = (\theta_{i1}, \ldots, \theta_{i4})^T$), while π denotes the relative proportion of motif segments (mixing proportion). Given the class indicator $Z_{ij} = 1$, X_i is assumed to be generated from a product-multinomial model characterized by Θ_j. Under this

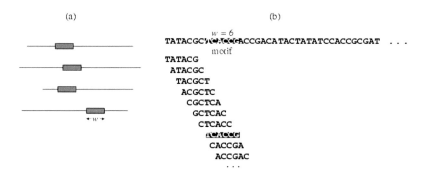

Fig. 16.1. (a) The basic motif model [23] and (b) the mixture model approximation [2].

setup, considering Z_{ij} as missing data, it is now possible to set up a standard EM algorithm to maximize the likelihood function $P(X \mid \Theta_1, \Theta_0, \pi)$ with respect to $(\Theta_1, \Theta_0, \pi)$.

A possible way to overcome the limitations of this oversimplified model, as suggested in Liu and Lawrence [26] and explained in more detail in the following section, is to recast the motif-finding problem as a problem of *segmenting* the sequences into two types of contiguous pieces, one described by the block-motif model (of a fixed length w) and the other by an iid model.

16.3.2 Dictionary Models for Motif Discovery

The dictionary model [5] is perhaps one of the first implementations of the aforementioned segmentation idea for motif discovery. In this model, one assumes that nature has a dictionary available, consisting of a list of d known words $\mathcal{D} = \{M_1, M_2, \ldots, M_d\}$. As a mathematical abstraction, we treat the whole observed data set as a single sequence, S. S is assumed to be generated by randomly drawing words from the dictionary according to a probability vector $\rho = (\rho(M_1), \ldots, \rho(M_d))$ and sequentially concatenating them together.

Since we cannot observe the actual words that are used to compose the data S, we need to sum over all possible segmentations of the sequences to get the likelihood function:

$$P(S \mid \rho) = \sum_{\mathcal{H}} \prod_{i=1}^{N(\mathcal{H})} \rho(S[H_i]) = \sum_{\mathcal{H}} \prod_{j=1}^{d} [\rho(M_j)]^{N_{M_j}(\mathcal{H})}, \qquad (16.1)$$

where $\mathcal{H} = (H_1, \ldots, H_k)$ is a partition of S so that each part H_i corresponds to a word in the dictionary, $N(\mathcal{H})$ is the total number of words in $\mathcal{H}$, and $N_{M_j}(\mathcal{H})$ is the number of occurrences of word type M_j in the partition. This can be viewed as a missing data problem where the partition $\mathcal{H}$ is missing; the summation over all $\mathcal{H}$ can be achieved recursively [26]. Let $\Phi_{i-1}(\boldsymbol{\rho})$ be the sum of all legitimate partitions for partial sequence $S_{[1:(i-1)]}$. Then,

$$\Phi_i(\boldsymbol{\rho}) = \sum_{j=1}^{W} \rho(S_{[(i-j):i]})\Phi_{i-j}, \tag{16.2}$$

where W is the length of the longest word in the dictionary. In other words, we check whether the last segment is a word from the dictionary for all possible word lengths j. To avoid minor complications, we assume that all the single letters (i.e., A, C, G, and T) are contained in the dictionary; if not, the above recursion needs to be modified slightly.

The maximum likelihood estimate (MLE) of $\boldsymbol{\rho}$ from model (16.1) can be found via a Newton–Raphson algorithm, since one can compute the derivative of the likelihood function (16.1) using a recursive procedure similar to (16.2). One can also employ an EM algorithm or a Gibbs sampler. More precisely, we can derive an estimating equation from (16.1) by taking derivatives with respect to ρ_i [5], the summations required in the estimating equation being computed recursively as in (16.2).

Bussemaker et al. [5] adopted a progressive strategy to estimate the unknown "dictionary" used by nature for constructing the genome. They start with the simplest dictionary consisting only of the $D = 4$ single-letter words, $\mathcal{D}^{(0)} = \{A, C, G, T\}$ and then iterate as follows: For a current dictionary consisting of D words, they find the MLE of the word usage frequencies, $\boldsymbol{\rho} = (\rho_1, \ldots, \rho_D)$, based on model (16.1); then, they consider whether any concatenation of a pair of the estimating words is overrepresented compared to what is expected by chance, and these new words are added to the current dictionary. This procedure is carried out iteratively until a stopping criterion is reached. The assumption that longer words are made up of overrepresented fragments may not be true, but this defect can be rectified by progressively considering words of increasing lengths. That is, for example, we may let the $(t + 1)st$ iteration of the dictionary, $\mathcal{D}^{(t+1)}$, be the union of $\mathcal{D}^{(t)}$ and all "significant" words of length $t + 1$. After introducing longer words, one can also remove some of the shorter words that appear to be parts of certain long words.

To generalize the model of Bussemaker et al. [5] to "fuzzy" words, Gupta and Liu [14] and Sabatti and Lange [32] introduce the idea of a *stochastic dictionary*, which consists of a collection of "stochastic words" each represented by a probabilistic word matrix, or exchangeably, a position-specific weight matrix (PWM). Each column of the PWM ($\boldsymbol{\Theta}$) gives the probabilities of finding each letter in that position of the corresponding stochastic word. For example, ACAGG and `GCAGA` may be two realizations, with probabilities 0.4328 and 0.0072 respectively, of the stochastic word characterized by the PWM

$$
\Theta = \begin{bmatrix}
A & 0.85 & 0.07 & 0.80 & 0.02 & 0.12 \\
C & 0.05 & 0.78 & 0.07 & 0.01 & 0.01 \\
G & 0.10 & 0.05 & 0.12 & 0.96 & 0.85 \\
T & 0.00 & 0.10 & 0.01 & 0.01 & 0.02
\end{bmatrix}.
$$

In the setting described above, the motif-finding problem reduces to inferring the form of the PWM and the likely locations of the stochastically varying words in the sequence, which can be carried out effectively under a Bayesian framework [14].

16.4 A Bayesian Approach to Motif Discovery

In this section, unless otherwise specified, we assume that the data set is a set of N unaligned DNA fragments. Let $S = (S_1, \ldots, S_N)$ denote the N sequences of the data set, where sequence S_i is of length L_i ($i = 1, \ldots, N$). Multiple instances of the same pattern in the data are referred to as motif *sites* or *elements* while different patterns are termed motifs. Motif type k (of, say, width w_k) is characterized by a PWM $\Theta_k = (\boldsymbol{\theta}_{k1}, \ldots, \boldsymbol{\theta}_{kw_k})$, where the J-dimensional ($J = 4$ for DNA) vector $\boldsymbol{\theta}_{ki} = (\theta_{ki1}, \ldots, \theta_{kiJ})^T$ represents the probabilities of occurrence of the J letters in column i ($i = 1, \ldots, w_k$). The corresponding letter occurrence probabilities in the *background* are denoted by $\boldsymbol{\theta}_0 = (\theta_{01}, \ldots, \theta_{0J})$. Let $\boldsymbol{\Theta} = \{\Theta_1, \ldots, \Theta_K\}$.

We assume for now that the motif widths, w_k ($k = 1, \ldots, K$), are known (this assumption will be relaxed later). The locations of the motif sites are unknown, and are denoted by an array of missing indicator variables $A = (A_{ijk})$, where $A_{ijk} = 1$ if position j ($j = 1, \ldots, L_i$) in sequence i ($i = 1, \ldots, N$) is the starting point of a motif of type k ($k = 1, \ldots, K$). For motif type k, we let $A_k = \{A_{ijk}\colon i = 1, \ldots, N; \ j = 1, \ldots, L_i\}$, that is, the indicator matrix for the site locations corresponding to this motif type, and define the alignment:

$$
S_1^{(A_k)} = \{S_{ij}\colon A_{ijk} = 1; i = 1, \ldots, N; \ j = 1, \ldots, L_i\},
$$

$$
S_2^{(A_k)} = \{S_{i(j+1)}\colon A_{ijk} = 1; i = 1, \ldots, N; \ j = 1, \ldots, L_i\},
$$

$$
\ldots
$$

$$
S_{w_k}^{(A_k)} = \{S_{i,j+w_k-1}\colon A_{ijk} = 1; i = 1, \ldots, N; \ j = 1, \ldots, L_i\}.
$$

In words, $S_i^{(A_k)}$ is the set of letters occurring at position i of all the instances of the type k motif.

In a similar fashion, we use $S^{(A^c)}$ to denote the set of all letters occurring in the background, where $S^{(A^c)} = S \setminus \bigcup_{k=1}^{K} \bigcup_{l=1}^{w_k} S_l^{(A_k)}$ (for two sets A, B, $A \subset B$, $B \setminus A \equiv B \cap A^c$). Further, let $\mathcal{C} : S \to \mathbb{Z}^4$ denote a "counting" function that gives the frequencies of the J letters in a specified subset of S. For example, if after taking the set of all instances of motif k, in the first column, we observe a total occurrence of 10 "A"s, 50 "T"s and no "C" or "G"s, $\mathcal{C}(S_1^{(A_k)}) = (10, 0, 0, 50)$. Assuming that the motif columns are independent, we have

$$[\mathcal{C}(S_1^{(A_k)}), \ldots, \mathcal{C}(S_{w_k}^{(A_k)}))] \sim \text{Product-Multinomial}[\Theta_k = (\boldsymbol{\theta}_{k1}, \ldots, \boldsymbol{\theta}_{kw_k})],$$

that is, the ith vector of column frequencies for motif k follows a multinomial distribution parameterized by θ_{ki}.

We next introduce some general mathematical notation. For vectors $\mathbf{v} = (v_1, \ldots, v_p)^T$, let us define $|\mathbf{v}| = |v_1| + \cdots + |v_p|$, and $\Gamma(\mathbf{v}) = \Gamma(v_1) \cdots \Gamma(v_p)$. Then the normalizing constant for a p-dimensional Dirichlet distribution with parameters $\boldsymbol{\alpha} = (\alpha_1, \ldots, \alpha_p)^T$ can be denoted as $\Gamma(|\boldsymbol{\alpha}|)/\Gamma(\boldsymbol{\alpha})$. For notational convenience, we will denote the inverse of the Dirichlet normalizing constant as $ID(\boldsymbol{\alpha}) = \Gamma(\boldsymbol{\alpha})/\Gamma(|\boldsymbol{\alpha}|)$. Finally, for vectors $\mathbf{v}$ and $\mathbf{u} = (u_1, \ldots, u_p)$, we use the shorthand $\boldsymbol{u}^{\boldsymbol{v}} = \prod_{i=1}^{p} u_i^{v_i}$.

The probability of observing S conditional on the indicator matrix A can then be written as

$$P(\boldsymbol{S} \mid \boldsymbol{\Theta}, \boldsymbol{\theta}_0, \boldsymbol{A}) \propto \boldsymbol{\theta}_0^{\mathcal{C}(S^{(A^c)})} \prod_{k=1}^{K} \prod_{i=1}^{w_k} \boldsymbol{\theta}_{ki}^{\mathcal{C}(S_i^{(A_k)})}.$$

For a Bayesian analysis, we assume a conjugate Dirichlet prior distribution for $\boldsymbol{\theta}_0$, $\boldsymbol{\theta}_0 \sim \text{Dirichlet}(\boldsymbol{\beta}_0)$, $\boldsymbol{\beta}_0 = (\beta_{01}, \ldots \beta_{0D})$, and a corresponding product-Dirichlet prior (i.e., independent priors over the columns) PD($\boldsymbol{B}$) for Θ_k ($k = 1, \ldots K$), where $\boldsymbol{B} = (\boldsymbol{\beta}_{k1}, \boldsymbol{\beta}_{k2}, \ldots \boldsymbol{\beta}_{kw_k})$ is a $J \times w_k$ matrix with $\boldsymbol{\beta}_{ki} = (\beta_{ki1}, \ldots \beta_{kiJ})^T$. Then the conditional posterior distribution of the parameters given A is

$$P(\boldsymbol{\Theta}, \boldsymbol{\theta} \mid \boldsymbol{S}, \boldsymbol{A}) \propto \boldsymbol{\theta}_0^{\mathcal{C}(S^{(A^c)})+\boldsymbol{\beta}_0} \prod_{k=1}^{K} \prod_{i=1}^{w_k} \boldsymbol{\theta}_{ki}^{\mathcal{C}(S_i^{(A_k)})+\boldsymbol{\beta}_{ki}}.$$

For the complete joint posterior of all unknowns $(\boldsymbol{\Theta}, \boldsymbol{\theta}, \boldsymbol{A})$, we further need to prescribe a prior distribution for A. In the original model [22], a single motif site per sequence with equal probability to occur anywhere was assumed. However, in the later model [27] that can allow multiple sites, a Bernoulli(π) model is proposed for motif site occurrence. More precisely, assuming that a motif site of width w can occur at any of the sequence positions, $1, 2, \ldots, L^* - w + 1$

in a sequence of length L^*, with probability π, the joint posterior distribution is

$$P(\boldsymbol{\Theta},\boldsymbol{\theta},\boldsymbol{A} \mid \boldsymbol{S}) \propto \theta_0^{\mathcal{C}(S^{(A^c)})+\boldsymbol{\beta}_0} \prod_{k=1}^{K}\prod_{i=1}^{w_k} \theta_{ki}^{\mathcal{C}(S_i^{(A_k)})+\boldsymbol{\beta}_{ki}} \pi^{|\boldsymbol{A}|}(1-\pi)^{L-|\boldsymbol{A}|}, \quad (16.3)$$

where $L = \sum_{i=1}^{N}(L_i - w)$ is the adjusted total length of all sequences and $|\boldsymbol{A}| = \sum_{k=1}^{K}\sum_{i=1}^{N}\sum_{j=1}^{L_i} A_{ijk}$. If we have reason to believe that motif occurrences are not independent, but occur as clusters (as in regulatory modules), we can instead adopt a prior Markovian model for motif occurrence [15, 38], which is discussed further in Section 16.6.

16.4.1 Markov Chain Monte Carlo Computation

Under the model described in (16.3), it is straightforward to implement a GS scheme to iteratively update the parameters, that is, sampling from $[\boldsymbol{\Theta}, \theta_0 \mid \mathcal{C}, \boldsymbol{A}]$, and impute the missing data, that is, sampling from $[\boldsymbol{A} \mid \mathcal{C}, \boldsymbol{\Theta}, \theta_0]$. However, drawing $\boldsymbol{\Theta}$ from its posterior at every iteration can be computationally inefficient. Liu et al. [27] demonstrated that *marginalizing* out $(\boldsymbol{\Theta}, \theta_0)$ from the posterior distribution can lead to much faster convergence of the algorithm [28]. In other words, one can use the Gibbs sampler to draw from the marginal distribution

$$p(\boldsymbol{A} \mid \boldsymbol{S}, \pi) = \int\int p(\boldsymbol{\Theta}, \theta_0 \mid \boldsymbol{S}, \boldsymbol{A}, \pi) p(\boldsymbol{A}) p(\boldsymbol{\Theta}, \theta_0) \, d\boldsymbol{\Theta} d\theta_0, \quad (16.4)$$

which can be easily evaluated analytically.

If π is unknown, one can assume a beta prior distribution Beta(α_1, α_2) and marginalize out π from the posterior, in which case $p(\boldsymbol{A} \mid \boldsymbol{S})$ can be derived from (16.4) by altering the last term in (16.4) to the ratio of normalizing constants for the Beta distribution, $B(|\boldsymbol{A}| + \alpha_1, L - |\boldsymbol{A}| + \alpha_2)/B(\alpha_1, \alpha_2)$. Based on (16.4), Liu et al. [27] derived a *predictive updating* algorithm for $\boldsymbol{A}$, which is to iteratively sample each component of $\boldsymbol{A}$ according to the predictive distribution

$$\frac{P(A_{ijk} = 1 \mid \boldsymbol{S})}{P(A_{ijk} = 0 \mid \boldsymbol{S})} = \frac{\pi}{1-\pi} \prod_{l=1}^{w_k}\left(\frac{\hat{\boldsymbol{\theta}}_{kl}}{\hat{\boldsymbol{\theta}}_0}\right)^{\mathcal{C}(S_{i,j+l,k})}, \quad (16.5)$$

where the posterior means are $\hat{\boldsymbol{\theta}}_{kl} = \dfrac{\mathcal{C}\left(S_l^{(A_k)}\right)+\boldsymbol{\beta}_{kl}}{|\mathcal{C}\left(S_l^{(A_k)}\right)+\boldsymbol{\beta}_{kl}|}$ and $\hat{\boldsymbol{\theta}}_0 = \dfrac{\mathcal{C}\left(S^{(A^c)}\right)+\boldsymbol{\beta}_0}{|\mathcal{C}\left(S^{(A^c)}\right)+\boldsymbol{\beta}_0|}$.

Under the model specified above, it is also possible to implement a "partition-based" DA approach [14] that is motivated by the recursive algorithm used in

Auger and Lawrence [1]. The DA approach samples A jointly according to the conditional distribution

$$P(A \mid \Theta, S) = \prod_{i=1}^{N} P(A_{iL_i} \mid \Theta, S) \prod_{j=1}^{L_i-1} P(A_{ij}|A_{i,j+1}, \ldots, A_{iL_i}, S, \Theta).$$

At a position j, the current knowledge of motif positions is updated using the conditional probability $P(A_{ij} \mid A_{i,j+1} \ldots A_{iL_i}, \Theta)$ (backward sampling), with $A_{i,j-1} \ldots A_{i1}$ marginalized out using a forward summation procedure (an example will be given in Section 16.6.1.2). In contrast, at each iteration, GS iteratively draws from the conditional distribution, $P(A_{ijk}|A \setminus A_{ijk}, S)$, iteratively visiting each sequence position i, updating its motif indicator conditional on the indicators for other positions. The Gibbs approach tends to be "sticky" when the motif sites are abundant. For example, once we have set $A_{ijk} = 1$ (for some k), we will not be able to allow segment $S_{[i,j+1:j+w_k]}$ to be a motif site. The DA method corresponds to a *grouping* scheme (with A sampled together), whereas the GS corresponds to a *collapsing* approach (with Θ integrated out). Both have been shown to improve upon the original scheme [28].

16.4.2 Scoring Functions and Bayesian Optimization

In motif discovery problems, the predictions of interest often correspond to the estimated maximizer A^* of the posterior probability $P(A \mid S)$, rather than the posterior average. In this regard, BioProspector [29] attempts to find a fast approximate estimate of A by slightly altering the Gibbs search strategy. From (16.5), an approximate posterior "scoring" function is derived as

$$\phi(A) = \frac{\log(|A|)}{w} \sum_{i=1}^{w} \sum_{j=1}^{J} \hat{\theta}_{ij} \log \frac{\hat{\theta}_{ij}}{\theta_{0j}}.$$

When using the current weight matrix to scan the sequence, all segments whose scores $\phi(\cdot)$ exceed a "high" threshold are automatically called a motif site, while those that are between the high and a "low" threshold are given a chance to be sampled into the set of sites. The low threshold is started as 0 and increased gradually during iterations to a suitable level. Jensen and Liu [18] present an optimization algorithm that provides (i) a more accurate scoring function approximation of (16.5) and (ii) a simulated annealing procedure to optimize this function.

16.5 Extensions of the Product-Multinomial Motif Model

Unknown motif width. In the following discussion, for simplicity of notation, we assume a single motif type Θ of width w. Previously, w was assumed to be known and fixed; we may instead view w as an additional unknown model parameter. Jointly sampling from the posterior distribution of (A, Θ, w) is difficult as the dimensionality of Θ changes with w. One way to update (w, Θ) jointly would be through a reversible jump procedure [12] – however, note that we can again integrate out Θ from the posterior distribution to avoid a dimensionality change during the updating. By placing an appropriate prior distribution $p(w)$ on w (a possible choice is a Poisson(λ)), we can update w using a Metropolis step. Using a Beta(α_1, α_2) prior on π, the marginalized posterior distribution of interest is $P(A, w \mid S)$,

$$\propto ID(\mathcal{C}(S^{(A^c)}) + \boldsymbol{\beta}_0) \prod_{i=1}^{w} \frac{ID(\mathcal{C}(S_i^{(A)}) + \boldsymbol{\beta}_i)}{ID(\boldsymbol{\beta}_i)} \frac{B(|A| + \alpha_1, L - |A| + \alpha_2)}{B(\alpha_1, \alpha_2)} p(w).$$

The product-multinomial model used for Θ is a first approximation to a realistic model for TFBSs. In empirical observations, it has been reported that certain specific features often characterize functional binding sites. We mention here a few extensions of the primary motif model that have been recently implemented to improve the performance of motif discovery algorithms.

Variations of the product multinomial assumption. The product multinomial model assumes that all columns of a weight matrix are independent – however, it has been observed that about 25% of experimentally validated motifs show statistically significant positional correlations. Zhou and Liu [41] extend the independent weight matrix model to including one or more correlated column pairs, under the restriction that no two pairs of correlated columns can share a column in common. For example, if columns 1 and 5 are correlated, 2 and 3 can be, but 1 and 2 cannot. A Metropolis–Hastings step is added in the Gibbs sampler [27] that deletes or adds a pair of correlated column at each iteration. Again, the posterior distribution can be collapsed over Θ during the Metropolis–Hastings step to avoid a parameter space of varying dimensions for different numbers of correlated columns. Barash et al. [3] proposed a Bayesian tree-like network to model the possible correlation structure among all the positions within a TF model. Zhao et al. [40] described a permuted Markov model – they assume that an unobserved permutation has acted on the positions of all the motif sites and that the original ordered positions can be described by a Markov chain. Thus, mathematically, the model of Zhou and Liu [41] is a subcase of Zhou and Liu [41], which is, in turn, a subcase of Barash et al. [3].

It has been observed that real TFBSs are not uniformly conserved over all positions – the conserved positions often occur as a group at one or two regions over the motif, since contacts between proteins and the DNA are likely to occur over a few bases at a time (more conservation indicates a higher chance of contact). In the hope that incorporation of this positional trend is more likely to find the correct motif, Kechris et al. [19] use a prior distribution that "penalizes" deviations from a conserved profile. Instead of using a Dirichlet distribution as a prior for the motif column probabilities θ, they instead use a normal or double exponential prior, for example, $p(\theta) \propto e^{-\sum_{i=1}^{4} |\theta_i - \beta_i|}$. To update parameters of the model, they developed an EM algorithm in which the M-step was slightly modified from Lawrence and Reilly [23] to reflect the change in the prior.

16.6 HMM-Type Models for Regulatory Modules

Motif predictions for high eukaryotes (e.g., human, mouse, dog, etc.) are more challenging than that for simpler organisms such as yeast and bacteria. Some of the reasons are (i) large sections of low-complexity regions (repeat sequences), (ii) weak motif signals, (iii) sparseness of signals compared to entire region under study – binding sites may occur as far as 2,000–3,000 bases away from the transcription start site, either upstream or downstream, and (iv) motifs occurring in clusters, varying in order or composition between sequences. In complex eukaryotes, regulatory proteins often work in combination to regulate target genes, and their binding sites have often been observed to occur in spatial clusters, or *cis-regulatory modules* (CRMs; Figure 16.2). One approach to locating CRMs is by predicting novel motifs and looking for co-occurrences [34]. However, since individual motifs in the cluster may not be well conserved, such an approach often leads to a large number of false negatives. Our strategy is to first use existing de novo motif-finding algorithms and TF databases to compose a list of putative binding motifs, $\mathcal{D} = \{\Theta_1, \ldots, \Theta_D\}$, where D is in the range of 50–100, and then simultaneously update these motifs and estimate the posterior probability for each of them to be included in the CRM.

Let S denote the set of n sequences with lengths $L_1, L_2, \ldots, L_n$, respectively, corresponding to the upstream regions of n coregulated genes. We assume that the CRM consists of K different kinds of TFs with distinctive PWMs. Both the PWMs and K are unknown and need to be inferred from the data. In addition to the indicator variable A defined in Section 16.4, we define a new variable $a_{i,j}$, which denotes the location of the jth site (irrespective of motif type) in the ith sequence. Let $a = \{a_{ij}; i = 1, \ldots, n; \ j = 1, \ldots, L_i\}$. Associated with

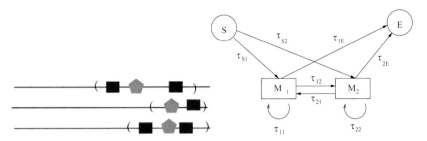

Fig. 16.2. Graphical illustration of a CRM.

each site is its *type* indicator $T_{i,j}$, with $T_{i,j}$ taking one of the K values (Let $T = (T_{ij})$). Note that the specification (a, T) is essentially equivalent to A.

Next, we model the dependence between $T_{i,j}$ and $T_{i,j+1}$ by a $K \times K$ probability transition matrix τ. The distance between neighboring TFBSs in a CRM, $d_{ij} = a_{i,j+1} - a_{i,j}$, is assumed to follow $Q(; \lambda, w)$, a geometric distribution truncated at w, that is, $Q(d; \lambda, w) = (1 - \lambda)^{d-w} \lambda \quad (d = w, w + 1, \ldots)$. The distribution of nucleotides in the *background* sequence a multinomial distribution with unknown parameter $\rho = (\rho_A, \ldots, \rho_T)$.

Next, we let u be a binary vector indicating which motifs are included in the module, that is, $u = (u_1, \ldots u_D)^T$, where

$$u_j = \begin{cases} 1, & \text{if the } j\text{th motif type is present in the module,} \\ 0, & \text{otherwise.} \end{cases}$$

By construction, $|u| = K$. Thus, the information regarding K is completely encoded by u. In light of this notation, the set of PWMs for the CRM is defined as $\Theta = \{\Theta_j : u_j = 1\}$. Since now we restrict our inference of CRM to a subset of $\mathcal{D}$, the probability model for the observed sequence data can be written as

$$P(S \mid \mathcal{D}, \tau, u, \lambda, \rho) = \sum_a \sum_T P(S \mid a, T, \mathcal{D}, \tau, u, \lambda, \rho) P(a \mid \lambda) P(T \mid a, \tau).$$

From the above likelihood formulation, we need to simultaneously estimate the optimal u and the parameters $(\mathcal{D}, \tau, \lambda, \rho)$. To achieve this, we first prescribe a prior distribution on the parameters and missing data:

$$P(\mathcal{D}, \tau, u, \lambda, \rho) = f_1(\mathcal{D} \mid u) f_2(\tau \mid u) f_3(\rho) g_1(u) g_2(\lambda).$$

Here the $f_i(\cdot)$'s are (product) Dirichlet distributions. Assuming each u_i takes the value 1 with a prior probability of π (i.e., π is the prior probability of including a motif in the module), $g_1(u)$ represents a product of D Bernoulli(π) distributions, and $g_2(\lambda)$, a generally flat Beta distribution. More precisely, we assume a priori that $\Theta_i \sim \prod_{j=1}^{w} \text{Dirichlet}(\boldsymbol{\beta}_{ij})$ (for $i = 1, \ldots, D$); $\boldsymbol{\rho} \sim \text{Dirichlet}(\boldsymbol{\beta}_0)$; $\lambda \sim \text{Beta}(a, b)$. Given $\boldsymbol{u}$ (with $|\boldsymbol{u}| = K$), each row of $\boldsymbol{\tau}$ is assumed to follow an independent Dirichlet. Let the ith row $v_i|\boldsymbol{u} \sim \text{Dirichlet}(\boldsymbol{\alpha}_i)$, where $i = 1, \ldots, K$.

Let $\Omega = (\mathcal{D}, \boldsymbol{\tau}, \lambda, \boldsymbol{\rho})$ denote the full parameter set. Then the posterior distribution of Ω has the form

$$P(\Omega, \boldsymbol{u} \mid S) \propto P(S \mid \boldsymbol{u}, \Omega) f_1(\mathcal{D} \mid \boldsymbol{u}) f_2(\boldsymbol{\tau} \mid \boldsymbol{u}) f_3(\boldsymbol{\rho}) g_1(\boldsymbol{u}) g_2(\lambda). \quad (16.6)$$

A GS approach was developed in Thompson et al. [38] to infer the CRM from a special case of the posterior distribution (16.6) with fixed $\boldsymbol{u}$. Given the flexibility of the model and the size of the parameter space for an unknown $\boldsymbol{u}$, it is unlikely that a standard MCMC approach can converge to a good solution in a reasonable amount of time. If we ignore the ordering of sites $\boldsymbol{T}$ and assume components of $\boldsymbol{a}$ to be independent, this model is reduced to the original motif model in Section 16.4, which can be updated through the previous Gibbs or DA procedure.

16.6.1 A Hybrid EMC–DA Approach

With a starting set of putative binding motifs $\mathcal{D}$, we simultaneously modify these motifs and estimate the posterior probability for each of them to be included in the CRM through iterations of the following Monte Carlo sampling steps: (i) Given the current collection of motif PWMs (or sites), sample motifs into the CRM by evolutionary Monte Carlo (EMC); (ii) Given the CRM configuration and the PWMs, update the motif site locations through DA; and (iii) Given motif site locations, update the corresponding PWMs and other parameters.

16.6.1.1 Evolutionary Monte Carlo for Module Selection

It has been demonstrated that the EMC method is effective for sampling and optimization with functions of binary variables [25]. Conceptually, we should be able to apply EMC directly to select motifs comprising the CRM, but a complication here is that there are many continuous parameters such as the Θ_j's, λ, and $\boldsymbol{\tau}$. We cannot just fix these parameters (as in the usual Gibbs sampler) and update the CRM composition because some of them vary in dimensionality when a putative motif in $\mathcal{D}$ is included or excluded from the CRM. We therefore have to integrate out the continuous parameters Θ and $\boldsymbol{\tau}$ analytically and condition on variables $\boldsymbol{a}$ and $\boldsymbol{T}$ when updating the CRM composition. Let $\Omega^{(u)} = (\Theta, \boldsymbol{\rho}, \boldsymbol{\tau}, \lambda)$ denote the set of all parameters in the model, for a fixed $\boldsymbol{u}$. Then, the marginalized conditional posterior probability for a module configuration $\boldsymbol{u}$ is

$$P(\boldsymbol{u}\,|\,\boldsymbol{a},\boldsymbol{T},\boldsymbol{S})\propto\pi^{|\boldsymbol{u}|}(1-\pi)^{D-|\boldsymbol{u}|}\int P(\boldsymbol{S}\,|\,\boldsymbol{a},\boldsymbol{T},\Omega^{(u)})P(\Omega^{(u)}\,|\,\boldsymbol{u})d\Omega^{(u)}, \quad (16.7)$$

where only Θ and τ are dependent on $\boldsymbol{u}$; and $\boldsymbol{a}$ and $\boldsymbol{T}$ are the sets of locations and types, respectively, of all putative motif sites (for all the D motifs in $\mathcal{D}$). Thus, only when the indicator u_i for the weight matrix Θ_i is 1, do its site locations and types contribute to the computation of (16.7). When we modify the current $\boldsymbol{u}$ by excluding a motif type, its site locations and corresponding motif type indicators are removed from the computation of (16.7).

For EMC, we need to prescribe a set of temperatures, $t_1 > t_2 > \cdots > t_M = 1$, one for each member in the population. Then, we define

$$\phi_i(\boldsymbol{u}_i) \propto \exp[\log P(\boldsymbol{u}_i \mid \boldsymbol{a}, \boldsymbol{T}, \boldsymbol{S})/t_i],$$

and $\phi(\boldsymbol{U}) \propto \prod_{i=1}^{M} \phi_i(u_i)$. The "population" $\boldsymbol{U} = (\boldsymbol{u}_1, \ldots, \boldsymbol{u}_M)$ is then updated iteratively using two types of moves: *mutation* and *crossover*.

In the mutation operation, a unit $\boldsymbol{u}_k$ is randomly selected from the current population and mutated to a new vector $\boldsymbol{v}_k$ by changing the values of some of its bits chosen at random. The new member $\boldsymbol{v}_k$ is accepted to replace $\boldsymbol{u}_k$ with probability $\min(1, r_m)$, where

$$r_m = \phi_k(\boldsymbol{v}_k)/\phi_k(\boldsymbol{u}_k).$$

In the crossover step, two individuals, $\boldsymbol{u}_j$ and $\boldsymbol{u}_k$, are chosen at random from the population. A crossover point x is chosen randomly over the positions 1 to D, and two new units $\boldsymbol{v}_j$ and $\boldsymbol{v}_k$ are formed by switching between the two individuals the segments on the right side of the crossover point. The two "children" are accepted into the population to replace their parents $\boldsymbol{u}_j$ and $\boldsymbol{u}_k$ with probability $\min(1, r_c)$, where

$$r_c = \frac{\phi_j(\boldsymbol{v}_j)\phi_k(\boldsymbol{v}_k)}{\phi_j(\boldsymbol{u}_j)\phi_k(\boldsymbol{u}_k)}.$$

If rejected, the parents are kept unchanged. On convergence, the samples of $\boldsymbol{u}_M$ (for temperature $t_M = 1$) follow the target distribution (16.7).

16.6.1.2 Sampling Motif Sites $\boldsymbol{A}$ through Recursive DA

The second part of the algorithm consists of updating the motif sites conditional on a CRM configuration (i.e., with $\boldsymbol{u}$ fixed). For simplicity, we describe the method for a single sequence $S = (s_1, \ldots, s_L)$; the same procedure is repeated for all sequences in the data set. For simplicity of notation, we assume that all motifs are of width w. For fixed $\boldsymbol{u}$, let $F(i, j, k, \boldsymbol{u}) = P(s_{[i,j,k]} \mid \Omega^{(u)}, \boldsymbol{u})$ denote the probability of observing the part of the sequence S from position i to j, with a motif of type k $\{k \in \mathcal{D}: u_k = 1\}$ occupying positions from $j - w + 1$ to j ($k = 0$ denotes the background). Let $K = \sum_{k=1}^{D} u_k$ denote the number of motif types in the module. For notational simplicity, let us assume that $\boldsymbol{u}$ represents the set of the first K motifs, indexed 1 through K. Since the motif site updating step is *conditional* given $\boldsymbol{u}$, we drop the subscript $\boldsymbol{u}$ from $F(i, j, k, \boldsymbol{u})$ in the remaining part of the section.

In the *forward summation* step, we recursively calculate the probability of different motif types ending at a position j of the sequence

$$
F(1, j, k) = \left[\sum_{i < j} \sum_{l=1}^{K} F(1, i, l)\tau_{l,k}\, Q(j - i - w; \lambda, w) + P(s_{[1, j-w, 0]} | \boldsymbol{\rho}) \right]
$$
$$
\times\, F(j - w + 1, j, k).
$$

By convention, the initial conditions are $F(0, 0, k) = 1$ ($k = 0, 1, \dots, K$) and $F(i, j, k) = 0$ for $j < i$ and $k > 0$. In the *backward sampling* step, we use Bayes theorem to calculate the probability of motif occurrence at each position, starting from the end of the sequence. If a motif of type k ends at position i in the sequence, the probability that the next motif further ahead in the sequence spans position $(i' - w + 1)$ to i' $(i' \le i - w)$ and is of type k' is

$$
P(A_{\cdot,i'-w+1,k'} = 1 \mid S, \Omega, A_{\cdot,i-w+1,k} = 1)
$$
$$
= \frac{F(1, i', k')\, P(s_{[i'+1, i-w, 0]} | \boldsymbol{\rho})\, F(i - w + 1, i, k)\, Q(i - i' - w; \lambda, w)\, \tau_{k',k}}{F(1, i, k)}.
$$

The required expressions have all been calculated in the forward sum.

16.6.1.3 Sampling Parameters from Posterior Distributions

Given the motif type indicator $\boldsymbol{u}$ and the motif position and type vectors $\boldsymbol{a}$ and T, we now update the parameters $\Omega = (\boldsymbol{\Theta}, \boldsymbol{\rho}, \boldsymbol{\tau}, \lambda)$ by a random sample from their joint conditional distribution. Since conjugate priors have been assumed for all parameters, their conditional posterior distributions are also of the same form and are straightforward to simulate from. For example, the posterior of Θ_i will be $\prod_{j=1}^{w}$ Dirichlet($\boldsymbol{\beta}_{ij} + \boldsymbol{n}_{ij}$), where $\boldsymbol{n}_{ij}$ is a vector containing the counts of the four nucleotides at the jth position of all the sites corresponding to motif type i. For those motifs that have not been selected by the module (i.e., with $u_i = 0$), the corresponding Θ's still follow their prior distribution. Similarly, the posterior distribution of $\boldsymbol{\rho}$ is Dirichlet($\boldsymbol{\beta}_0 + \boldsymbol{n}_0$), where $\boldsymbol{n}_0$ denotes the frequencies for the four nucleotides in the *background* sequence.

For updating $\boldsymbol{\tau}$, we note that if $\boldsymbol{m}_{ij}$ $\{i, j \in \mathcal{D}: u_i = u_j = 1\}$ denotes the number of transitions from PWM type i to j (when i and j are both included

Table 16.1. *Error Rates for Module Prediction Methods*

Method	MEF	MYF	SP1	SRF	Total	SENS	SPEC	TSpec
EM	0	1	21	0	161	0.14	0.14	0.20
BioProspector	6	1	8	1	155	0.10	0.10	0.36
GS	6	6	2	1	84	0.10	0.25	0.44
GS^{p*}	14	14	4	6	162	0.25	0.23	0.60
EMC–DA	12	12	5	7	180	0.23	0.20	0.67
EMC–DA^{p*}	17	13	8	10	108	0.31	0.44	0.80
True	**32**	**50**	**44**	**28**	**154**	–	–	–

Note: The Total column shows the total number of sites predicted. There are 154 true sites. *SENS* (sensitivity) $\equiv \frac{(\#\text{predicted true positives})}{(\#\text{true positives})}$; SPEC (specificity) $\equiv \frac{(\#\text{predicted true positives})}{\#\text{predicted sites}}$; TSpec: Total specificity, defined as the fraction of the predicted motif types that "correspond" to known motifs (match in at least 80% of all positions). The Gibbs sampler (GS) requires the total number of motif types to be specified (set equal to 5). GS^{p*} denotes the GS using a strong informative prior, EMC–DA^{p*} denotes using prior information from the JASPAR database. Rounded averages over five runs of each algorithm are recorded.

in the module), then the posterior distribution of v_i is Dirichlet($\alpha_i + m_i$). Let the distance between consecutive sites on sequence i ($i = 1, \ldots, n$) be $d_{ij} = a_{i,j+1} - a_{ij}$, where each d follows $Q(\,;\lambda, w)$, a geometric(λ) distribution truncated at w. Let $d = \sum_{i=1}^{n} \sum_{j=1}^{|A_i|-1} d_{ij}$ be the total length of sequence covered by the CRMs, where $|A_i|$ is the total number of sites in sequence i, and $|A'| = \sum_{i=1}^{n}(|A_i| - 1)$. Then the posterior distribution of λ is Beta($a + |A'|, b + d - w|A'|$).

16.6.2 A Case Study

We compared the performance of EMC–DA with EM- and GS-based methods in an analysis of mammalian skeletal muscle regulatory sequences [38]. The raw data consist of upstream sequences of lengths up to 5,000 bp each corresponding to 24 orthologous pairs of genes in the human and mouse genomes – each of the sequences being known to contain at least one experimentally reported TFBS corresponding to one of five motif types: MEF, MYF2, SRF, SP1, and TEF. Following the procedure of Thompson et al. [38], we aligned the sequences for each orthologous pair (human and mouse) and retained only the parts that shared a percent identity greater than 65%, cutting down the sequence search space to about 40% of the original sequences.

Using BioProspector, EM (MEME), and AlignAce (Gibbs sampler for independent motifs), we obtained initial sets of 100 motifs including redundant ones.

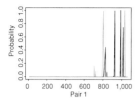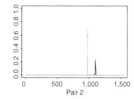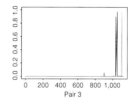

Fig. 16.3. Posterior probability of sampling sites in human–rodent sequence pairs. The light and dark lines correspond to the MEF2 and MYF motif; the horizontal axes denote the site location on sequences.

The top-scoring 10 motifs from BioProspector and MEME respectively contained two and three matches to the true motif set (of five), whereas AlignAce found none. The Gibbs sampler under a module model [38] found two matches in general, but could find two others with a more detailed and precise prior input (the number of sites per motif and motif abundance per sequence), which is generally unavailable in real applications. The best scoring module configuration from EMC–DA contained three of the true five, MYF, MEF2, and SP1, and two uncharacterized motifs. There are few TEF sites matching the reported consensus in these sequences, and they were found by none of the algorithms.

The relative error rates for the algorithms could be compared in this case as we had exact knowledge of each of the experimentally determined TFBSs. Table 16.1 shows that EMC–DA significantly cuts down the percentage of false positives in the output, compared to the methods that do not adjust for positional clustering of motifs. We next tested whether it is beneficial to choose a subset of motifs from the eukaryotic motif database [33] as the starting motif set for EMC–DA. This time, EMC–DA can find four out of five expected motifs. Figure 16.3 shows the posterior probability of site occurrence over the first three aligned sequence pairs, indicating a strong evidence of clustering. For multiple runs of EMC–DA with different starting seeds, there was no noticeable difference in the results over a wide range of prior settings.

16.7 Model Selection through a Bayesian Approach

One of the basic questions that arise in motif discovery is whether the patterns "discovered" from the sequence data by these algorithms are "real." Although the biological relevance of such findings generally needs further biological experimentation, we can at least try to assess the significance of the predictions from a statistical viewpoint.

As a Bayesian model selection problem, it is of interest to assess whether the sequence data should be better explained by model $\mathcal{M}_1$, which assumes the

Table 16.2. *Comparison of Model Selection Criteria for Three Data Sets from Bacillus subtilis (BS), yeast (Y), and E. coli (EC)*

TF	Order	logMAP	BIC	AIC	KLI	Motif consensus	Count
SigA	1	−326.27	185.01	258.26	4.10	TTTTTT	186
(BS)	2	−192.02	163.2	309.69	4.07	TGAAAA	94
	3	**263.31**	**2.48**	**148.98**	**5.70**	TTGACA	40
	4	**90.19**	**101.46**	**247.95**	**4.91**	TATAAT	41
GAL	1	**20.3**	**−130.74**	**43.45**	**11.52**	GGAGCACTTTCCTCCGA	16
(Y)	2	−20.26	−259.75	88.62	9.97	AGCACGCAACTTGCAAA	6
	3	−49.26	−341.15	7.23	11.44	GGGTGCCTGTGCCATGG	5
	4	−12.53	−398.98	−50.61	9.10	TTTTTTTTTTTTTTGAA	16
CRP	1	**2.27**	**−167.93**	**17.8**	**10.70**	TTATTTGAACGAGGTCACACTT	11
(EC)	2	−7.53	−394.14	−22.67	10.83	GGATCATATGTTGTGTGAAATA	5
	3	−19.33	−401.54	−30.07	9.44	ATTTATAAACATTTAAAATCGT	8
	4	−1.99	−360.39	11.08	10.63	TGTATTGATGTGTCTTACGAAA	5

Note: "Order" represents the order in which the motif was found using the method of Gupta and Liu [14]. Experimentally confirmed motifs are highlighted in boxes. For all data sets, the MAP score decreased after the true motif was found [BIC: Bayes Information Criterion; AIC: Akaike Information Criterion; KLI: Kullback-Leibler Information].

existence of a nontrivial motif, than by $\mathcal{M}_0$, which says that the sequences are generated entirely from a background model (e.g., an i.i.d. or Markov model). The Bayes factor, which is the ratio of the marginal likelihoods under the two models, can be computed as

$$\frac{p(S \mid \mathcal{M}_1)}{p(S \mid \mathcal{M}_0)} = \frac{\sum_A \int_\theta p(A, S, \theta \mid \mathcal{M}_1)d\theta}{\int_\theta p(S, \theta \mid \mathcal{M}_0)d\theta} = \frac{\sum_A p(A, S \mid \mathcal{M}_1)}{p(S \mid \mathcal{M}_0)}. \quad (16.8)$$

The individual additive terms in the numerator of (16.8) consist of ratios of products of gamma functions. To evaluate this sum exhaustively over all partitions involves prohibitive amounts of computation. A lower bound for (16.8) is $p(A^*, S \mid \mathcal{M}_1)/p(S \mid \mathcal{M}_0)$, where A^* is the maximizer of the ratio. This bound, called the maximum a posteriori score (denoted by MAP(A^*)), can be used as a model selection criterion which can be tracked along with the Gibbs or DA iterations. As a frequentist evaluation of its performance, we have elsewhere [13] shown that the MAP asymptotically attains several desirable properties. For example, with a single motif type (width w) having occurrence probability π, under mild conditions, the MAP score selects the correct model, with the performance of the MAP improving as w and π increases (Table 16.2).

16.8 Discussion: Motif Discovery Beyond Sequence Analysis

TFBS prediction remains an important unsolved problem in molecular biology. The availability of massive amounts of genomic data, such as multispecies genome sequence, gene expression microarray, and the physical structure of DNA, has thrown up a huge challenge to computational scientists to develop investigative tools to infer biological function. In this chapter we have mainly demonstrated how Bayesian statistical models can be used to capture significant aspects of genomic sequence data and lead to more accurate motif predictions. Using the Bayesian approach naturally leads to a host of flexible Monte Carlo based algorithms that can deal with high-dimensional integration and multimodality problems effectively. The Bayesian framework also provides us with a basic infrastructure for hierarchically modeling dependence and for dealing with nuisance parameters without leading to overwhelming analytical complexity. Finally, the Bayesian paradigm allows a "learning" capability so that "historical" data can be used in modeling a new, but similar problem. This can be important in building prior distributions based on partial information for known motifs, improving estimation of novel motifs.

It is becoming increasingly clear that sequence information alone is insufficient for accurate motif predictions (being especially true for complex genomes). An important aspect of further development of motif discovery tools is the efficient integration of multiple sources of genomic data, with the aim of refining and improving predictions.

16.8.1 Cross-species Phylogenetic Information

When multi-species sequence information is available, it is often seen that using multiple alignment [10] and restricting motif search to regions having a high sequence similarity improves the specificity of motif predictions. Thompson et al. [38] use this strategy to simultaneously search for motifs in aligned pairs of regulatory sequences from the human and mouse genomes, significantly improving predictions. It is still a challenge to efficiently incorporate more complete evolutionary information such as a phylogenetic tree of sequence divergence [11] in probabilistic motif models.

16.8.2 Chromatin Structure Information

The precise control of transcription in eukaryotes depends on the binding of TFs to promoter regions on DNA. Although in general practice, TF–DNA binding is represented as a one-dimensional process, in reality, binding occurs in three-dimensional space. DNA is neither static nor one-dimensional – much of DNA is wrapped around certain proteins called histones in a specific pattern, and binding is most likely to occur at the regions of exposed DNA [24]. For a given TF, there may be many potential TFBSs conserved in sequence, scattered throughout the genome of an organism; however, only a subset of these is actually active. As more experimental data become available (e.g., from chromatin immunoprecipitation or ChIP-chip experiments), knowledge of DNA structure holds a huge potential to aid in motif discovery.

16.8.3 Further Incorporation of Gene Expression Information

A highly successful tactic for computational motif prediction is to cluster genes based on their expression profiles, and search for motifs in the sequences upstream of tightly clustered genes. When noise is introduced into the cluster through spurious correlations, however, such an approach may result in many false positives. A filtering method based on the specificity of motif occurrences has been shown to effectively eliminate false positives [17]. An iterative procedure for simultaneous gene clustering and motif finding has been suggested [16], but no effective algorithm has been implemented to demonstrate its advantage. Two methods for TFBM discovery via the association of gene expression values with motif abundance have been proposed by Bussemaker et al. [6] and Keles et al. [20]. These first conduct word enumeration and then use regression to check whether the genes whose upstream sequences contain a set of words have significant changes in their expression. Conlon et al. [7] provide an algorithm to further utilize gene expression or ChIP-chip information to help motif discovery. They first use an algorithm such as BioProspector, MEME, or MDscan [30] to report a large set of putative motifs, and then do a linear stepwise regression to select candidates that correlate with the microarray expression data (Tadesse et al. [36] later present a Bayesian version). However, these methods still face drawbacks such as the inappropriateness of the linearity assumption, high-dimensionality, and difficulties in using multiple microarray data sets simultaneously. Surmounting such challenges and finding effective ways to integrate multiple data sources into motif discovery is likely to hold the future key to accurate inference in biological systems.

Bibliography

[1] Auger, I. E. and Lawrence, C. E. (1989). Algorithms for the optimal identification of segment neighborhoods. *Bull. Math. Biol.*, 51(1):39–54.

[2] Bailey, T. and Elkan, C. (1994). Fitting a mixture model by expectation maximization to discover motifs in biopolymers. In *Proceedings of the Second International Conference on Intelligent Systems for Molecular Biology*, pp. 28–36.

[3] Barash, Y., Elidan, G., Friedman, N., and Kaplan, T. (2003). Modeling dependencies in protein-DNA binding sites. In *RECOMB Proceedings*, pp. 28–37.

[4] Bellhouse, D. R. (2004). The Reverend Thomas Bayes, FRS: A biography to celebrate the tercentenary of his birth. *Statist. Sci.*, 19(1):3–43.

[5] Bussemaker, H. J., Li, H., and Siggia, E. D. (2000). Building a dictionary for genomes: Identification of presumptive regulatory sites by statistical analysis. *Proc. Natl. Acad. Sci. U.S.A.*, 97(18):10096–10100.

[6] Bussemaker, H. J., Li, H., and Siggia, E. D. (2001). Regulatory detection using correlation with expression. *Nat. Genet.*, 27:167–174.

[7] Conlon, E. M., Liu, X. S., Lieb, J. D., and Liu, J. S. (2003). Integrating regulatory motif discovery and genome-wide expression analysis. *Proc. Natl Acad. Sci. U.S.A.*, 100(6):3339–3344.

[8] Dabrowiak, J. C., Goodisman, J., and Ward, B. (1997). Quantitative DNA footprinting. *Methods Mol. Biol.*, 90:23–42.

[9] Dempster, A. P., Laird, N. M., and Rubin, D. B. (1977). Maximum likelihood from incomplete data via the EM algorithm. *J. Roy. Stat. Soc. B*, 39(1):1–38.

[10] Durbin, R., Eddy, S., Krogh, A., and Mitchison, G. (1998). *Biological Sequence Analysis*. Cambridge University Press, Cambridge, UK.

[11] Graur, D. and Li, W. H. (2000). *Fundamentals of Molecular Evolution*, Chapter 4. Sinauer Associates, Sunderland.

[12] Green, P. J. (1995). Reversible jump MCMC and Bayesian model determination. *Biometrika*, 82:711–732.

[13] Gupta, M. (2003). *Stochastic Models for Sequence Pattern Discovery*. PhD thesis, Harvard University.

[14] Gupta, M. and Liu, J. S. (2003). Discovery of conserved sequence patterns using a stochastic dictionary model. *J. Am. Stat. Assoc.*, 98(461):55–66.

[15] Gupta, M. and Liu, J. S. (2005). De-novo cis-regulatory module elicitation for eukaryotic genomes. *Proc. Nat. Acad. Sci. U.S.A.*, 102(20):7079–7084.

[16] Holmes, I. and Bruno, W. (2000). Finding regulatory elements using joint likelihoods for sequence and expression profile data. *Proc. Int. Conf. Intell. Syst. Mol. Biol.*, 8:202–210.

[17] Hughes, J. D., Estep, P. W., Tavazoie, S., and Church, G. M. (2000). Computational identification of cis-regulatory elements associated with groups of functionally related genes in *Saccharomyces cerevisiae. J. Mol. Biol*, 296(5):1205–1214.

[18] Jensen, S. T. and Liu, J. S. (2004). Biooptimizer: A Bayesian scoring function approach to motif discovery. *Bioinformatics*, 20(10):1557–1564.

[19] Kechris, K. J., van Zwet, E., Bickel, P. J., and Eisen, M. B. (2004). Detecting DNA regulatory motifs by incorporating positional trends in information content. *Genome Biol.*, 5(7):R50.

[20] Keles, S., van der Laan, M., and Eisen, M. B. (2002). Identification of regulatory elements using a feature selection method. *Bioinformatics*, 18(9):1167–1175.

[21] Kellis, M., Patterson, N., Endrizzi, M., Birren, B., and Lander, E. (2003). Sequencing and comparison of yeast species to identify genes and regulatory elements. *Nature*, 423:241–254.

[22] Lawrence, C. E., Altschul, S. F., Boguski, M. S., Liu, J. S., Neuwald, A. F., and Wootton, J. C. (1993). Detecting subtle sequence signals: A Gibbs sampling strategy for multiple alignment. *Science*, 262(5131):208–214.

[23] Lawrence, C. E. and Reilly, A. A. (1990). An expectation–maximization (EM) algorithm for the identification and characterization of common sites in biopolymer sequences. *Proteins*, 7:41–51.

[24] Lee, C. K., Shibata, Y., Rao, B., Strahl, B., and Lieb, J. (2004). Evidence for nucleosome depletion at active regulatory regions genome-wide. *Nat. Genet.*, 36(8):900–905.

[25] Liang, F. and Wong, W. H. (2000). Evolutionary Monte Carlo: Applications to c_p model sampling and change point problem. *Stat. Sin.*, 10:317–342.

[26] Liu, J. S. and Lawrence, C. (1999). Bayesian inference on biopolymer models. *Bioinformatics*, 15:38–52.

[27] Liu, J. S., Neuwald, A. F., and Lawrence, C. E. (1995). Bayesian models for multiple local sequence alignment and Gibbs sampling strategies. *J. Am. Stat. Assoc.*, 90:1156–1170.

[28] Liu, J. S., Wong, W. H., and Kong, A. (1994). Covariance structure of the Gibbs sampler with applications to the comparisons of estimators and augmentation schemes. *Biometrika*, 81:27–40.

[29] Liu, X., Brutlag, D. L., and Liu, J. S. (2001). Bioprospector: Discovering conserved DNA motifs in upstream regulatory regions of co-expressed genes. In *Pacific Symposium on Biocomputing*, pp. 127–138.

[30] Liu, X., Brutlag, D. L., and Liu, J. S. (2002). An algorithm for finding protein-DNA binding sites with applications to chromatin-immunoprecipitation microarray experiments. *Nat. Biotechnol.*, 20(8):835–839.

[31] Neuwald, A. F., Liu, J. S., and Lawrence, C. E. (1995). Gibbs motif sampling: Detection of bacterial outer membrane protein repeats. *Protein Sci.*, 4:1618–1632.

[32] Sabatti, C. and Lange, K. (2002). Genomewide motif identification using a dictionary model. *IEEE Proc.*, 90:1803–1810.

[33] Sandelin, A., Alkema, W., Engström, P., Wasserman, W., and Lenhard, B. (2004). JASPAR: An open access database for eukaryotic transcription factor binding profiles. *Nucleic Acids Res.*, 32(D):91–94.

[34] Sinha, S. and Tompa, M. (2002). Discovery of novel transcription factor binding sites by statistical overrepresentation. *Nucleic Acids Res.*, 30:5549–5560.

[35] Stormo, G. D. and Hartzell, G. W. (1989). Identifying protein-binding sites from unaligned DNA fragments. *Proc. Natl. Acad. Sci. U.S.A.*, 86:1183–1187.

[36] Tadesse, M. G., Vannucci, M., and Lio, P. (2004). Identification of DNA regulatory motifs using Bayesian variable selection. *Bioinformatics*, 20(16):2553–2561.

[37] Tanner, M. and Wong, W. H. (1987). The calculation of posterior distributions by data augmentation. *J. Am. Stat. Assoc.*, 82:528–550.

[38] Thompson, W., Palumbo, M. J., Wasserman, W. W., Liu, J. S., and Lawrence, C. E. (2004). Decoding human regulatory circuits. *Genome Res.*, 10:1967–1974.

[39] Tupler, R., Perini, G., and Green, M. (2001). Expressing the human genome. *Nature*, 409(6822):832–833.

[40] Zhao, X., Huang, H., and Speed, T. P. (2004). Finding short DNA motifs using permuted Markov models. In *RECOMB Proceedings*, pp. 68–75.

[41] Zhou, Q. and Liu, J. S. (2004). Modeling within-motif dependence for transcription factor binding site predictions. *Bioinformatics*, 20(6):909–916.

[42] Zhou, Q. and Wong, W. H. (2004). Cismodule: De novo discovery of cis-regulatory modules by hierarchical mixture modeling. *Proc. Natl. Acad. Sci. U.S.A.*, 101(33):12114–12119.

17

Identification of DNA Regulatory Motifs and Regulators by Integrating Gene Expression and Sequence Data

DEUKWOO KWON
National Cancer Institute

SINAE KIM
University of Michigan

DAVID B. DAHL
Texas A&M University

MICHAEL SWARTZ
Texas A&M University and University of Texas M.D. Anderson Cancer Center

MAHLET G. TADESSE
University of Pennsylvania

MARINA VANNUCCI
Texas A&M University

Abstract

We discuss methods to identify DNA regulatory elements by exploiting the correlation between sequence data and gene expression. We start by reviewing the contribution of M. G. Tadesse et al. (Identification of DNA regulatory motifs using Bayesian variable selection. *Bioinformatics*, **20** (2005), 2553–2561) in the use of Bayesian methods for variable selection for the identification of binding sites for regulatory factors. We then propose an extension of their model to include gene regulators. Although the modeling frameworks for variable selection has been extensively studied in the literature, their application in genomic studies for the identification of regulatory elements represents a novel contribution. We report performances of the methodologies on the well-studied regulatory systems of *Saccharomyces cerevisiae* under heat shock.

17.1 Introduction

The study of gene regulation plays an important role in understanding gene expression. A biological understanding of this complicated process motivates the techniques for analyzing and modeling gene expression and gene regulation.

333

Fundamental principles of genetics are transcription (the process of encoding information in DNA as mRNA) and translation (the process of making proteins from mRNA). Microarrays measure the abundance of mRNA and, thus, describe gene expression at the transcription level. Understanding how transcription is regulated in the cell can provide insights into developing rich models for analyzing microarrays.

The mechanisms that control gene transcriptions consist of many different classes of proteins and classes of DNA sequences [10]. The proteins involved, known as *trans-acting factors* or *transcription factors*, interact with control points of DNA sequences known as *cis-acting regulatory sequences*. In eukaryotic systems, such as human cells and yeast, RNA polymerase II is solely responsible for transcribing DNA to mRNA. This polymerase requires multiple sets of cis-acting regulatory sequences. Therefore, gene transcription is the result of multiple transcription factors binding these cis-acting regulatory sequences. The transcription factors contain structural *motifs* that are designed to recognize and bind the cis-regulatory sequences of DNA [1, 10]. The term *motif* is also sometimes associated with the particular sequence in the cis-acting regulatory sequence that the transcription factor binds to. A *regulator* is a molecule that affects gene regulation, either activating or repressing it. Regulators can be either signal modules from outside the cell or proteins (such as transcription factors and protein kinases) which are themselves products of genes regulated by a whole set of other proteins. In this chapter we refer to the expression of regulators as the expression levels of the genes that code for such regulators. Therefore, the regulation of gene expression involves a network of genes that code for transcription factors, which bind to cis-regulatory sequences, which in turn bind to motifs, and thereby induce the expression of the genes.

An example can be useful to understand gene regulation: Suppose that the expression of gene B is regulated by transcription factor A that binds to the cis-regulatory sequence for gene B, and transcription factor A is a protein coded for by gene A. Since gene A codes for the protein that regulates gene B, gene A can be referred to as a regulator gene. In this example, for simplicity, we have described it as a simple, one-to-one process. In reality, many genes can be coregulated by the same small set of transcription factors, especially if these genes have a common biological purpose. Therefore, examining a set of coregulated genes can reveal the motifs in the cis-regulatory sequences.

Many of the popular statistical methods for motif detection are based on clustering genes by similar expression profiles. DNA microarrays in fact provide a simple and natural vehicle for exploring the regulation of thousands of genes and their interactions. Methods such as CONSENSUS, MEME, Gibbs Motif sampler, and AlignACE identify sets of genes that may be coregulated by clustering genes based on expression levels. Clustering-based methods however have some drawbacks. In particular, it is not always true that coregulated genes have similar expression profiles, a fact that can introduce false positives in the motifs detection approaches. An improvement on these methods is the REDUCE algorithm [4] that further refines the sets of candidate motifs by using linear models to exploit the correlation between sequences data and expression level.

Other approaches for studying transcriptional regulation utilize probabilistic models, such as networks. Segal et al. [19] modeled coregulated genes into *modules* as functions of small sets of regulators that coordinate certain genes whose products perform a specific function in the cell. Accounting for the activity of regulators in the model improves prediction. In Segal et al. [20], the authors suggest a probabilistic model that combines sequence data with gene expression to model transcriptional and regulatory modules. Recently, Middendorf et al. [17] developed a learning algorithm, called MEDUSA, based on a classification model that predicts the up- and downregulation of genes using motif information and the expression patterns of potential regulators as covariates for the classification model. They code the information as a binary matrix indicating whether a motif is present or not and whether a regulator is up- or downregulated.

In this chapter we describe two applications of methods for Bayesian variable selection to the identification of regulatory elements. In Section 17.2, we provide background information for the model formulation and data processing. In Section 17.3, we review the work of Tadesse et al. [21] in the context of linear regression models relating gene expression data to large sets of candidate motifs. In Section 17.4, we propose an extension of their model to sets of predictors that include regulators. This is similar in spirit to the approach of Middendorf et al. [17]. With respect to their work, however, we model gene expressions and pattern scores, rather than discretized values that indicate up- or downregulation and presence or absence. In addition, instead of a classification model, we employ a linear regression setting with variable selection methods to detect sets of motifs and regulators that act together to affect the target gene expression. Section 17.5 presents some concluding remarks.

17.2 Integrating Gene Expression and Sequence Data

Motif detection involves searching for DNA patterns that are overrepresented in the upstream regions of a set of coregulated genes. Several computational algorithms have been developed for this task. Some algorithms are based on word-enumeration approaches [22], others are based on probability-based models [14, 15], and still others are based on dictionary models [3, 11]. A detailed account of the different methods can be found in the contribution of Gupta and Liu [12] to this edited volume.

Computational methods for motifs detection require a set of coregulated genes, which can be determined experimentally or computationally. A common approach consists of clustering high-throughput gene expression data and searching the upstream regions of each cluster for shared sequence patterns. This approach, however, often leads to large lists of candidate motifs. Bussemaker et al. [4] and Keleş et al. [13] have proposed methods to refine the search for biologically meaningful motifs by considering linear models that relate the expression data to the counts of each motif present in such candidate lists. Conlon et al. [7] have considered similar models where the gene expression is regressed on scores of candidate motifs, rather than simple counts. Scores are obtained by using MDScan [16], an algorithm that makes use of word-enumeration and position-specific probability matrix updating techniques. Conlon and collaborators have also proposed the use of stepwise selection to identify pattern scores that most correlate with the gene expression. Tadesse et al. [21] have investigated the alternative use of Bayesian variable selection techniques to select pattern scores. Their methodology is summarized in Figure 17.1. The methods employ stochastic search methods that perform a more thorough search of the model space and hence might potentially pick up motifs that can be missed by stepwise methods. In the next section we review the contribution of Tadesse et al. [21] and describe an application to cDNA microarrays on the transcriptional response of *Saccharomyces cerevisiae* to heat shock. Next, we propose an adaptation of the model by Tadesse and collaborators to sets of predictors that include regulators.

In both modeling frameworks described next we will define sets of predictors as pattern scores computed using the software Motif Regressor [7] via MDScan [16]. The algorithm starts by enumerating each segment of width w (seed) in the top t sequences. For each seed, it looks for w-mers with at least n base pair matches in the t sequences. These are used to form a motif matrix and the highest scoring seeds are retained, based on a semi-Bayesian scoring function

$$\frac{\log(x_n)}{w} \left[\sum_{i=1}^{w} \sum_{j=A}^{T} p_{ij} \log(p_{ij}) - \frac{1}{x_n} \sum_{\text{all segments}} \log(p_0(s)) \right],$$

where x_n is the number of n-matches aligned in the motif, p_{ij} is the frequency of nucleotide j at position i of the motif matrix, and $p_0(s)$ is the probability of generating the n-match s from the background model. The updating step is done iteratively by scanning all w-mers in the set of sequences used for

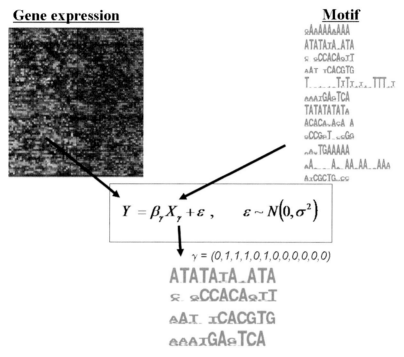

Fig. 17.1. Graphical representation of the methodology of Tadesse et al. [21]: Expression levels are regressed on a large list of candidate motif scores. Bayesian variable selection methods are used to locate sets of motifs that best predict changes in gene expression. (See color plate 17.1.)

refinement and adding in or removing from the weight matrix segments that increase the score. This is repeated until the alignment stabilizes.

17.3 A Model for the Identification of Regulatory Motifs

Our goal is to identify regulatory motifs among the overrepresented nucleotide patterns obtained as described above. This is accomplished by fitting a linear regression model relating gene expression levels (Y) to pattern scores (X), and using a Bayesian variable selection method to select motifs that best predict the expression. Motif pattern scores are calculated in terms of number of sites and degree of matching with each gene. The pattern score of motif m for gene g is given by

$$X_{gm} = \log_2 \left[\sum_{s \in S_{wg}} \frac{P(s \text{ from } \theta_m)}{P(s \text{ from } \theta_0)} \right],$$

where θ_m is the probability matrix of motif m of width w, θ_0 is the transition probability matrix for the background model, and S_{wg} is the set of all w-mers in the upstream sequence of gene g [7].

Variable selection is achieved by writing the regression model as

$$\mathbf{Y} = \mathbf{X}_\gamma \beta_\gamma + \varepsilon, \quad \varepsilon \sim N(0, \sigma^2 I) \tag{17.1}$$

with γ a vector of binary indicators for the exclusion and inclusion of the single variables (here motifs) [2, 9]. A prior is specified on γ, typically independent Bernoulli's on the single elements with common probability $\pi = p_{\text{prior}}/p$, where p_{prior} is the number of variables expected a priori to be included in the model. Conjugate priors can be specified for the model parameters

$$\beta_\gamma \sim N(0, c\,\sigma^2 \{\mathbf{X}'_\gamma \mathbf{X}_\gamma\}^{-1})$$
$$\sigma^2 \sim \text{Inv-}\chi^2(a, b), \tag{17.2}$$

where $\text{Inv-}\chi^2(a, b)$ indicates the scaled-inverse-χ^2 distribution. The hyperparameters a, b, and c need to be suitably specified. Here, columns of $\mathbf{X}$ and $\mathbf{Y}$ are assumed to be mean-centered.

Posterior inference is performed on γ only by integrating out the model parameters. Stochastic search Markov chain Monte Carlo (MCMC) techniques can be employed to look for sets of variables with high posterior probabilities. These methods visit a sequence of models that differ successively by one or two variables. At each iteration a new γ vector is generated from the current one by one of the following two moves:

(i) Add or delete one variable from γ^{old}
(ii) Swap the inclusion status of two variables in γ^{old}.

The new candidate γ^{new} is accepted with probability

$$\min \left\{ 1, \frac{f(\gamma^{\text{new}} | \mathbf{X}, \mathbf{Y})}{f(\gamma^{\text{old}} | \mathbf{X}, \mathbf{Y})} \right\}. \tag{17.3}$$

The MCMC samples lead to an estimate of γ as either the model with largest joint posterior probability or the marginal model consisting of those γ_j's with marginal posterior probability larger than a chosen cutoff value.

17.3.1 Application

We briefly describe an application of the methodology to cDNA microarray experiments that explore the transcriptional responses of the budding yeast *S. cerevisiae* [8] to heat shock caused by temperature increase. The other data consist of the organism genome sequences and related information, such as the start/stop position and orientation of each open reading frame (ORF). These were obtained from the NCBI's FTP site (ftp://ftp.ncbi.nih.gov/genomes/). The details of this and other applications can be found in Tadesse et al. [21]. That paper also reports a simulation study and comparisons to existing methods.

The model regresses the expression levels on the pattern scores. Motif Regressor [7] can be used to generate a large list of candidate motifs and calculate the matching scores for each gene. In the application presented here, sequences up to 800 bp upstream were extracted, shortening them, if necessary, to avoid overlap with adjacent ORFs. For genes with negative orientation, this was done by taking the reverse complement of the sequences. The search was restricted to the top 20 upregulated and top 20 downregulated genes. The top 50 upregulated and top 50 downregulated genes were used for refinement. The intergenic regions were extracted and used as background models. Nucleotide patterns of length 5–12 bp were considered with up to 30 distinct candidates for each width. This process resulted in a set of around 400 patterns.

Priors were specified by taking $p_{\text{prior}} = 20$ and setting $a = 3$ and b to be commensurate with the variability of the data. To assess the sensitivity of the results, three different values of the hyperparameter c were considered. For every regression model, two MCMC chains were run for 100,000 iterations each. One of the chains was started with 10 and the other with 100 randomly selected γ_j's set to 1. The sets of motifs visited by the two MCMC chains were pooled together. The normalized posterior probabilities of each distinct visited set were computed, together with the marginal posterior probabilities, $p(\gamma_j = 1|\mathbf{X}, \mathbf{Y})$, for the inclusion of single nucleotide patterns.

Table 17.1 reports motifs selected by the "best" model and ordered according to their marginal probabilities. Selections that are robust to the choice of c, that is, motifs that showed up in the best model of all MCMC analyses run with different values of c, are represented with two asterisks, and those that appeared in two of the three MCMC analyses have a single asterisk. Selected motifs explained approximately 16% of the expression variability in response to heat stress. Some of the selected motifs were experimentally known to be related to stress. Others were novel and constituted a set of promising candidates for future experimental work. Nucleotide patterns that match known motifs appear in the tables with bold characters, along with the associated binding site or a reference. Among the selected motifs, some contained matches to three well-known stress-related motifs: STRE, M3A, and M3B. STRE is known to respond to general environmental stress and to positively regulate transcription [18]. M3A and M3B had previously been found in genes repressed under environmental stress and act by slowing down cell growth [8]. Some patterns

Table 17.1. *Selection of Motifs: Selected Motifs Ordered
According to Their Marginal Posterior Probability*

Selected	Known	p
WTAAGGGAK**		1.0000
T**GAAA****	M3A	1.0000
ACCYT**GAAA****	M3A	0.9999
T**CYAGAA**TRTT**	Cliften et al.	0.9998
GGCAGGAMA**		0.9991
HYCCWTMCAT**		0.9991
W**ARGGG****	STRE	0.9987
M**GATGAG**ATGAR**	M3B	0.9985
GM**GATGAG**MWT**	M3B	0.9839
GAADRAA**AGGGR****	STRE	0.9739
GCCCC*		0.9573
A**GGGRG**SGAAD*	STRE	0.9251
GCWCATCCACC		0.8441
CMAACAAAS		0.8195
GSCCKGSWA		0.5308
A**RGGGG**SGGR*	STRE	0.5136
AMRWGCCAGAA		0.4364

Note: Selections that are robust to the choice of the hyperparameter c are shown with asterisks. Characters in bold correspond to
matches between known and discovered motifs. IUPAC codes are used
for degenerate nucleotides: K = G/T; M = A/C; R = A/G; S = C/G;
Y = C/T; W = A/T; B = C/G/T; D = A/G/T; H = A/C/T; V = A/C/G;
N = A/C/G/T.

that overlap with the stress-related motifs found by Cliften et al. [6] using
comparative genomics were also selected.

17.4 Identification of Regulatory Motifs and Regulators

We now present a novel application of the model where predictors include sets
of regulators. To fix our notation, we assume there are G genes, E experiments,
M motifs, and R regulators. Let $y_{e,g}$ be the expression level of a target gene g
from experiment e. Then we have

$$\mathbf{Y} = (y_{1,1}, \ldots, y_{1,G}, y_{2,1}, \ldots, y_{2,G}, \ldots, y_{E,1}, \ldots, y_{E,G}). \qquad (17.4)$$

Each gene has a set of associated motif pattern scores. Genes across experiments
share same regulators while the expression levels of regulators is dependent on
the experiment. We therefore have a motif score matrix, $\mathbf{X}$, with G rows and
M columns and an expression matrix for the regulators, $\mathbf{Z}$, with E rows and R

columns. The design matrix for our linear regression model is defined in terms of Kronecker products as

$$W = [j(E) \otimes X, Z \otimes j(G)], \tag{17.5}$$

where $j(n)$ is a column vector of ones having length n. The resulting matrix W has $G \times E$ rows and $M + R$ columns. A linear regression model with response Y and predictors W is then defined as

$$Y = W\beta + \varepsilon, \tag{17.6}$$

where $\varepsilon \sim N(0, \sigma^2 I)$.

17.4.1 Application

We exemplify our model using the data from Gasch et al. [8]. The data set consists of cDNA microarray experiments measuring gene expression in *S. cerevisiae* under various environmental stress conditions. The data set has a total of 6,110 genes and 173 experiments. Here we focus on the experiments under heat shock by temperature increase.

In our study we used the processed data available at www.cs.columbia. edu/compbio/geneclass. There were 29 experiments that involved temperature changes. We focused on the $E = 15$ heat shock experiments from 25 to 37°C. As described in Section 17.2, the computational tools for motif search require a set of coregulated genes. We used hierarchical clustering with complete linkage to locate a set of genes with similar expression patterns across the 15 experiments. These "coregulated" genes were used by MotifRegressor to search for overrepresented nucleotide patterns and led to the identification of 432 motifs. For each of these motifs, we calculated their scores in each of $G = 1,326$ regulated genes provided by Middendorf et al. [17]. In addition, we obtained from the Web site cited above the expression profiles of $R = 456$ potential regulators.

We used different c values ($c = 4, 25$, and 100) and ran two MCMC chains with 200,000 iterations and different initial number of selected variables (10 and 50). We pooled chains together and computed the normalized posterior probabilities of distinct visited sets. We also computed the marginal posterior probabilities, $p(\gamma_j = 1 | W, Y)$, for the inclusion of motifs and regulators.

Table 17.2 reports motifs selected by the "best" model and ordered according to their marginal probabilities. Selections that are robust to the choice of c (i.e., motifs that showed up in the best model of all MCMC analyses run with different values of c) are represented with two asterisks, and those that appeared in two of the three MCMC analyses have a single asterisk.

Table 17.2. *Selection of Motifs and Regulators: Selected Motifs Ordered According to Their Marginal Posterior Probability*

Selected	Factor	Known	Function	p
TTTCA**	SWI4	**TTTC**GCG	Transcription factor that participates in the SBF complex (SWI4p-SWI6p) for regulation at the cell cycle box element	1.000
CCCCTTA**	STRE	TM**AGGGG**N	Controls expression of genes in response to heat shock and DNA damage	0.957
GMGATGMSCA**	GCN4	RTGA**CTCAT**	Increases after starvation for various amino acids or purines	0.948
CTCTCTTKTKT**	STF	GT**MAACAA**	Stabilizes and facilitates the formation of the complex between mitochondrial ATP synthase and its intrinsic inhibitor protein	0.766
TCAKCTCATCGC**	GCN4	RTGA**CTCAT**	Increases after starvation for various amino acids or purines	0.6819
GCWCGCA*	MBF	A**CGC**GT	Mediates GCN4-dependent transcriptional activation	0.6624
AGRGMAAAGGAG**	HSF	**AGAAN**	Heat shock transcription factor – necessary for recovery from heat shock	0.568
SAGCCTG*	UME6	TCGGC**GGCTA**	Required for glucose repression of FOX3; involved in nitrogen repression and induction of meiosis	0.563
CKACCCT	STRE	TM**AGGGG**N	Controls expression of genes in response to heat shock and DNA damage	0.466

Note: Selections that are robust to the choice of the hyperparameter c are shown with asterisks.

Table 17.3. *Selection of Motifs and Regulators:*
Selected Regulators Ordered According to Their
Marginal Posterior Probability

Regulator	p	Known
YJL187C**	0.489	SWE1
YGL099W**	0.228	LSG1
YLR433C**	0.097	CNA1
YGR123C**	0.095	PPT1
YIL154C**	0.038	IMP2'
YIR023W*	0.028	DAL81
YLR336C**	0.013	SGD1
YNL309W	0.013	STB1

Note: Selections that are robust to the choice of the hyperparameter c are shown with asterisks.

We compiled the table by looking at the motif sequences in both directions as well as the different possibilities for ambiguous nucleotides. We searched for matches in the TRANSFAC database and also compared them with several published papers that have looked at regulatory motifs for *S. cerevisiae*. Nucleotide patterns that match known motifs appear in the table with bold characters, along with the associated binding sites and factors. A brief description of their function is also given. As in the previous application, some of the selected motifs were experimentally known to be related to stress. Others were novel and constituted a set of promising candidates for future experimental work.

Table 17.3 reports results on the selection of the regulators. Our novel finding here is the SWE1 (YJL187C) regulator, that ranked at the top in all simulations we ran with different c values. This regulator has not been previously identified by other methods. According to Ciliberto et al. [5], SWE1 is known to be a mitosis inhibitor protein kinase. It is involved in the morphogenesis checkpoint that arrests the cell cycle at the G2-M transition when bud formation is impaired, perhaps due to environmental stimuli such as heat or osmotic shock. The cell cycle delay induced by the morphogenesis checkpoint requires Swe1p. When bud formation is impaired, SWE1 is stabilized and active. Among the other regulators we selected, PPT1 and LSG1 are known to relate to severe heat shock and have been identified also by Middendorf et al. [17]. Also, from Segal et al. [19] we notice that PPT1 is related to GCN4, which appears in the list of selected motifs. CNA1, Calcineurin A, is a Ca^{2+}/calmodulin-regulated protein phosphatase that regulates Crz1p, a known stress-response transcription

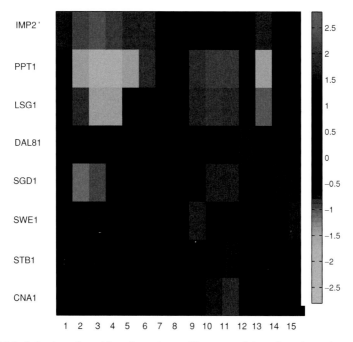

Fig. 17.2. Selection of motifs and regulators: Heatmap of the selected regulators over the 15 experiments under consideration. (See color plate 17.2.)

factor. Figure 17.2 shows the activity of the selected regulators over the 15 experiments. Many of them exhibit a change in expression over some portion of the experiments.

17.5 Conclusion

We have discussed methods to identify DNA regulatory elements by exploiting the correlation between sequence data and gene expression. In particular we have reviewed the work of Tadesse et al. [21] who used Bayesian methods for variable selection for the identification of binding sites for regulatory factors. We have also presented an extension of this model to include gene regulators and showed applications to regulatory systems of *S. cerevisiae* under heat shock.

In the extended model, only the main effects of motifs and regulators are considered. It may be biologically interesting to consider statistical interactions between motifs and regulators. A model containing interactions between motifs and regulators will result in a design matrix W with $M + R + M * R$ columns and, therefore, may present computational challenges for typical values of M and R. Of course, the prior of the regression coefficient β would also need to be modified to ensure that main effects are not eliminated in the presence of interactions.

Acknowledgments

Tadesse and Vannucci are supported by NIH/NHGRI grant R01HG003319. Vannucci is also supported by NSF CAREER award DMS-0093208. Michael Swartz is supported by NCI grant CA90301.

Bibliography

[1] Alberts, B., Johnson, A., Lewis, J., Raff, M., Robers, K. and Walter, P. (2002). *Molecular Biology of the Cell*. Garland Science: New York.

[2] Brown, P.J., Vannucci, M. and Fern, T. (1998). Multivariate Bayesian variable selection and prediction. *Journal of the Royal Statistical Society, Series B*, **60**, 627–641.

[3] Bussemaker, H.J., Li, H. and Siggia, E.D. (2000). Building a dictionary for genomes: Identification of presumptive regulatory sites by statistical analysis. *Proceedings of the National Academy of Science*, **97**, 10096–10100.

[4] Bussemaker, H.J., Li, H. and Siggia, E.D. (2001). Regulatory element detection using correlation with expression. *Nature Genetics*, **27**, 167–171.

[5] Ciliberto, A., Novak, B. and Tyson, J.J. (2003). Mathematics model of the morphogenesis checkpoint in budding yeast. *Journal of Cell Biology* **163**, 1243–1254.

[6] Cliften, P., Sudarsanam, P., Desikan, A., Fulton, F., Fulton, B., Majors, J., Waterston, R., Cohen, B.A. and Johnston, M. (2003). Finding functional features in *Saccharomyces* genomes by phylogenetic footprinting. *Science*, **301**, 71–76.

[7] Conlon, E.M., Liu, X.S., Lieb, J.D. and Liu, J.S. (2003). Integrating regulatory motif discovery and genome-wide expression analysis. *Proceedings of the National Academy of Science*, **100**, 3339–3344.

[8] Gasch, A.P., Spellman, P.T., Kao, C.M., Carmel-Harel, O., Eisen, M.B. Storz, G., Botstein, D. and Brown, P.O. (2000). Genomic expression programs in the response of yeast cells to environmental changes. *Molecular Biology of the Cell*, **11**, 4241–4257.

[9] George, E.I. and McCulloch, R.E. (1993). Variable selection via Gibbs sampling. *Journal of the American Statistical Association*, **88**, 881–889.

[10] Griffiths, A.J., Miller, J.H., Suzuki, D.T., Lewontin, R.C. and Gelbart, W.M. (1996). *An Introduction to Genetic Analysis*. W.H. Freeman and Company: New York.

[11] Gupta, M. and Liu, J.S. (2003). Discovery of conserved sequence patterns using a stochastic dictionary model. *Journal of the American Statistical Association*, **98**, 55–66.

[12] Gupta, M. and Liu, J.S. (2006). Bayesian modeling and inference for sequence motif discovery. In *Bayesian Inference for Gene Expression and Proteomics*,

K.A. Do, P. Müller and M. Vannucci (Eds.). New York: Cambridge University Press (this book).

[13] Keleş, H., van der Laan, M. and Eisen, M.B. (2002). Identification of regulatory elements using a feature selection method. *Bioinformatics*, **18**, 1167–1175.

[14] Lawrence, C.E., Altschul, S.R., Boguski, M.S., Liu, J.S., Neuwald, A.F. and Wootton, J.C. (1993). Detecting subtle sequence signals: A Gibbs sampling strategy for multiple alignment. *Science*, **262**, 208–214.

[15] Liu, J.S., Neuwald, A.F. and Lawrence, C.E. (1995). Bayesian models for multiple local sequence alignment and Gibbs sampling strategies. *Journal of the American Statistical Association*, **90**, 1156–1170.

[16] Liu, X.S., Brutlag, D.L. and Liu, J.S. (2002). An algorithm for finding protein-DNA binding sites with applications to chromatin-immunoprecipitation microarray experiments. *Nature Biotechnology*, **20**, 835–839.

[17] Middendorf, M., Kundaje, A., Wiggins, C., Freund, Y. and Leslie, C. (2004). Predicting genetic regulatory response using classification. *Bioinformatics*, **20**, 1232–1240.

[18] Schmitt, A.P. and McEntee, K. (1996). Msn2p, a zinc finger DNA-binding protein, is the transcriptional activator of the multistress response in *Saccharomyces cerevisiae*. *Proceedings of the National Academy of Science USA*, **93**, 5777–5782.

[19] Segal, E., Shapira, M., Regev, A., Botstein, D., Koller, D. and Friedman, N. (2003a). Module networks: Identifying regulatory modules and their condition-specific regulators from gene expression data. *Nature Genetics*, **34**, 166–176.

[20] Segal, E., Yelensky, R. and Koller, D. (2003b). Genome-wide discovery of transcriptional modules from DNA sequence and gene expression. *Bioinformatics*, **19**, i273–i282.

[21] Tadesse, M.G., Vannucci, M. and Liò, P. (2005). Identification of DNA regulatory motifs using Bayesian variable selection. *Bioinformatics*, **20**, 2553–2561.

[22] van Helden, J., André, B. and Collado-Vides, J. (1998). Extracting regulatory sites from the upstream region of yeast genes by computational analysis of oligonucleotide frequencies. *Journal of Molecular Biology*, **281**, 827–842.

18

A Misclassification Model for Inferring Transcriptional Regulatory Networks

NING SUN AND HONGYU ZHAO

Yale University School of Medicine

Abstract

One major goal in biological research is to understand how genes are regulated through transcriptional regulatory networks. Recent advances in biotechnology have generated enormous amounts of data that can be utilized to better achieve this goal. In this chapter, we develop a general statistical framework to integrate different data sources for transcriptional regulatory network reconstructions. More specifically, we apply measurement error models for network reconstructions using both gene expression data and protein–DNA binding data. A linear misclassification model is used to describe the relationship between the expression level of a specific gene and the binding activities of the proteins (transcription factors) that regulate this gene. We propose Markov chain Monte Carlo method for statistical inference based on this model. Extensive simulations are conducted to evaluate the performance of this model and assess the sensitivity of its performance when the model parameters are misspecified. Our simulation results suggest that our approach can effectively integrate gene expression data and protein–DNA binding data to infer transcriptional regulatory networks. Lastly, we apply our model to jointly analyze gene expression data and protein–DNA binding data to infer transcriptional regulatory networks in the yeast cell cycle.

18.1 Introduction

Understanding gene regulations through the underlying transcriptional regulatory networks (referred as TRNs in the following) is a central topic in biology. A TRN can be thought of as consisting of a set of proteins, genes, small modules, and their mutual regulatory interactions. The potentially large number of components, the high connectivity among various components, and the transient stimulation in the network result in great complexity of TRNs. With the rapid advances of molecular technologies and enormous amounts of data being collected, intensive efforts have been made to dissect TRNs using data generated from the state-of-the-art technologies, including gene expression data and other data types. The computational methods include gene clustering (e.g., Eisen et al. 1998), Boolean networks (e.g., Akutsu et al. 2000; Shmulevich et al. 2002), Bayesian networks (e.g., Friedman et al. 2000; Hartemink et al. 2002; Hartemink 2005), differential equation systems (e.g., Gardner et al. 2003; Tegnér et al. 2003), information integration methods (e.g., Bar-Joseph et al. 2003; Gao et al. 2004), and other approaches. For recent reviews, see de Jong (2002) and Sun and Zhao (2004). As discussed in our review (Sun and Zhao 2004), although a large number of studies are devoted to infer TRNs from gene expression data alone, such data only provide very limited amount of information. On the other hand, other data types, such as protein–DNA interaction data (which measure the binding targets of each transcription factor, denoted by TF in our following discussion, through direct biological experiments), may be much more informative and should be combined together for network inference.

In this chapter, we describe a Bayesian framework for TRN inference based on the combined analysis of gene expression data and protein–DNA interaction data. The statistical properties of our approach are investigated through extensive simulations, and our method is then applied to study TRNs in the yeast cell cycle.

18.2 Methods

In this chapter, we model a TRN as a bipartite graph: a one-layer network where a set of genes are regulated by a set of TFs. The TFs bind to the regulatory regions of their target genes to regulate (activate or inhibit) their transcription initiation, which is a principal mode of regulating the expression levels of many, if not most, genes (Carey and Smale 1999). Because the number of genes largely exceeds the number of TFs in any organism, there is combinatorial control of the TFs on genes. That is, for a given gene, its expression level is controlled by the joint actions of its regulators. Two well-known facts on the joint actions of TFs include cooperativity, which in the context of protein–DNA interaction refers to two or more TFs engaging in protein–protein interaction stabilizing each other's binding to DNA sequences, and transcriptional synergy, which refers to the interacting effects among the Polymerase II general transcriptional machinery and the multiple TFs on controlling transcription levels. In our previous work (Zhao et al. 2003), we assumed that the expression level of a specific gene is controlled through the additive effects of its regulators.

Liao et al. (2003) applied Hill's equation for the cooperative TF bindings on the regulatory regions of their target genes and the first-order kinetics for the rate of gene transcription. Under a quasi-steady-state assumption, they proved that the relative gene expression level has a linear relationship with the relative activities of the TFs that bind on the gene's regulatory region. In this chapter, we extend our previous work (Zhao et al. 2003) to fully incorporate gene expression data and protein–DNA binding data to infer TRNs. Before the discussion of our model, we first give a brief overview of the protein–DNA binding data used in our method.

As the primary goal of TRN inference is to identify the regulatory targets of each TF, the most direct biological approach is to experimentally identify the targets of various TFs. Many different biological methodologies are available to serve this purpose. The large-scale chromatin immunoprecipitation microarray data (ChIP-chip data) provide the in vivo measurements on TFs and DNA binding (e.g., Ren et al. 2000; Lee et al. 2002). In our study, the protein–DNA binding data thus collected are viewed as one measurement of the TRN with certain level of measurement errors due to biological and experimental errors, for example, physical binding is not equivalent to regulation. We use the ChIP-chip data collected by Lee et al. (2002) as the data source for protein–DNA binding. These data represent a continuous measurement of the binding strength between each TF and its potential targets, and a p value is derived based on replicated experiments to assess the statistical significance of binding. In the following, the inferred binding p values between a TF and its potential target genes are converted into binary observations using a significance level cutoff of 0.05. That is, for all TF–gene pairs whose p value is below 0.05, we denote the observation as 1, representing evidence for binding, and for those pairs whose p value is larger than 0.05, we denote the observation as 0, representing not sufficient evidence for binding. The reason that we utilize protein–DNA binding data is because we believe that the information from such data serves as a close measurement for the true underlying TRN.

In our previous work (Zhao et al. 2003), we treated protein–DNA binding data as representing the true underlying network, and used a linear model to describe the relationship between the transcript amounts of the genes considered and their regulators' activities. In our current work, we extend this linear model to incorporate potential errors associated with protein–DNA binding data to integrate three components that are biologically important in transcription regulation, namely, the TRN as characterized by the covariate (or design) matrix in the linear model, protein regulation activities as defined by the predictors in the model, and gene expression levels as defined by the response variables. We propose a misclassification model to simultaneously

extract information from protein–DNA binding data and gene expression data
to reconstruct TRNs.

18.2.1 Model Specification

Our model relating gene expression levels, TRNs, and TF activities can be
described through three submodels:

- A linear regression model relating gene expression levels with the true underlying TRNs and regulators' activities;
- A misclassification model relating the true underlying networks and the
  observed protein–DNA binding data;
- Prior distribution on the TRNs.

The hierarchical structure of our graphical model is summarized in Figure 18.1 and we describe each component in detail in the following. Note
that measurement error models have been advocated in other contexts in the
literature (e.g., Richardson and Gilks, 1993).

18.2.1.1 The First Submodel: The Linear Regression Model

Let N denote the number of genes and M denote the number of TFs related to
the regulation of these genes. We consider a total of T microarray experiments,
which may represent a time-course study, or different knock-out experiments.
We focus on time-course experiments in our following discussion, where t
represents a specific time point. The observed gene expression levels at time
t, $\mathbf{Y}_t$, are the vector of N expression levels normalized over all time points for
each gene i and serve as the response variable in the linear model (18.1) with
the following form:

$$\mathbf{Y}_t = \mathbf{X}\boldsymbol{\beta}_t + \boldsymbol{\epsilon}_t, \tag{18.1}$$

$$\epsilon_{it} \sim N\left(0, \sigma_t^2\right), \tag{18.2}$$

where $\mathbf{X}$ represents the true TRN, $\boldsymbol{\beta}_t$ represents the time-dependent regulator
activities of the M TFs, and $\boldsymbol{\epsilon}_t$ represents the errors that are associated with
gene expression measurements. In matrix $\mathbf{X}$, each row corresponds to a gene
and each column corresponds to a TF, and the (i, j)th entry is 1 if the jth TF
regulates the ith gene, and the value is 0 otherwise. Because our primary interest
is to infer the TRN, the overall objective is to infer the values in this matrix,
either 0 or 1.

This model states that (1) the expression level of a gene is largely controlled
by the additive regulation activities of its regulators, (2) the same regulator has

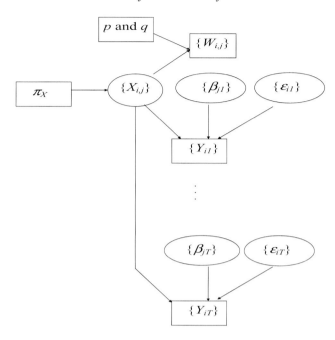

Fig. 18.1. The hierarchical structure of the misclassification model discussed in this chapter. The unknown parameters are in the ovals, and the known parameters are in the rectangles. Y_{it} is log-transformed relative gene expression value of gene i at time t. β_{jt} is the log-transformed relative TF activity of TF j at time t. ε_{it} represents the error associated with gene expression data. $\{X_{ij}\}$ is the TRN. $\{W_{ij}\}$ is the observed binding matrix with a false-positive rate of q and a false-negative rate of p. π_X is the prior distribution for TRN, $\mathbf{X}$, in the exposure model.

the same relative effect on all its targets, (3) the TRN is identical across all time points, and (4) the errors associated with gene expression measurements have the same distribution across all the genes. We note that these assumptions are simplistic and may provide only a first-order approximation to reality. The limitations and modifications of these assumptions are discussed in the Discussion section.

Since protein–DNA binding data are often obtained from a mixture of biological samples across all the time points, for example, the asynchronized cells, they measure an averaged protein–DNA binding over cell cycles. Although we may use the time-course gene expression data to investigate the fluctuation of the network over time, the information at one time point may not be sufficient for statistical inference (see results in the simulation study in the following). Therefore, we make the assumption that the network is time independent and combine the information across time points. Consequently, the variation of the response variable, gene expression, across time points is accredited to the change in the activities of the TFs, $\boldsymbol{\beta}_t$.

18.2.1.2 The Second Submodel: The Misclassification Model

In our model setup, both the true and observed covariates are binary, where 0 corresponds to no regulation and 1 corresponds to regulation. We assume the following model [(18.3)–(18.6)]:

$$P(W_{ij} = 1 | X_{ij} = 1) = 1 - p, \tag{18.3}$$

$$P(W_{ij} = 0 | X_{ij} = 1) = p, \tag{18.4}$$

$$P(W_{ij} = 0 | X_{ij} = 0) = 1 - q, \tag{18.5}$$

$$P(W_{ij} = 1 | X_{ij} = 0) = q, \tag{18.6}$$

where the values of p and q are the false-negative and false-positive rates of the protein–DNA interaction data. In practice, these values may be directly estimated from some control experiments, and thus we treat these parameters as known. In the case these values are not precisely known, we can study the robustness of their misspecifications on statistical inference. Note that the false-positive and false-negative rates may be gene-TF-specific, therefore, our assumption here represents an approximation to reality that may need further extension in future studies. The binary matrix $\mathbf{W}$ serves as the measurement for the true TRN $\mathbf{X}$.

18.2.1.3 The Third Submodel: The Exposure Model

For this submodel, we need to specify the prior distribution of the regulatory matrix $\mathbf{X} = \{X_{ij}\}$. We assume that the X_{ij} are independent and have an identical Bernoulli distribution with parameter π_X. For a given true network $\mathbf{X}$, the value of π_X can be calculated from the data. When $\mathbf{X}$ is unknown and $\mathbf{W}$ serves as the surrogate of $\mathbf{X}$, π_X is a model parameter that needs to be specified.

18.2.2 MCMC Algorithm for Statistical Inference

In our model setup, a large number of unknown parameters $\{\mathbf{X}, \boldsymbol{\beta}_t, \sigma_t^2\}$ need to be inferred based on the observations $\mathbf{Y}_t, t = 1, \ldots, T$, and $\mathbf{W}$. We propose to use the Gibbs sampler for statistical inference. The Gibbs sampler is alternated between two steps: (1) sample $\{\boldsymbol{\beta}_t, \sigma_t^2\}$ conditional on $\mathbf{X}$, and (2) sample

$\mathbf{X}$ conditional on $\{\boldsymbol{\beta}_t, \sigma_t^2\}$. These two steps are described in detail in the following.

Given current estimate $\widehat{\mathbf{X}}$, the model reduces to a standard linear regression model. The parameters $\{\boldsymbol{\beta}_t, \sigma_t^2\}$ are sampled through (18.7) and (18.8) (Gelman et al. 1995):

$$\sigma_t^2 \sim Inv - \chi^2(df, s_t^2), \tag{18.7}$$

$$\boldsymbol{\beta}_t \sim N(\widehat{\boldsymbol{\beta}}_t, \mathbf{V}_\beta \sigma_t^2), \tag{18.8}$$

where $df = N - M$, $\mathbf{V}_\beta = (\widehat{\mathbf{X}}^T \widehat{\mathbf{X}})^{-1}$, $\widehat{\boldsymbol{\beta}}_t = \mathbf{V}_\beta \widehat{\mathbf{X}}^T \mathbf{Y}_t$, and s_t is the sample standard deviation.

Given current estimates of $\{\boldsymbol{\beta}_t, \sigma_t^2\}$, we individually update the TRN for each gene. If there are M TFs, there are a total of $K = 2^M$ possible joint patterns among the TFs to jointly regulate a specific gene. The likelihood L_{ik} for each pattern k can be evaluated as

$$L_{ik} = L_{ik}^X + L_{ik}^Y + \text{constant}, \tag{18.9}$$

where

$$L_{ik}^X = n_1 \log \pi_X + n_{11} \log(1 - p) + n_{10} \log p + n_0 \log(1 - \pi_X) \\ + n_{01} \log q + n_{00} \log(1 - q), \tag{18.10}$$

$$L_{ik}^Y = {}^* - \sum_{t=1}^{T} \frac{(Y_{it} - \widehat{Y_{ikt}})^2}{2\sigma_t^2}. \tag{18.11}$$

In the above expression, L_{ik}^X and L_{ik}^Y represent the likelihood contributions from the protein–DNA binding data and the expression data, respectively. In the expression for L_{ik}^X, n_{so} represents the number of TF–gene pairs whose true regulation is s and the observed binding is o, where the value of s (or o) is 0 or 1. For example, n_{11} corresponds to the number of pairs whose true regulation and observed binding are both 1. In addition, $n_1 = n_{10} + n_{11}$, and $n_0 = n_{00} + n_{01}$. The expression for L_{ik}^Y represents the likelihood component derived from gene expression data across all time points. After evaluating the log-likelihood for all the patterns, we sample one pattern based on the following multinomial distribution:

$$\widehat{\mathbf{X}}_i \sim \text{multinomial}\left(1, \frac{\exp(L_{ik})}{\sum_{k=1}^{K} \exp(L_{ik})}\right). \tag{18.12}$$

Therefore, in updating $\mathbf{X}$, our algorithm does an exhaustive search over all possible network patterns for each gene, and sample a specific pattern based on the relative likelihood of all possible networks. We repeat this for each of the N genes to obtain the updated $\widehat{\mathbf{X}}$ for the next iteration.

Based on the sampled parameter values, we can derive the posterior distributions for all the unknown parameters. For example, we can obtain the inferred TRN describing the binding between the jth TF and the ith gene through the marginal posterior distribution, that is, the proportion of samples for which the value of X_{ij} is 1. These posterior probabilities can then be used to infer the presence or absence of regulation through specifying a cutoff value (e.g., 0.5).

18.2.3 Data Analysis and Simulation Setup

As our simulation model is based on the real data to be analyzed, we describe the data sources first. According to the literature, we select eight cell cycle TFs, namely Fkh1, Fkh2, Ndd1, Mcm1, Ace2, Swi5, Mbp1, and Swi4. Based on protein–DNA interaction data reported in Lee et al. (2002), we obtain a binary binding matrix for these regulators and all yeast genes by applying a threshold of 0.05 onto the p values reported by Lee and colleagues. We then remove those genes with no in vivo binding evidence with any of the eight TFs from the binding matrix, and further focus only on yeast cell cycle genes defined by Spellman et al. (1998). These steps result in a total of 295 genes to be analyzed, and the observed protein–DNA binding matrix has a dimension of 295 (genes) by 8 (TFs). For gene expression data, we use the α arrest cell cycle data with 18 time points collected by Spellman et al. (1998).

Now we describe our simulation setup to evaluate the performance of our proposed procedure. In our simulation model, we need to specify (1) true TRN, (2) true protein regulation activities, (3) false-positive and false-negative rates in the observed binding matrix, and (4) measurement errors associated with microarray data. We consider all 295 genes used in the real data analysis, and select five TFs (Fkh2, Mcm1, Ace2, Mbp1, and Swi4, which control gene expression at the four cell cycle stages) in our simulations to simplify the analysis. For the specification of the "true" TRN in our simulations, we use the observed binding data to represent the true TRN. As for TF activity specifications, we estimate the activities of the chosen five TFs from the linear regression model using the above true TRN and the expression levels of all 295 genes at each time point. The estimated activity levels of the five TFs over 18 time points are shown in Figure 18.2. As for false-positive and false-negative rates, we vary their levels from 0.1 to 0.9 to examine their effects on statistical inference. Finally, we assess the effect of the measurement variation associated with microarray data on statistical inference. For the majority of

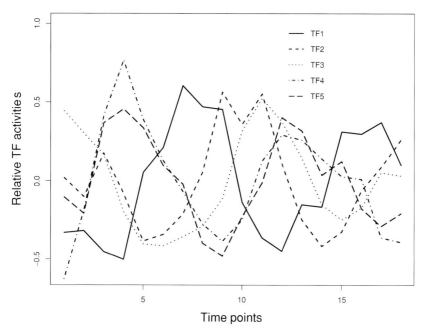

Fig. 18.2. The inferred activities of five transcription factors vary over 18 time points. Two of the five transcription factors share similar profiles, which may lead to an identifiability problem of the model. However, our results show that the slight difference between the TF activities prevent the problem.

simulations, we assume that the microarray data are collected from 18 time points as in Spellman et al. (1998). In one case, we vary the number of time points available to investigate the effect of the number of time points on statistical inference.

18.3 Simulation Results

18.3.1 Convergence Diagnosis of the MCMC Procedure

Based on our simulation runs, we generally find good mixing of the proposed MCMC procedure. Both the traces of the parameter values and the autocorrelations of the parameter curves indicate that a burn-in run of 1,000 iterations out of 10,000 iterations is stable enough to obtain reliable posterior distributions. The posterior distributions of the five TF activities (β_t) and measurement errors from microarrays σ_t^2 at a time point from one simulated data set are shown in Figure 18.3. We also investigate the effect of the initial network (covariate matrix) on MCMC results. When the measurement errors in gene expression

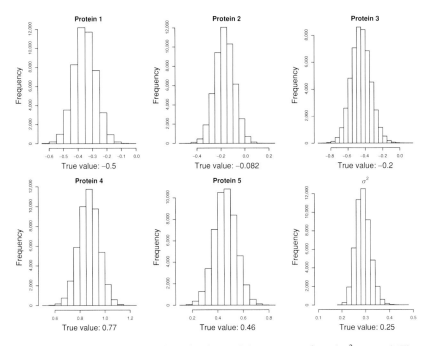

Fig. 18.3. The posterior distributions for the model parameters β_t and σ_t^2 at $t = 4$. The standard deviations of these posterior distributions are 0.075, 0.078, 0.092, 0.077, 0.091, and 0.027, respectively.

data are low, the MCMC procedure has good convergence regardless of the initial network. In general, the observed protein–DNA binding data provide a good starting point for statistical inference.

In our model specification, there are two types of errors: the errors associated with the measured gene expression levels (responses, denoted by σ) and those associated with the observed protein–DNA binding data (denoted by p and q). In order to systematically investigate the effect of both types of errors, we consider seven pairs of p and q as $(0.1, 0.1), (0.2, 0.2), (0.2, 0.4), (0.4, 0.2), (0.3, 0.3), (0.4, 0.4)$, and $(0.5, 0.5)$. For each pair of p and q values, we simulate the observed protein–DNA binding data as well as gene expression data under 22 different σ values, ranging from 0.001 to 1.5. For each specification of the 22 $\times$ 7 $= 154$ sets of parameter values, we simulate data sets consisting of protein–DNA interaction data and gene expression data. Each data set is analyzed through our proposed MCMC approach with a burn-in of 1,000 iterations and a further run of 5,000 iterations. The posterior distribution for each unknown parameter is summarized and compared to the true underlying network. We use a cutoff of 0.5 to infer the presence or absence of regulations between

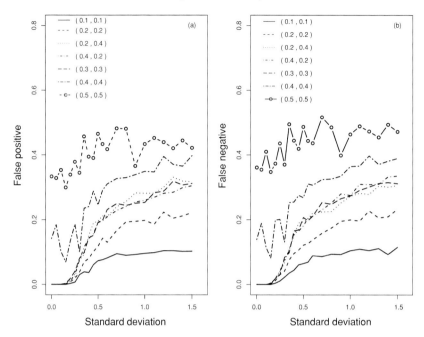

Fig. 18.4. The false-positive and false-negative rates of the inferred network. The x-axis is the standard deviation in gene expression data, while the y-axis is either the false-positive rate or false-negative rate of the posterior network with respect to the true regulatory network. Different lines correspond to different levels of assumed quality of protein–DNA binding data.

TFs and genes. The inferred network is then compared to the true network to calculate the proportion of false-positive and false-negative inferences for each TF–gene pair. The overall false-positive and false-negative rates are then estimated through the average of all TF–gene pairs across all the simulated data sets. The results are summarized in Figure 18.4. In Figure 18.4(a), we plot the false-positive rates for the inferred network. As can be seen from this figure, the false-positive rates for the inferred network increase as σ, p, and q increase. The false-negative rates for the inferred networks show a similar pattern. The major feature is that the information from gene expression data may significantly improve the estimation on **X**. When σ is small and p and q are not too high, there is a very good chance that the true network can be recovered from the joint analysis of gene expression data and protein–DNA binding data. For example, with 30% false-positive and 30% false-negative rates, when σ is less than 0.2, the whole network may be fully recovered. Even when σ is large, the false-positive rates in the inferred network using both binding data and gene expression data still outperform those in the observed protein–DNA

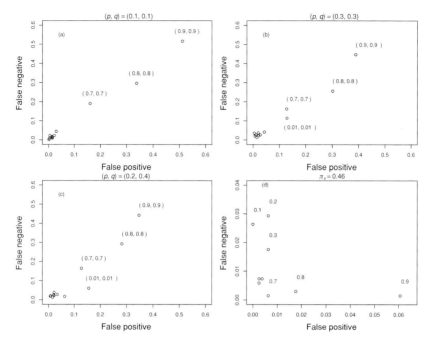

Fig. 18.5. The effects of misspecifying model parameters p, q, and π_X on the inferred network. The standard deviation of the simulated gene expression data is 0.2. The real values of parameters (p, q) or π_X are indicated in the title of each plot. In (a)–(c), the true value of π_X is 0.46, but (p, q) are specified as (0.9, 0.9), (0.8, 0.8), (0.7, 0.7), (0.6, 0.6), (0.5, 0.5), (0.4, 0.4), (0.3, 0.3), (0.2, 0.2), (0.1, 0.1), (0.05, 0.05), (0.01, 0.01), and (0.05, 0.4). For (d), the values of (p, q) are (0.1, 0.1), but π_X is specified at various levels: 0.1, 0.2, 0.3, 0.4, 0.46, 0.5, 0.6, 0.7, 0.8, and 0.9.

binding data. The results for the false-negative rates as shown in Figure 18.4(b) show similar patterns.

18.3.2 Misspecification of the Model Parameters p, q, and π_X

In the results summarized above, we assume that the true values of p and q are precisely known. However, their exact values may not be accurately inferred. Therefore, we conduct simulation experiments to examine the performance of the proposed procedure when the values of p and q are misspecified. In this set of simulations, we simulate data from three sets of p and q values: (0.1, 0.1), (0.3, 0.3), and (0.2, 0.4). For each simulated data set under a given set of parameter values, we perform statistical analysis under different sets of specifications for p and q, including (0.9, 0.9), (0.8, 0.8),

(0.7, 0.7), (0.6, 0.6), (0.5, 0.5), (0.4, 0.4), (0.3, 0.3), (0.2, 0.2), (0.1, 0.1), (0.05, 0.05), (0.01, 0.01), and (0.05, 0.4). Throughout these simulations, we assume $\sigma = 0.2$. The performance of our procedure in terms of false-positive and false-negative rates is summarized in Figures 18.5(a) to 18.5(c). These results suggest that the statistical inference is robust to the misspecification of the parameters p and q when the specified values are not too distinct from the true parameter values. We observe similar patterns for other values of σ.

As another parameter that needs to be specified in our approach is the prior probability π_X, we further investigate the performance of our approach when π_X is misspecified. The true value of π_X is about 0.46 (683/(295 × 5), where there are 683 regulation pairs in the protein–DNA binding data) in the given true network **X**, but we consider 0.1, 0.2, 0.3, 0.4, 0.46, 0.5, 0.6, 0.7, 0.8, and 0.9 in our analysis. The results are summarized in Figure 18.5(d). Compared to the results for p and q, the statistical inference is more sensitive to the value of π_X. However, when the specified parameter value is reasonably close to the true value, our approach generally yields robust estimates.

Overall, our simulation studies suggest that misspecifications of model parameters p, q, and π_X within a reasonable range will not substantially affect the statistical inference of the true network.

18.3.3 Effect of the Number of Experiments Used in the Inference

In the above simulations, we simulated data from 18 time points and used all of them in the inference of the underlying network. In this subsection, we consider the effect of the number of time points on the inference. For this set of simulations, we simulate the protein–DNA binding data by fixing the values of p and q at 0.1, selecting the value of σ at 0.001, 0.2, and 0.5, and varying the number of time points used in the analysis from 1 to 18. When there is little error associated with gene expression data (i.e. $\sigma = 0.001$), the data at one time point can carry enough information to fully recover the true network. With increasing σ values, the number of time points affects the results on the inferred network (Figure 18.6). When σ is 0.2, our previous results show that there is a significant improvement of the inferred network from the binding data. As more time points are included in the analysis, we observe more accurate inference of the underlying network. When σ is 0.5, the improvement of the inferred network from the binding data is still obvious but limited due to too much noise in gene expression data.

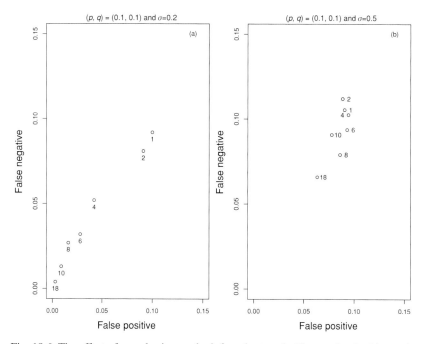

Fig. 18.6. The effect of sample size on the inferred network. The number besides each symbol indicates the number of the time points used in the simulated gene expression data. The value of π_X is 0.46, and the values of other parameters are indicated in the title of each plot.

18.4 Application to Yeast Cell Cycle Data

In this section, we apply our method to jointly analyze gene expression data from 295 genes over 18 time points (Spellman et al. 1998) and protein–DNA binding data of Fkh1, Fkh2, Ndd1, Mcm1, Swi5, Ace2, Mbp1, and Swi4 (Lee et al. 2002). We consider eight sets of model parameters for $\{p, q, \pi_X\}$: $\{0.1, 0.1, 0.5\}$, $\{0.2, 0.2, 0.5\}$, $\{0.2, 0.1, 0.5\}$, $\{0.1, 0.2, 0.5\}$, $\{0.2, 0.2, 0.4\}$, $\{0.2, 0.2, 0.6\}$, $\{0.1, 0.1, 0.4\}$, and $\{0.1, 0.1, 0.6\}$. For each set of parameter specifications, we run MCMC with a burn-in of 1,000 runs and an additional 5,000 runs to obtain the posterior distributions for the parameters of interest. The overall inference is based on the average posterior probabilities over the eight model parameter settings, which yield similar results among different settings.

The posterior distributions of the protein activities for the eight TFs and the σ at every time point are summarized in Table 18.1. The average value of σ across 18 time points is about 0.55. Based on our simulation studies, at this level of expression errors, the incorporation of gene expression data should improve the inference of TRNs.

Table 18.1. *The Estimated Regulation Activities*
of the Transcription Factors and σ

Time	Fkh1	Fkh2	Ndd1	Mcm1	Ace2	Swi5	Mbp1	Swi4	σ
1	0.09	−0.81	−0.55	0.54	1.84	−0.29	−0.79	−0.27	0.88
	±0.13	±0.12	±0.13	±0.13	±0.14	±0.13	±0.12	±0.12	
2	−0.36	−1.00	0.24	0.28	1.18	−0.46	−0.18	−0.01	0.75
	±0.11	±0.11	±0.11	±0.11	±0.13	±0.12	±0.10	±0.11	
3	−0.53	−0.63	0.14	0.09	0.98	−0.35	1.43	0.06	0.66
	±0.10	±0.10	±0.10	±0.10	±0.14	±0.11	±0.09	±0.10	
4	−0.34	−0.31	−0.25	−0.29	0.17	−0.42	1.86	0.27	0.58
	±0.08	±0.09	±0.09	±0.08	±0.13	±0.10	±0.07	±0.08	
5	0.73	0.12	−0.62	−0.63	0.26	−0.67	0.79	0.13	0.54
	±0.07	±0.08	±0.08	±0.07	±0.09	±0.08	±0.07	±0.08	
6	0.72	0.20	−0.42	−0.49	−0.17	−0.49	0.28	−0.04	0.6
	±0.08	±0.08	±0.09	±0.08	±0.10	±0.09	±0.08	±0.08	
7	1.31	0.16	0.41	−0.61	−0.07	−0.55	−0.28	−0.28	0.53
	±0.08	±0.09	±0.08	±0.08	±0.10	±0.09	±0.08	±0.08	
8	0.44	0.18	0.61	0.01	−0.47	−0.31	−0.43	−0.57	0.44
	±0.06	±0.06	±0.06	±0.06	±0.08	±0.07	±0.06	±0.06	
9	0.17	0.09	1.03	0.58	−0.46	−0.00	−0.57	−0.74	0.5
	±0.07	±0.07	±0.07	±0.07	±0.09	±0.08	±0.07	±0.07	
10	−0.27	−0.48	0.81	0.47	−0.54	1.11	−0.39	−0.42	0.57
	±0.07	±0.08	±0.07	±0.07	±0.10	±0.08	±0.07	±0.07	
11	−0.90	0.02	−0.01	0.79	−0.32	1.23	0.13	0.08	0.75
	±0.10	±0.11	±0.11	±0.10	±0.13	±0.12	±0.10	±0.11	
12	−1.07	0.22	−0.29	0.14	−0.45	0.93	0.56	0.65	0.44
	±0.07	±0.06	±0.07	±0.06	±0.08	±0.07	±0.07	±0.06	
13	−0.20	0.44	−0.82	−0.28	−0.15	0.35	0.16	0.63	0.45
	±0.07	±0.07	±0.07	±0.06	±0.08	±0.07	±0.06	±0.06	
14	−0.35	0.42	−0.68	−0.37	−0.31	−0.08	−0.31	0.52	0.45
	±0.06	±0.07	±0.07	±0.07	±0.08	±0.07	±0.06	±0.06	
15	0.44	0.68	−0.61	−0.51	−0.08	−0.32	−0.44	0.38	0.44
	±0.06	±0.07	±0.07	±0.06	±0.08	±0.07	±0.06	±0.07	
16	0.09	0.59	−0.10	−0.16	−0.58	−0.04	−0.45	0.13	0.6
	±0.08	±0.08	±0.08	±0.08	±0.10	±0.09	±0.07	±0.08	
17	0.26	0.26	0.46	−0.02	−0.27	−0.08	−0.71	−0.26	0.62
	±0.08	±0.09	±0.09	±0.08	±0.10	±0.09	±0.07	±0.08	
18	−0.20	−0.15	0.66	0.48	−0.57	0.44	−0.63	−0.26	0.57
	±0.08	±0.09	±0.09	±0.08	±0.10	±0.10	±0.07	±0.08	

18.5 Discussion

In this chapter, we have developed a misclassification model to integrate gene expression data and protein–DNA binding data to infer TRNs. Compared to other models, our model (1) integrates gene expression data and protein–DNA binding data through a consistent framework, (2) considers misclassifications

associated with protein–DNA binding data explicitly, and (3) consists of a flexible model structure. The systematic simulation results indicate that this model
performs well in TRN reconstruction, when the measurement errors associated
with gene expression data and (more importantly) protein–DNA binding data
are within reasonable ranges. For example, in the case of less than 30–40%
false-positive and false-negative rates in the observed binding data, our method
may significantly reduce both types of errors in the inferred network when the
standard deviation in gene expression measurements is around 0.5 or less. In
all the cases, the inclusion of gene expression data leads to improved inference
of the underlying network compared to that solely based on the binding data
even when the measurement error in gene expression data is very high.

Simulation studies suggested that (1) protein–DNA binding data can serve
as a good starting point in the proposed MCMC procedure, and (2) the larger
the number of gene expression data sets used, the more accurate we expect our
procedure performs. Therefore, in general, when the number of TFs increases,
we hope to collect more samples on relevant gene expressions. More samples
can be achieved by increasing the number of experimental conditions or the
number of replicates per experimental condition or both. The advantage of
increasing the number of experimental conditions is that more variations of TF
activity profiles can be introduced so as to better infer the underlying network.
However, more parameters are needed to specify the model for the additional
conditions. We also need to be cautious on how to pool the experiments to infer
the TRN, for example, a time-invariant TRN may not hold when using data under drastically different experimental conditions. The advantage of increasing
the number of replicates per condition is that errors associated with measured
gene expression levels can be reduced at each point without introducing more
model parameters. In this study, the replicates were not included in the model
setup; however, the flexible structure of our model allows an easy incorporation
of such information.

In our simulation studies, we have investigated the sensitivity of our method
when some of the model parameters are misspecified, including the prior distribution on the network connections and our belief on the quality of protein–DNA
binding data. We found that the method is not sensitive to the misspecifications
of these parameters unless they are drastically different from the true values. In
the analysis of yeast cell cycle data, we considered eight sets of model parameters and observed general agreements. In practice, we may take a full Bayesian
approach to inferring the network through averaging inferred networks under
certain prior distributions for the model parameters.

As discussed above, although we have treated the observed protein–DNA
binding data as a 0–1 variable, the observed data are, in fact, continuous.

Our model can be modified within the measurement model framework so that the measured and true covariate values are continuous. To specify the prior distribution for the covariates, we may use normal mixtures or more sophisticated models.

In our model setup, we assume that all the TFs act additively to affect the transcription levels of their target genes and this linear relationship between the normalized expression levels and TF activities is a key assumption for this model. Because of the complexity in transcription regulation, such as synergistic effects among TFs, a linear model can serve as an approximation at best. Nevertheless, linear models have been used in this context by various authors (e.g., Bussemaker et al. 2001; Liu et al. 2002; Wang et al. 2002; Gao et al. 2004). Similar to yeast data, protein–DNA binding data are available for human (e.g., Boyer et al. 2005). Since the mechanisms of TRN remains unknown, especially for human, our model can serve as a tool to jointly use gene expression and protein–DNA binding in understanding TRNs in human.

To conclude, we note that our model can be extended in different ways to be more comprehensive and better represent the underlying biological mechanisms. For example, the linear form of the model can be extended to incorporate nonlinear interactions among different TFs; the replicates per experiment can be considered into the model to improve the data quality; more prior information or more sophisticated statistical models can be used to construct the prior distribution of the network (π_X). In addition, our general framework has the potential to integrate more data types into the model, such as sequence data and mRNA decay data.

Acknowledgment

This work was supported in part by NSF grant DMS-0241160.

Bibliography

T. Akutsu, S. Miyano, S. Kuhara, "Inferring qualitative relations in genetic networks and metabolic pathways," *Bioinformatics*, 16(8): 727–734, 2000.

Z. Bar-Joseph, G.K. Gerber, T.I. Lee, N.J. Rinaldi, J.Y. Yoo, F. Robert, D.B. Gordon, E. Fraenkel, T.S. Jaakkola, R.A. Young, D.K. Gifford, "Computational discovery of gene modules and regulatory networks," *Nature Biotechnology*, 21(11): 1337–1342, 2003.

L.A. Boyer, T.I. Lee, M.F. Cole, S.E. Johnstone, S.S. Levine, J.P. Zucker, M.G. Guenther, R.M. Kumar, H.L. Murray, R.G. Jenner, D.K. Gifford, D.A. Melton, R. Jaenisch, R.A. Young, "Core transcriptional regulatory circuitry in human embryonic stem cells," *Cell*, 122(6): 947–956, 2005.

H.J. Bussemaker, H. Li, E.D. Siggia, "Regulatory element detection using correlation with expression," *Nature Genetics*, 27(2): 167–171, 2001.

M. Carey, S.T. Smale, *Transcriptional Regulation in Eukaryotes*, Cold Spring Harbor Laboratory Press, Cold Spring Harbor, NY, 1999.

H. de Jong, "Modeling and simulation of genetic regulatory systems: A literature review," *Journal of Computational Biology*, 9(1): 67–103, 2002.

M.B. Eisen, P.T. Spellman, P.O. Brown, D. Botstein, "Cluster analysis and display of genome-wide expression patterns," *Proceedings of the National Academy of Sciences USA*, 95(25): 14863–14868, 1998.

N. Friedman, M. Linial, I. Nachman, D. Pe'er, "Using Bayesian networks to analyze expression data," *Journal of Computational Biology*, 7(34): 601–620, 2000.

F. Gao, B.C. Foat, H.J. Bussemaker, "Defining transcriptional networks through integrative modeling of mRNA expression and transcription factor binding data," *BioMed Central Bioinformatics*, 5(1): 31, 2004.

T.S. Gardner, D. di Bernardo, D. Lorenz, J.J. Collins, "Inferring genetic networks and identifying compound mode of action via expression profiling," *Science*, 301(5629): 102–105, 2003.

A. Gelman, J.B. Carlin, H.S. Stern, D.B. Rubin, *Bayesian Data Analysis*, CRC Press, Boca Raton, FL, 1995.

A.J. Hartemink, "Reverse engineering gene regulatory networks," *Nature Biotechnology*, 23: 554–555, 2005.

A.J. Hartemink, D.K. Gifford, T.S. Jaakkola, R.A. Young, "Combining location and expression data for principled discovery of genetic regulatory network models," *The Pacific Symposium on Biocomputing*, 7: 437–449, 2002.

T.I. Lee, N.J. Rinaldi, F. Robert, D.T. Odom, Z. Bar-Joseph, G.K. Gerber, N.M. Hannett, C.T. Harbison, C.M. Thompson, I. Simon, J. Zeitlinger, E.G. Jennings, H.L. Murray, D.B. Gordon, B. Ren, J.J. Wyrick, J.B. Tagne, T.L. Volkert, E. Fraenkel, D.K. Gifford, R.A. Young, "Transcriptional regulatory networks in *Saccharomyces cerevisiae*," *Science*, 298(5594): 799–804, 2002.

J.C. Liao, R. Boscolo, Y.L. Yang, L.M. Tran, C. Sabatti, V.P. Roychowdhury, "Network component analysis: Reconstruction of regulatory signals in biological systems," *Proceedings of the National Academy of Sciences* USA, 100(26): 15522–15527, 2003.

X.S. Liu, D.L. Brutlag, J.S. Liu, "An algorithm for finding protein–DNA binding sites with applications to chromatin-immunoprecipitation microarray experiments," *Nature Biotechnology*, 20(8): 835–839, 2002.

B. Ren, F. Robert, J.J. Wyrick, O. Aparicio, E.G. Jennings, I. Simon, J. Zeitlinger, J. Schreiber, N. Hannett, E. Kanin, T.L. Volkert, C.J. Wilson, S.P. Bell, R.A. Young, "Genome-wide location and function of DNA binding proteins," *Science*, 290(5500): 2306–2309, 2000.

S. Richardson, W.R. Gilks, "Conditional independence models for epidemiological studies with covariate measurement error," *Statistics in Medicine*, 12: 1703–1722, 1993.

I. Shmulevich, E.R. Dougherty, S. Kim, W. Zhang, "Probabilistic Boolean networks: A rule-based uncertainty model for gene regulatory networks," *Bioinformatics*, 18(2): 261–274, 2002.

P.T. Spellman, G. Sherlock, M.Q. Zhang, V.R. Iyer, K. Anders, M.B. Eisen, P.O. Brown, D. Botstein, B. Futcher, "Comprehensive identification of cell cycle-regulated genes of the yeast *Saccharomyces cerevisiae* by microarray hybridization," *Molecular Biology of the Cell*, 9(12): 3273–3297, 1998.

N. Sun, H. Zhao, "Genomic approaches in dissecting complex biological pathways," *Pharmacogenomics*, 5(2): 163–179, 2004.

J. Tegnér, M.K. Yeung, J. Hasty, J.J. Collins, "Reverse engineering gene networks: Integrating genetic perturbations with dynamical modeling," *Proceedings of the National Academy of Sciences USA*, 100(10): 5944–5949, 2003.

W. Wang, J.M. Cherry, D. Botstein, H. Li, "A systematic approach to reconstructing transcription networks in *Saccharomyces cerevisiae*," *Proceedings of the National Academy of Sciences USA*, 99(26): 16893–16898, 2002.

H. Zhao, B. Wu, N. Sun, "DNA-protein binding and gene expression patterns," in *Science and Statistics: A Festschrift for Terry Speed*, *IMS Lecture Notes-Monograph Series*, Vol. 40, pp. 259–274, 2003.

19

Estimating Cellular Signaling from Transcription Data

ANDREW V. KOSSENKOV
Fox Chase Cancer Center

GHISLAIN BIDAUT
University of Pennsylvania

MICHAEL F. OCHS
Fox Chase Cancer Center

Abstract

Cells initiate responses to the external environment and internal state through a complex network of signaling pathways composed of many multipurpose proteins. Errors within these signaling networks play a major role in disease progression, so determining signaling activity is crucial in understanding many diseases, including cancer. The changes in these pathways lead to multiple responses within cells, including induction of transcription, allowing the use of microarray data for interpretation of signaling activity. However, linking transcriptional changes to signaling pathways is complicated by the multipurpose nature of proteins, the overlap of signaling pathways, the presence of routine background transcription of housekeeping genes, and the lack of correlation between transcript and protein levels. In order to recover estimates of signaling from microarray data, several steps are required, including (1) modeling of signaling pathways and their links to transcription factors, (2) analysis of transcription factor and transcription complex binding sites in the genome, (3) use of Bayesian methods to extract overlapping transcriptional signatures, and (4) determination of the appropriate dimensionality for analysis. Here we present an approach using simplistic network models, existing databases of transcription factors, and Bayesian Decomposition to demonstrate the methodology.

19.1 Introduction

Many methods have been developed to model biological processes and extract information from transcriptional data, and this review cannot fully cover all such methods. The goal will be instead to provide an overview of the key issues to resolve in estimating signaling changes when working with transcriptional data, as provided by GeneChips and microarrays.

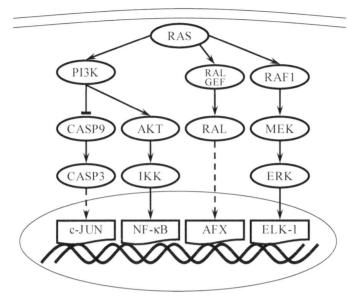

Fig. 19.1. RAS signaling. The transcriptional response of activation of the RAS protein depends on activity in proteins that are either activated downstream of RAS (AKT, RAL, MEK) or repressed due to RAS (CASP9). Activation of a full signaling pathway results in activation of specific transcription factors, leading to transcription of a set of genes.

19.1.1 Signaling Networks and Transcription

Signaling networks provide cells with the ability to initiate complex responses to the external environment and internal state. Changes in signaling pathways lead to multiple responses within cells, which comprise many different potential changes, including modification of enzymatic activity [10], triggering of multiple different pathways through activation of proteins by phosphorylation or cleavage [13], and, of primary interest here, induction of transcription [37]. The pathways generally interact through cross-talk, forming networks that generate complex responses [22].

Because of the central role of signaling in controlling cellular behavior, the development and progression of cancer, as well as many other diseases, often involves disruption of the cellular signaling networks [20, 24]. Because of the extreme underlying biological complexity of these pathways, observed cancers arise from a myriad of different cellular malfunctions [8, 27]. An analysis must address this inherent biological complexity.

An example of this complexity is given in Figure 19.1, which is modified from [9] with additional information from BioCarta (see below for details on the BioCarta database). Figure 19.1 provides a reduced and highly simplified view of the critical RAS signaling network (for a more complete view of the network see Figure 2 in [11] and the review in [24]). The RAS signaling protein is a cytosolic protein that undergoes posttranslational modification leading to its being bound to the membrane and capable of initiating signaling. As Figure 19.1 shows, RAS interacts with many downstream signaling proteins, including PI3K, a well-connected node linking many signals, RAF, which activates the ERK pathway important in cell growth, and RAL, through RALGEF and CASPASE9, both of which play critical roles in apoptosis (i.e., programmed cell death). The final points in each pathway (i.e., c-JUN, NFκB, AFX, and ELK-1) are transcription factors that initiate transcription of overlapping sets of genes.

19.1.2 Biological Issues in the Analysis of Gene Expression

One of the standard assumptions within many analyses of transcriptional data is that the function of a gene identified through standard biological studies can be assumed to be initiated if the mRNA for that gene is detected. Unfortunately, studies that have looked at mRNA and protein level correlations suggest that this is not the case, since the correlation excluding highly expressed structural and housekeeping genes is only about 0.36 [14, 15]. Since signaling proteins are both produced at very low levels and require significant transport and posttranslational modification to enter the active state, the correlation of mRNA levels and activities for signaling proteins is likely to be significantly less than even this low level.

Interpreting the activity within the pathways of Figure 19.1 from transcriptional data therefore requires estimation of the activity of the individual transcription factors as downstream indicators of signaling activity, rather than the use of mRNA species encoding signaling proteins as upstream indicators. Unfortunately, the majority of genes regulated by these factors have not been identified, and additional regulators of the genes also remain poorly delineated. This leaves the problem of identifying overlapping signatures of transcription factor activity (i.e., patterns of expression that explain part of the behavior of a gene) without the knowledge of how many such signatures exist or whether any individual gene may be uniquely linked to a single factor.

In addition, what is not shown in Figure 19.1 cannot be ignored. While the transcription factors shown may represent the proteins of interest for a study, additional factors are active at all times in living cells. These factors initiate transcription of genes encoding proteins required for cellular metabolism, ongoing protein and biochemical synthesis, and other housekeeping functions, so that the signals of interest always exist in a background of unknown and varying

Table 19.1. *Genes Regulated by Transcription Factors in Figure 19.1*

Transcription factor	Regulated genes
AFX	BCL6, IGFBP-1, RBL2
ELK-1	B-ACT, C-FOS, EGR2, ELK1, NOS3, TNFA
NFκB	COL1A2, F8, GRO2, GROA, ICAM-1, IFNB, IFNG, IL-2, IL-2Rα, IL-6, MCP1, p53, RANTES, SELE, TNFA, TNFB, TNFRSF6
c-JUN	4F2HC, ANF, ATF3, BCL2A1, GLOB-B, CD11c, C-JUN, CYCD1, ET-1, FN, GJA1, IFNβ, IL-2, IL-5, KRT16, MMP1, MSH2, MT-IIA, p53, ENK, RANTES, SELE, TNFA, TSG-6, TSHB, uPA, VIP

transcription. In addition, as noted above, genes generally encode proteins that are active in multiple biological functions, so that genes are not transcribed uniquely in response to a single transcription factor. For example, as can be seen in Table 19.1, even for the limited pathways in Figure 19.1, transcription of TNFA is initiated by ELK-1, c-JUN, and NFκB. [Note that for each gene in Table 19.1, TRANSFAC provides evidence codes, as all genes are not equally reliably linked to the transcription factors.] In effect, we are faced with unknown overlap in transcriptional response, incomplete models of signaling pathways, and incomplete knowledge of the links between genes and the transcription factors that regulate them.

19.1.3 Modeling Signaling Networks

The ideal method of interpreting a successfully disentangled set of transcriptional signatures would be to create a model of all cellular protein networks (signaling and metabolic), chemical fluxes, and transcriptional behavior. Unfortunately such a model is well beyond current technology and knowledge. Presently, a number of potential approaches are being taken to model cellular networks, focused primarily on genetic networks with some work on protein interactions as well [36].

Perhaps the most widely used network model is a Bayesian network, which is a form of a directed acyclic graph (DAG) with transition probabilities governing how nodes evolve. This has been used to model the transcriptional response of a genetic network, deriving relations between genes from microarray data [16]. These models are data-driven and reconstruct the relationship between expression levels of genes, creating networks that can couple microarray data and proteomic data together.

Another computational approach has been to use probabilistic Boolean networks (PBNs) to predict genetic networks [43]. Boolean networks have a useful feature for signaling, in that each node is either active (1) or inactive (0), which can abstract the primary measurement of interest in signaling, whether or not the signaling protein is activating downstream targets. PBNs extend Boolean networks by having probabilistic transition rules, making them more appropriate to stochastic processes such as protein interactions. PBNs also have the advantage of allowing estimation of node transitions (i.e., signaling protein activity) using Markov chains [43].

A recent development is the derivation of signaling networks from perturbative experiments where phosphoantibody measurements are made [40]. This approach uses Bayesian networks to reconstruct signaling from protein measurements. While this method is focused on signaling, it relies on both perturbations and the availability of highly targeted phosphoantibodies, instead of transcriptional response measurements that can be made globally. Such antibodies remain limited and have issues with specificity, and the experiments desired are often untenable in vivo and are certainly impossible in humans.

Another approach to determining networks has been the large-scale determination of protein interactions, generating networks determining links between proteins. While this has been useful for determination of overall structure, for instance showing that protein networks appear to follow scale-free structures typical in robust networks [1, 21], these studies do not lead to determination of the arrows defining how one protein affects another. In signaling, this is critical, since one protein may serve as an activator of another protein, while a second protein may be an inhibitor of the same protein. These protein interaction studies may be useful for identifying potential partners; however, the false positive problem remains in addition to the problem of arrows [47].

In addition, one can approach the problem of modeling by creating full biochemical models that include rate constants, dissociation rates, diffusion, and transport [2, 41]. These models are useful for exploring parameters of interest to the problem of signaling [28]; however, the present state of knowledge does not allow these models to reflect physiologically relevant networks. Nevertheless, one key development of these models has been the demonstration of the validity of using a modular view [6]. This permits models such as that shown in (19.1) to be used when interpreting overall signaling activity from transcriptional data.

19.2 Bayesian Decomposition

The issue of overlapping transcriptional response signatures requires an analysis that can identify patterns within the data that are nonorthogonal, since many biological processes are strongly overlapping both in time and between samples. Essentially, the basis vectors that describe the transcriptional response of a pathway or a group of pathways activated or deactivated simultaneously within an experiment form the natural bases for describing the biological response. As noted above, the patterns of interest (i.e., those related to the signaling pathways) will be joined by patterns arising from transcription due to ongoing normal metabolic processes and cellular maintenance. As such, one can expect that the set of expression changes of interest will comprise one or a few multiple patterns (i.e., basis vectors) present within the data. The transcriptional data from a study, such as a time course following perturbation or measurements across multiple subjects, can be viewed then as arising from a matrix multiplication,

$$a_{ji} = \sum_{p=1}^{N_p} f_{jp} p_{pi} + \epsilon_{ji} = m_{ji} + \epsilon_{ji}, \qquad (19.1)$$

where a_{ji} is the measured average relative expression level for the jth gene in the ith condition, m_{ji} is the modeled average relative expression level for the jth gene in the ith condition, f_{jp} is the amount of pattern p that is included in the model for gene j, p_{pi} is the fractional level of expression in pattern p under condition i (relative to the other conditions), and ϵ_{ji} is the error or misfit of the model to the data for the expression of the jth gene in the ith condition, which under ideal circumstances is a random error. However, if the number of patterns is incorrectly estimated or if systematic error remains in the data, this term can include nonrandom components.

Since equation (19.1) is mathematically degenerate, allowing multiple solutions, a Bayesian Markov chain Monte Carlo (MCMC) procedure [17, 30] is used to identify the **f** and **p** matrices that best explain the observed data. In general, a single solution may not exist; however, in practice when the number of data points (elements of **a**) significantly exceeds the number of parameters, then a single solution (i.e., monomodal distributions at each element in **f** and **p** allowing a reasonable estimate of the mean and variance) can often be recovered. At a maximum, the number of elements of **f** and **p** will be the number of parameters. However, if correlations can be identified a priori in the **f** and **p** matrices, then the number of parameters can be significantly lower. The algorithm proposes solutions to equation (19.1) by assuming that the elements of **f** and **p** arise from an underlying mixture model. Let Ψ generically denote an element of **f** and **p**, then

$$\Psi = \sum_{w} K_w \Phi_w. \qquad (19.2)$$

provides a method of encoding prior knowledge of correlations within kernels, K_w, operating on a family of measures, Φ_w [44]. This permits multiple matrix elements to vary in a coordinated fashion. The algorithm incorporates a domain for creation, destruction, and modification of flux elements that are mapped to the $\mathbf{f}$ and $\mathbf{p}$ matrices using the convolution functions in equation (19.2), which is detailed in [37]. In the present work, each row of $\mathbf{p}$ can be viewed as measuring flux through a set of pathways, indicating the strength of a transduced signal as measured by the transcriptional response. Each associated element of $\mathbf{f}$ will be the relative level of expression for each gene related to the associated pathways. Ideally the convolution functions would encode full transcriptional response from transcription factors, but such data is not yet available.

MCMC simulation is implemented as a Gibbs sampler that requires relative probability estimates between points in the posterior distribution. The posterior is evaluated as proportional to the likelihood, which is easily determined by comparing the model to the data, times the prior, which is the probability of the model independent of the data. Inserting the $\mathbf{f}$ and $\mathbf{p}$ matrices in Bayes' equation and ignoring the normalization integral, $p(\mathbf{a})$ (the marginal probability), generates the posterior distribution used by Bayesian decomposition,

$$p(\mathbf{f}, \mathbf{p}|\mathbf{a}) \propto p(\mathbf{a}|\mathbf{f}, \mathbf{p}) \, p(\mathbf{f}, \mathbf{p}), \qquad (19.3)$$

where $p(\mathbf{a}|\mathbf{f}, \mathbf{p})$ gives the likelihood and $p(\mathbf{f}, \mathbf{p})$ gives the prior. The sampling from the posterior distribution and the encoding of the prior are done using a customized form of the Massive Inference (TM) Gibbs sampler (Maximum Entropy Data Consultants, Cambridge, England) [44]. For the work presented here, the prior encodes only positivity of expression (ratios are positive) and an Occam's razor preference for minimal structure. Other implementations have encoded prior information in class association [25, 32] and coregulation information gathered through transcription factor databases [26].

Assuming a normal error distribution, the log-likelihood, L, is given by

$$L = -\sum_{j=1}^{J} \sum_{i=1}^{I} \left\{ \frac{1}{2\sigma_{ji}^2} \left(a_{ji} - \sum_{p=1}^{N_p} f_{jp} p_{pi} \right)^2 \right\}, \qquad (19.4)$$

where σ_{ji} is the standard deviation for the expression measurement of the jth gene in the ith condition. Although other likelihoods could be encoded, in our experience, a normal error model has been adequate. For any change to the model, the change in the log-likelihood can be calculated by inserting the change in equation (19.4) and subtracting the result from equation (19.4). For a change $\delta\mathbf{p}$ at matrix element $[x, y]$ in the $\mathbf{p}$ matrix, for example, the change in the log-likelihood is

$$\delta L\left(\delta p_{xy}\right) = -\sum_{j=1}^{J}\left\{2\Delta_{jy}f_{jx}\delta p_{xy} + \frac{1}{2\sigma_{jy}^2}f_{jx}^2\delta p_{xy}^2\right\}, \qquad (19.5)$$

with

$$\Delta_{ji} = \frac{1}{2\sigma_{ji}^2}\left\{a_{ji} - \sum_{p}^{N_p}f_{jp}p_{pi}\right\} \qquad (19.6)$$

defining the normalized mismatch between the model and data at each point. A similar equation applies for any change in the $\mathbf{f}$ matrix. In addition, the prior probability is included in determining the transition probability for the step in the Markov chain. In order to simplify the calculations, simultaneous changes in $\mathbf{f}$ and $\mathbf{p}$ are not permitted, since allowing such changes would require evaluation of terms involving $\delta\mathbf{f}\delta\mathbf{p}$. Note that barring these changes does not prevent the system from reaching any state and should have no effect on the final result, since the sampler can move $\delta\mathbf{p}$ followed by $\delta\mathbf{f}$ and reach the same point. The algorithm presently calculates the mean and variance at each matrix element, although more complex analyses of the samples could be performed.

19.3 Key Biological Databases

The analysis described below relies on detailed knowledge of a number of key biological components within cells. This information has been generated over many decades of study. Several databases exist that can be queried to retrieve data on signaling pathways, transcription factors and the genes they regulate, consensus binding sites for transcription factors, and protein–protein interactions that may be useful in interpreting inconsistencies in predictions of signaling activity that arise in analysis. In all cases the data within these resources must be viewed as a mixture of highly reliable annotations for well-studied genes and proteins mixed with tentative assignments of function or interaction for less well studied ones. A few Web accessible data resources are listed in Table 19.2.

There are two main repositories of pathway information which include known signaling pathways, as well as metabolic pathways. The first is the Kyoto Encyclopedia of Genes and Genomes (KEGG), which includes signaling pathways for many organisms from yeast through humans, as well as information on metabolic, biosynthetic, degradation, and other pathways [23]. The KEGG system allows interactive highlighting of signaling components

Table 19.2. Web Resources

Resource	URL
KEGG	http://www.genome.ad.jp/kegg/pathway.html
BioCarta	http://www.biocarta.com/genes/allpathways.asp
TRANSFAC	http://www.biobase.de/pages/products/transfac.html
PAINT	http://www.dbi.tju.edu/dbi/tools/paint/
WebGestalt	http://genereg.ornl.gov/webgestalt/
SGD	http://www.yeastgenome.org/

within a simple schematic presentation of the network information, which is used by some Web tools for interpretation of the results of microarray analyses [46]. The second database is the BioCarta pathways database, provided openly by BioCarta, Inc. (San Diego, CA), that includes signaling pathways for mouse and human, as well as many other cellular pathways similar to those in the KEGG database. The BioCarta pathways are presented as high-quality figures that indicate some aspects of protein structure; however, they do not allow interactive annotation.

Both databases must be used somewhat carefully. Signaling pathways are known to be cell-type-dependent, and the literature contains numerous examples of contradictory claims for network structure. The databases will also sometimes miss a key published and accepted component of the pathways. For example, the KEGG pathway for the yeast signaling pathways fails to include the direct activation by a G-protein coupled receptor of the MAPK cascade leading to the mating response, despite the publication of this mode of activation in a review [39].

The systems for transcription factor identification from groups of genes comprise two different approaches. The first contains curated lists of genes that are believed to be regulated by specific known transcription factors, including the gene, the consensus transcription factor binding sequence, and the evidence for the claim. The primary database is TRANSFAC [29], although there are many databases specific to organisms or included in organism-specific genome databases. The second type uses information in these databases together with genomic data to predict potential transcription factors for sets of genes based on the presence of binding sites at a higher than expected rate in the upstream regions of the genes. For instance, PAINT relies on information from TRANSFAC on consensus binding sequences to guide searching for binding sites shared by many genes in a group, such as a cluster from an analysis [45]. Finding a significantly enhanced set of binding sites is then taken as evidence for activity of the corresponding transcription factor. In addition, tools exist to

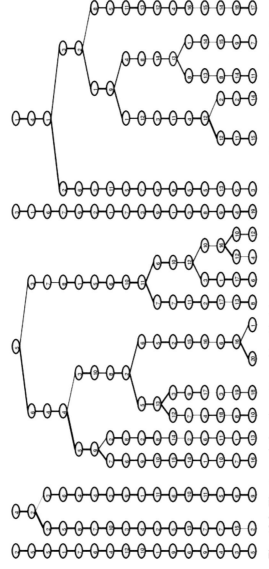

Fig. 19.2. The tree relating the patterns identified by Bayesian decomposition as the number of posited patterns increased from 5 to 20. The thickness of the connecting line indicates the correlation coefficient (thicker is closer to 1), while the numbers in each node are merely used for linking patterns in the **p** matrix to genes in the **f** matrix. (See color plate 19.2.)

look for potential binding sites independent of known transcription factor sites, for instance AlignACE [18]; however, for the approach here linking back to a transcription factor is critical.

19.4 Example: Signaling Activity in *Saccharomyces cerevisiae*

Here we demonstrate the methodology using the the Rosetta compendium, which provides a large set of replicated measurements of expression in 300 separate deletion mutants or chemically treated cultures of *S. cerevisiae* [19]. The data were downloaded from Rosetta Inpharmatics and filtered to remove experiments where less than two genes underwent threefold changes and to remove genes that did not change by threefold across the remaining experiments. The resulting data set contains 764 genes and 228 conditions. The Rosetta gene-specific error model provides an estimate of the uncertainty based on the replicates and 63 replications of control cultures [19].

The analysis proceeds by application of Bayesian Decomposition [33, 37, 38] positing many different potential numbers of transcriptional signatures or patterns, estimation of the correct dimensionality for interpretation by a consistency argument, and linking of the patterns to signaling pathways through transcription factors. This then allows inference of the activity of signaling pathways and proteins in specific conditions. The analysis here summarizes the results presented previously [4].

19.4.1 Bayesian Decomposition Analysis

Bayesian Decomposition was applied multiple times to the reduced Rosetta data set, with each application positing a different number of patterns (i.e., transcriptional signatures), from 3 to 30. A tree was constructed using ClutrFree [5]. First, each analysis was represented as a tree level, beginning with the experiment positing three patterns. Second, the next level was compared to the previous level by calculating the Pearson correlation between all nodes at the first level and all at the second level. Third, connections were made from the highest to the lowest correlation, with nodes removed from the process as they were connected. Each remaining node was connected to the node at the previous level that gave the highest Pearson correlation coefficient. This was repeated for each additional level, until the full tree was constructed (see Figure 19.2, where results for 5–20 patterns are shown). The first issue to resolve in this analysis is the correct number of patterns, equivalent to identifying the appropriate number of basis vectors (rows of **p**) needed to reconstruct the data (**a**).

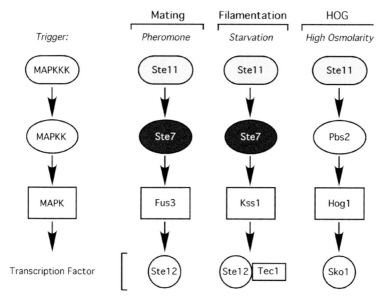

Fig. 19.3. Schematic view of three MAPK modules that regulate mating, filamentous growth, and high-osmolarity glycerol signaling pathways in the yeast *Saccharomyces cerevisiae*. Activation of these pathways is determined by the state of the cell and exposure to external signals.

In order to determine the dimensionality, we calculated the persistence of a gene within the branches defined in Figure 19.2. The persistence is defined by the number of consecutive times a gene appears within a branch given its presence in a node at the present level. We conjectured that once we exceeded the correct number of basis vectors, genes would be able to move more easily between patterns (i.e., nodes) due to mathematical degeneracy as the number of patterns increased (i.e., as we move down the tree), leading to a reduction in the average persistence. The persistence as we increase the number of basis vectors showed a significant drop between 15 and 16 basis vectors, suggesting 15 as the correct dimensionality for interpretation of the data.

19.4.2 Transcription Factors

The next step in the analysis is to relate the transcriptional signatures identified in the analysis at 15 dimensions with the transcription factors of interest in the experiment. Figure 19.3 shows the signaling pathways in *S. cerevisiae* as three separate MAPK cascades [42]. The network actually uses the MAPKKK protein Ste11p for all pathways and the MAPKK protein Ste7p for both mating and filamentation responses. In addition, the Ste12p transcription factor is required for both mating and filamentation; however, in filamentation the coactivator Tec1p is required. [Note: for yeast the suffix p indicates the protein and the name without the p the gene.]

In order to identify which patterns relate to different transcription factors, each pattern is explored for enhancement in gene ontology (GO) [3]. This is approached in two ways using ClutrFree [5]. First, the enhancement is calculated as

$$E = \frac{N_{\text{patt}}^{\text{term}} / N_{\text{patt}}}{N_{\text{data}}^{\text{term}} / N_{\text{data}}} \tag{19.7}$$

where $N_{\text{patt}}^{\text{term}}$ is the number of genes with the GO term in the pattern, N_{patt} is the number of genes in the pattern, $N_{\text{data}}^{\text{term}}$ is the number of genes with the GO term in the full data set, and N_{data} is the number of genes in the full data set. Second, a hypergeometric test of overrepresentation of ontology terms in each pattern is performed. The enhancement provides a useful simple estimate for exploration, while the hypergeometric test insures that terms with few genes are not erroneously highlighted. However, because genes encode proteins with multiple functions, an ontology term may appear significant in a pattern when the reason for association of some genes with the pattern is not due to that specific function. Enhancement calculations allow a quick overview of terms that may be related to processes, and it is the overall combination of terms that provide insight. Here we use the MIPS ontology for yeast to assign biological processes to genes [31]. The GO analysis allows each pattern to be interpreted in terms of how likely it is to be related to signaling activity of interest to minimize the amount of effort in the next step. Alternatively, one could immediately move to link the individual genes associated with the patterns to transcription factors as detailed below.

For this analysis, patterns 13 and 15 show significant enhancement in several GO terms (enhancement given first for pattern 13, then for pattern 15): mating type determination ($E = 6.3, E = 7.2$), mating ($E = 6.1, E = 5.7$), meiosis ($E = 2.9$, not enhanced), filamentation (not enhanced, $E = 2.9$), and development ($E = 6.1, E = 5.7$), among other terms including several for signal transduction. These enhancements suggest that patterns 13 and 15 are related to mating or filamentation signaling pathway activity. No enhancement is seen in any pattern that suggests activity of the high-osmolarity glycerol pathway; however, this is not surprising since the cultures are all grown in rich medium, and the yeast are unlikely to require proteins useful in high-osmolarity conditions.

Focusing on patterns 13 and 15, the individual genes that are highly associated with the patterns can be explored for information on whether they are regulated by Ste12p or the Ste12p–Tec1p complex through use of information in the Saccharomyces Genome Database [7]. Since Bayesian Decomposition provides an amplitude of assignment for each gene with each pattern, the genes can be ranked in order of strength of association with a pattern. For pattern 13, the top 10 genes are (with M indicating known function in mating and S indicating known to be regulated by Ste12p) Fig1 (M), Prm6 (M, S), Fus1 (M, S), Ste2 (M, S), Aga1 (M), Fus3 (M, S), Pes4, Prm1 (M, S), a hypothetical ORF, Bar1 (M). This provides strong support for linking pattern 13 to activation of Ste12p. [As noted previously, many genes have not been fully elucidated as to function with even fewer having been fully studied in terms of known transcriptional regulation, so that having 5 of 10 genes known to be regulated by Ste12p is quite strong evidence.] For pattern 15, 7 of the top 10 genes are transposable element genes involved in gene rearrangement. The other three genes include Prm5, which encodes a protein of unknown function, and two hypothetical ORFs. Little is known about the genes directly regulated by the Ste12p–Tec1p complex; however, it is known that activation of transposable elements is necessary for filamentous growth [34, 35], so pattern 15 is likely the filamentation response signature and thus linked to activation of the Ste12p–Tec1p complex.

19.4.3 Inference on Signaling

From the transcription factors, we can infer activity of the previous protein in the pathway using Figure 19.3. For instance, for pattern 13, we infer that Fus1p has activated Ste12p, that therefore Ste7p has activated Fus1p, that Ste11p has activated Ste7p, and on to other factors not shown here linking to a membrane receptor. For pattern 15, we get activation of Ste11p and Ste7p as well; however, we do not get activation of Fus3p, instead get activation of Kss1p. In reality, life can be more complex even in yeast, as in certain conditions Kss1p has been noted to substitute for Fus3p in the mating pathway. Nevertheless, this approach allows prediction of specific signaling activity from microarray data.

19.4.4 Validation

The Rosetta data set also provides a way to validate this approach, at least for *S. cerevisiae*. The inferences on signaling have relied only on the gene lists contained in the **F** matrix. If the transcription factors have been correctly identified and linked to signaling pathways, any mutant that eliminates a key gene encoding a signaling protein, as noted in the previous section, must eliminate the presence of the pattern (13 or 15), since that pattern is the transcriptional response induced by activation of the pathway. The pathway clearly cannot be activated if a required signaling protein is not present.

Pattern 13 shows near-zero signal (i.e., is absent) for the deletion mutants of Ste11, Ste7, Fus3, and Ste12, while being present for the deletion mutant of Tec1, which is the transcriptional cofactor for filamentation response. This is exactly as expected for the mating pathway, as all signaling proteins in the cascade and the transcription factor necessary to generate the transcriptional response related to the mating signal do not contain the pattern. For pattern 15, the response is very similar. The signal is near zero for deletion mutants of Ste11, Ste7, and Ste12. The Fus3 deletion mutant shows a signal for pattern 15, as appropriate, while the Fus3,Kss1 double deletion mutant does not (there is no Kss1 single deletion mutant in the data set). However, the Tec1 deletion mutant shows no signal for pattern 15, indicating that Tec1p is required for filamentation [34]. Together the presence and absence of patterns for these mutants, and for others detailed in [4], demonstrate that the transcriptional signatures for two strongly overlapping signaling pathways can be separated by this approach.

19.5 Conclusion

Many diseases, including cancer, develop because of errors in signaling, and newer therapeutics specifically target proteins involved in cellular signaling. However, these therapeutics are not always effective, both in human studies and in model organisms. Microarrays provide one of the first truly global measurements of biological functional response, so that use of transcriptional data offers a chance to identify key points of failure for therapeutics and key proteins required for disease progression. However, identification of signaling protein activity is problematic due to the complexity of the biological system and the limitations of the data.

Here we have demonstrated an approach that relies on models of signaling pathways and their links to transcription factors identified through decades of research in molecular biology, use of Bayesian methods to extract overlapping transcriptional signatures that can be linked to transcription factors through annotations, and inference from the transcription factors back to the signaling pathways. In this simplistic approach, which does not require a full network model, the recovery of activity within *S. cerevisiae* is demonstrated. The key components permitting this recovery are the identification of overlapping transcriptional signatures using Bayesian Decomposition, estimation of dimensionality by ClutrFree, and the linking of these signatures to transcription factors using GO and the SGD database.

As this methodology is extended into higher organisms, the signaling networks increase significantly in complexity, so that the simple approach of moving from transcription factor activity to signaling proteins will require modification. As noted in the introduction, a great deal of work has been done on modeling networks. Importantly, work by Kholodenko and colleagues [6] suggests that much of the biochemical complexity can be abstracted away, so that relatively simple PBNs may be able to provide enough complexity to recover significant biological behavior. As noted above, PBNs have the additional advantage of being mappable to Markov chains, permitting the efficient computational methods already developed to be applied to the problem [12].

The use of Bayesian Decomposition to identify transcriptional signatures in mammalian cells has already been successfully accomplished [25, 32]. While estimation of dimensionality remains an issue, as with estimation of the correct number of clusters in other approaches, ClutrFree provides one method of addressing this issue. Hopefully a stronger statistical approach will allow more reliable estimation in the future. Nevertheless, the key issue for extension now is likely to be creation of reasonable network models for inference and extension of data on transcription factors and the genes that they regulate. In addition, as proteomics technologies improve, it should become easier to get direct estimation of the phosphorylation state of some signaling proteins, which should improve inference on the network models.

Bibliography

[1] R. Albert, H. Jeong, and A. L. Barabasi. Error and attack tolerance of complex networks. *Nature*, 406(6794):378–382, 2000.

[2] M. Andrec, B. N. Kholodenko, R. M. Levy, and E. Sontag. Inference of signaling and gene regulatory networks by steady-state perturbation experiments: Structure and accuracy. *J Theor Biol*, 232(3):427–441, 2005.

[3] M. Ashburner, C. A. Ball, J. A. Blake, D. Botstein, H. Butler, J. M. Cherry, A. P. Davis, K. Dolinski, S. S. Dwight, J. T. Eppig, M. A. Harris, D. P. Hill, L. Issel-Tarver, A. Kasarskis, S. Lewis, J. C. Matese, J. E. Richardson, M. Ringwald, G. M. Rubin, and G. Sherlock. Gene ontology: Tool for the unification of biology. The gene ontology consortium. *Nat Genet*, 25(1):25–29, 2000.

[4] G. Bidaut, A. V. Kossenkov, and M. F. Ochs. Determination of strongly overlapping signaling activity from microarray data. *BMC Bioinformatics*, 7:99, 2006.

[5] G. Bidaut and M. F. Ochs. Clutrfree: Cluster tree visualization and interpretation. *Bioinformatics*, 20(16):2869–2871, 2004.

[6] F. J. Bruggeman, H. V. Westerhoff, J. B. Hoek, and B. N. Kholodenko. Modular response analysis of cellular regulatory networks. *J Theor Biol*, 218(4):507–520, 2002.

[7] K. R. Christie, S. Weng, R. Balakrishnan, M. C. Costanzo, K. Dolinski, S. S. Dwight, S. R. Engel, B. Feierbach, D. G. Fisk, J. E. Hirschman, E. L. Hong,

L. Issel-Tarver, R. Nash, A. Sethuraman, B. Starr, C. L. Theesfeld, R. Andrada, G. Binkley, Q. Dong, C. Lane, M. Schroeder, D. Botstein, and J. M. Cherry. Saccharomyces genome database (sgd) provides tools to identify and analyze sequences from *Saccharomyces cerevisiae* and related sequences from other organisms. *Nucleic Acids Res*, 32(Database issue):D311–D314, 2004.

[8] G. M. Cooper. *Elements of Human Cancer*. Jones and Bartlett Publishers, Boston, 1992.

[9] A. D. Cox and C. J. Der. Ras family signaling: Therapeutic targeting. *Cancer Biol Ther*, 1(6):599–606, 2002.

[10] J. Downward. The ins and outs of signalling. *Nature*, 411(6839):759–762, 2001.

[11] J. Downward. Targeting RAS signalling pathways in cancer therapy. *Nat Rev Cancer*, 3(1):11–22, 2003.

[12] W. R. Gilks, S. Richardson, and D. J. Spiegelhalter. *Markov Chain Monte Carlo in Practice*. Interdisciplinary statistics. Chapman & Hall, London, 1996.

[13] E. A. Golemis, M. F. Ochs, and E. N. Pugacheva. Signal transduction driving technology driving signal transduction: Factors in the design of targeted therapies. *J Cell Biochem Suppl*, 37 (Suppl):42–52, 2001.

[14] T. J. Griffin, S. P. Gygi, T. Ideker, B. Rist, J. Eng, L. Hood, and R. Aebersold. Complementary profiling of gene expression at the transcriptome and proteome levels in *Saccharomyces cerevisiae*. *Mol Cell Proteomics*, 1(4):323–333, 2002.

[15] S. P. Gygi, Y. Rochon, B. R. Franza, and R. Aebersold. Correlation between protein and MRNA abundance in yeast. *Mol Cell Biol*, 19(3):1720–1730, 1999.

[16] A. Hartemink, D. Gifford, T. Jaakkola, and R. Young. Using graphical models and genomic expression data to statistically validate models of genetic regulatory networks. In R. Altman, A. K. Dunker, L. Hunter, K. Lauderdale, and T. Klein, editors, *Pacific Symposium on Biocomputing 2001 (PSB01)*, pp. 422–433. World Scientific, New Jersey, 2001.

[17] W. K. Hastings. Monte Carlo sampling methods using Markov chains and their applications. *Biometrika*, 57:97–109, 1970.

[18] J. D. Hughes, P. W. Estep, S. Tavazoie, and G. M. Church. Computational identification of cis-regulatory elements associated with groups of functionally related genes in *Saccharomyces cerevisiae*. *J Mol Biol*, 296(5):1205–1214, 2000.

[19] T. R. Hughes, M. J. Marton, A. R. Jones, C. J. Roberts, R. Stoughton, C. D. Armour, H. A. Bennett, E. Coffey, H. Dai, Y. D. He, M. J. Kidd, A. M. King, M. R. Meyer, D. Slade, P. Y. Lum, S. B. Stepaniants, D. D. Shoemaker, D. Gachotte, K. Chakraburtty, J. Simon, M. Bard, and S. H. Friend. Functional discovery via a compendium of expression profiles. *Cell*, 102(1):109–126, 2000.

[20] T. Jacks and R. A. Weinberg. Taking the study of cancer cell survival to a new dimension. *Cell*, 111(7):923–925, 2002.

[21] H. Jeong, B. Tombor, R. Albert, Z. N. Oltvai, and A. L. Barabasi. The large-scale organization of metabolic networks. *Nature*, 407(6804):651–654, 2000.

[22] J. D. Jordan, E. M. Landau, and R. Iyengar. Signaling networks: The origins of cellular multitasking. *Cell*, 103(2):193–200, 2000.

[23] M. Kanehisa, S. Goto, S. Kawashima, and A. Nakaya. The kegg databases at genomenet. *Nucleic Acids Res*, 30(1):42–46, 2002.

[24] W. Kolch. Meaningful relationships: The regulation of the ras/raf/mek/erk pathway by protein interactions. *Biochem J*, 351 (Pt 2):289–305, 2000.

[25] A. Kossenkov, G. Bidaut, and M. F. Ochs. Genes associated with prognosis in adenocarcinoma across studies at multiple institutions. In K. Johnson and S. Lin, editors, *Methods of Microarray Data Analysis IV*, p. 239. Kluwer Academic, Boston, 2005.

[26] A. V. Kossenkov, G. Wang, and M. F. Ochs. Incorporating prior knowledge of transcription factor regulation in microarray analysis. Fox Chase Bioinformatics Technical Report, 2005.

[27] F. Macdonald and C. H. J. Ford. *Molecular Biology of Cancer*. BIOS Scientific Publishers, Ltd., Oxford, 1997.

[28] N. I. Markevich, J. B. Hoek, and B. N. Kholodenko. Signaling switches and bistability arising from multisite phosphorylation in protein kinase cascades. *J Cell Biol*, 164(3):353–359, 2004.

[29] V. Matys, E. Fricke, R. Geffers, E. Gossling, M. Haubrock, R. Hehl, K. Hornischer, D. Karas, A. E. Kel, O. V. Kel-Margoulis, D. U. Kloos, S. Land, B. Lewicki-Potapov, H. Michael, R. Munch, I. Reuter, S. Rotert, H. Saxel, M. Scheer, S. Thiele, and E. Wingender. Transfac: Transcriptional regulation, from patterns to profiles. *Nucleic Acids Res*, 31(1):374–378, 2003.

[30] N. Metropolis, A. Rosenbluth, M. Rosenbluth, A. Teller, and E. Teller. Equations of state calculations by fast computing machines. *J Chem Phys*, 21:1087–1091, 1953.

[31] H. W. Mewes, C. Amid, R. Arnold, D. Frishman, U. Guldener, G. Mannhaupt, M. Munsterkotter, P. Pagel, N. Strack, V. Stumpflen, J. Warfsmann, and A. Ruepp. Mips: Analysis and annotation of proteins from whole genomes. *Nucleic Acids Res*, 32(Database issue):D41–D44, 2004.

[32] T. D. Moloshok, D. Datta, A. V. Kossenkov, and M. F. Ochs. Bayesian decomposition classification of the project normal data set. In K. F. Johnson and S. M. Ln, editors, *Methods of Microarray Data Analysis III*, pp. 211–232. Kluwer Academic, Boston, 2003.

[33] T. D. Moloshok, R. R. Klevecz, J. D. Grant, F. J. Manion, W. F. Speier IV, and M. F. Ochs. Application of Bayesian Decomposition for analysing microarray data. *Bioinformatics*, 18(4):566–575, 2002.

[34] A. Morillon, M. Springer, and P. Lesage. Activation of the kss1 invasive-filamentous growth pathway induces ty1 transcription and retrotransposition in *Saccharomyces cerevisiae*. *Mol Cell Biol*, 20(15):5766–5776, 2000.

[35] H. U. Mosch and G. R. Fink. Dissection of filamentous growth by transposon mutagenesis in *Saccharomyces cerevisiae*. *Genetics*, 145(3):671–684, 1997.

[36] Sun Ning and Hongyu Zhao. Genomic approaches in dissecting complex biological pathways. *Pharmacogenomics*, 5(2):163–179, 2004.

[37] M. F. Ochs. Bayesian decomposition. In G. Parmigiani, E. S. Garrett, R. A. Irizarry, and S. L. Zeger, editors, *The Analysis of Gene Expression Data: Methods and Software*. Springer Verlag, New York, 2003.

[38] M. F. Ochs, T. D. Moloshok, G. Bidaut, and G. Toby. Bayesian decomposition: Analyzing microarray data within a biological context. *Annals of the New York Academy of Sciences*, 1020:212–226, 2004.

[39] F. Posas, M. Takekawa, and H. Saito. Signal transduction by map kinase cascades in budding yeast. *Curr Opin Microbiol*, 1(2):175–182, 1998.

[40] K. Sachs, O. Perez, D. Pe'er, D. A. Lauffenburger, and G. P. Nolan. Causal protein-signaling networks derived from multiparameter single-cell data. *Science*, 308(5721):523–529, 2005.

[41] H. M. Sauro and B. N. Kholodenko. Quantitative analysis of signaling networks. *Prog Biophys Mol Biol*, 86(1):5–43, 2004.

[42] M. A. Schwartz and H. D. Madhani. Principles of map kinase signaling specificity in *Saccharomyces cerevisiae*. *Annu Rev Genet*, 38:725–748, 2004.

[43] I. Shmulevich, E. R. Dougherty, S. Kim, and W. Zhang. Probabilistic boolean networks: A rule-based uncertainty model for gene regulatory networks. *Bioinformatics*, 18(2):261–274, 2002.

[44] S. Sibisi and J. Skilling. Prior distributions on measure space. *Journal of the Royal Statistical Society, B*, 59(1):217–235, 1997.

[45] R. Vadigepalli, P. Chakravarthula, D. E. Zak, J. S. Schwaber, and G. E. Gonye. Paint: A promoter analysis and interaction network generation tool for gene regulatory network identification. *Omics*, 7(3):235–252, 2003.

[46] B. Zhang, S. Kirov, and J. Snoddy. Webgestalt: An integrated system for exploring gene sets in various biological contexts. *Nucleic Acids Res*, 33(Web Server issue):W741–W748, 2005.

[47] J. Zhong, H. Zhang, C. A. Stanyon, G. Tromp, and Finley, R. L., Jr. A strategy for constructing large protein interaction maps using the yeast two-hybrid system: Regulated expression arrays and two-phase mating. *Genome Res*, 13(12):2691–2699, 2003.

20

Computational Methods for Learning Bayesian Networks from High-Throughput Biological Data

BRADLEY M. BROOM
University of Texas M.D. Anderson Cancer Center
DEVIKA SUBRAMANIAN
Rice University

Abstract

Data from high-throughput technologies, such as gene expression microarrays, promise to yield insight into the nature of the cellular processes that have been disrupted by disease, thus improving our understanding of the disease and hastening the discovery of effective new treatments. Most of the analysis thus far has focused on identifying differential measurements, which form the basis of biomarker discovery. However, merely listing differentially expressed genes or gene products is not sufficient to explain the molecular basis of disease. Consequently, there is increasing interest in extracting more information from available data in the form of biologically meaningful relationships between the quantities being measured. The holy grail of such techniques is the robust identification of causal models of disease from data.

The goal of this chapter is to survey computational learning methods that extract models of altered interactions that lead to and occur in the diseased state. Our focus is on methods that represent biological processes as Bayesian networks and that learn these networks from experimental measurements of cellular activity. Specifically, we will survey computational methods for learning Bayesian networks from high-throughput biological data.

20.1 Introduction

Many diseases, especially cancers, involve the disruption or deregulation of many cellular processes. It is hoped that high-throughput technologies, such as gene expression microarrays – which provide a snapshot of the level of gene transcription occurring in a cell, for many thousands of genes – will yield insight into the nature of the affected processes, improve our understanding of the disease, and hasten the discovery of effective new treatments.

385

However, merely identifying differential measurements is not enough. For instance, numerous studies [1, 2, 5, 8, 10, 16, 20, 23–26, 31, 32] have identified hundreds of genes that are differentially expressed between tumor cells corresponding to prostate cancer of different grades and normal prostate cells. Yet our detailed understanding of the genetic and/or regulatory events that lead to the initiation and progression of prostate cancer remains incomplete. There is increasing evidence that disease progression in complex diseases, especially solid tumors, does not arise from an individual molecule or gene, but from complex interactions between a cell's numerous constituents and its environment [3].

Consequently, in addition to making inferences about the differential expression of individual measurements, such as gene and protein expression levels, there is increasing interest in learning the underlying relationships between the quantities being measured. For example, we might hope to obtain a network of dependencies between the differentially expressed genes. Such a network can help distinguish root causes from downstream effects of a cellular process disruption. The goal of this chapter is to survey computational learning methods for elucidating from high-throughput experimental measurements, insights into the nature of the altered interactions that lead to and occur in the diseased state.

Biological interaction networks (often called pathways) can be represented at several levels of abstraction ranging from network models which emphasize the fundamental components (genes and metabolic products) and connections between them (the L1 models as defined in [17]), to detailed differential equation models of the kinetics of specific reactions (the L2 models) [17, 18]. The choice of abstraction level is generally a function of the biological problem being addressed and the type and quantity of data available. For instance, models based on differential equations have been used for detailed modeling of specific molecular interactions when time series data for the concentrations of the various molecular components involved is available. Boolean networks approximate gene expression values as binary variables that are either on or off, and represent gene interactions as Boolean functions. Approaches based on Bayesian networks [12] and their generalizations allow representations of multiple valued discrete values as well as continuous quantities. Bayesian networks have a solid formal foundation in probability theory and naturally support reasoning about incomplete and noisy data. They have been used in a wide variety of models generated from gene expression data including [4, 13, 15, 27–29].

The following section introduces Bayesian networks and their use in modeling biological processes. Section 20.3 describes challenges that arise in learning Bayesian networks from high-throughput data. Section 20.4 presents methods for addressing these challenges. A complete example of structure learning from expression data is presented in Section 20.5. Section 20.6 concludes the chapter with a summary of the state-of-the art as well as open questions in the area.

20.2 Bayesian Networks

Bayesian networks are a compact graphical representation of the joint probability distribution over a set of random variables, $X_1, \ldots, X_n$. A variable X_i can represent the mRNA expression level of a gene, or expression level of a protein, or the activity level of a signaling molecule. Typically, continuous expression levels are discretized into two or more categories, for example, on/off for signaling activity and high/medium/low for enzyme levels, by the selection of appropriate thresholds. A Bayesian network specification has two components:

(i) A directed acyclic graph $G = (V, E)$ with a node set V corresponding to the random variables $X_1, \ldots, X_n$, and edge set E on these nodes. The edges reflect conditional independence assumptions made. A node is conditionally independent of all other nodes given its parents in the network.
(ii) A set θ of conditional probability distributions for each node in the graph G. These probability distributions are local, and are of the form $P(X_i|\text{Parents}_G(X_i))$.

The two components (G, θ) specify a unique distribution on the random variables $X_1, \ldots, X_n$.

$$P(X_1, \ldots, X_n) = \prod_{i=1}^{n} P(X_i|\text{Parents}_G(X_i))$$

Thus, unlike purely qualitative network models, Bayesian networks contain quantitative information in the form of conditional probabilities of variables given their parents in the network.

As an example, consider the portion of the PI3K/PTEN/AKT signaling pathway implicated in androgen-independent prostatic adenocarcinoma [14]. PI3 kinase generates the potent phospholipid PIP3 in the absence of PTEN. PIP3 is absent in quiescent cells, but is significantly upregulated following stimulation by growth and survival factors. PIP3 recruits AKT (a proto-oncoprotein), which is activated by two kinases: PDK1 and PDK2. Once activated, AKT suppresses apoptosis by phosphorylating and inactivating the pro-apoptotic proteins caspase-9 and BAD. A Bayesian network representation of this pathway is shown in Figure 20.1. The edges in the network topology mirror the causal mechanisms in this pathway, and the conditional probability

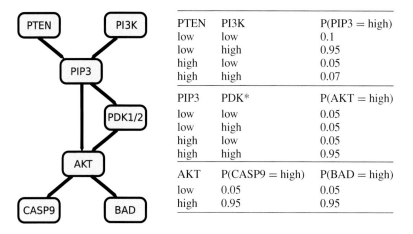

PTEN	PI3K	P(PIP3 = high)
low	low	0.1
low	high	0.95
high	low	0.05
high	high	0.07

PIP3	PDK*	P(AKT = high)
low	low	0.05
low	high	0.05
high	low	0.05
high	high	0.95

AKT	P(CASP9 = high)	P(BAD = high)
low	0.05	0.05
high	0.95	0.95

Fig. 20.1. The PI3K/PTEN/AKT signaling pathway represented as a Bayesian network.

distributions associated with the nodes reflect our understanding of how the individual components of the pathway work. The network topology makes a number of conditional independence assumptions explicit. For instance, the AKT levels are a function of its parents in the network: PIP3 and PDK12. The influence of other nodes on the levels of AKT is mediated through their effects on the levels of its parents. Thus,

$$P(AKT = high|PIP3, PDK12, PTEN, PI3K, CASP9, BAD) = P(AKT = high|PIP3, PDK12)$$

We say that AKT is conditionally independent of all other nodes in the network, given its parent nodes. The quantitative network parameters model the underlying processes. The first conditional probability table Pr (PIP3 = high|PTEN, PI3K) represents a stochastic process that turns on the levels of PIP3 when PTEN is underexpressed and there is plenty of PI3K available in the cell. The levels of caspase-9 and BAD respond directly to the level of AKT. AKT is activated by high levels of PIP3 and PDK12.

Bayesian networks are representations of the full joint distributions on their nodes. In our example network which has seven Boolean nodes, we would need $2^7 - 1 = 127$ parameters to fully specify the distribution. Our factored representation only requires 14 parameters. We can derive any probability of interest from this model. For example, using standard Bayesian network inference we can calculate that BAD levels are high when PTEN is suppressed and PIP3 levels are high, and low otherwise. Note that having elevated levels of PTEN is not sufficient to raise levels of BAD unless PIP3 is also present.

$$P(BAD = high|PTEN = low, PIP3 = high) = 0.824$$
$$P(BAD = high|PTEN = low, PIP3 = low) = 0.090$$
$$P(BAD = high|PTEN = high) = 0.138$$

We now turn to the problem of learning such networks from available data on cellular activity.

20.3 Learning Bayesian Networks

To learn a Bayesian network on variables $X_1, \ldots X_n$, we start with M measurements of these n variables in a data set

$$D = \{(X_1(1), \ldots X_n(1)), \ldots, (X_1(M), \ldots, X_n(M))\}$$

These measurements can be obtained from a variety of sources. One source is flow cytometry, where each measurement $(X_1(i), \ldots, X_n(i))$ is a set of n phosphorylated protein expression levels measured simultaneously in an individual cell. Flow cytometry easily yields thousands of data points ($M \approx$ 10,000). Using such data, Sachs et al. [27] automatically derived most of the traditionally described signaling relations among 11 ($n = 11$) signaling components in human immune system cells.

The data most commonly available at the current time are gene expression microarrays that simultaneously measure the level of mRNA transcription for tens of thousands of genes. For such data sets, $n \approx 12,500$, while the number of independent measurements M is very small; for example, $M = 100$ would be a fairly large study. This chapter concentrates on the issues raised by this kind of data, but many of the principles involved apply to other data types also.

The problem of learning Bayesian networks from data has been studied extensively over the past decade [13, 22]. Most approaches define a hypothesis space of potential network models and use the data to find ones that are most likely given the data. Learning a network model on a set $X_1, \ldots, X_n$ of variables entails inferring the graph of dependencies between them, as well as the parameters θ consisting of the local conditional probabilities: $P(X_i|Parents_G(X_i))$. If the graph structure G is known, the parameters θ can be estimated from the available data D by maximum likelihood estimation if M is large, or by Bayesian estimation, if M is small and priors on the parameter vector θ are available. The likelihood of the data D given parameter vector θ for a known structure G is

$$L(\theta; D) = P(D|\theta) = \prod_{i=1}^{M} P(X_1(i), \ldots, X_n(i))|\theta).$$

For maximum likelihood estimation, we estimate parameters θ^*_{ML} such that

$$\theta^*_{ML} = \text{argmax}_\theta L(\theta; D).$$

When the number of samples M is small, the above approach tends to overfit the model parameters to the available data. Bayesian methods reduce overfitting by representing and using available knowledge about the parameters in the form of a prior distribution $P(\theta)$. For example, if we had knowledge about how levels of AKT impacted the levels of caspase-9, then we can generate a prior distribution such as P(AKT = high|caspase_9 = high) = 0.8 and P(AKT = high|caspase_9 = low) = 0.2. The data D then serves to update the prior $P(\theta)$ to yield the posterior probability distribution $P(\theta|D)$. By Bayes rule,

$$P(\theta|D) = \frac{P(D|\theta)P(\theta)}{P(D)}.$$

Then, the estimated parameter θ^*_{MAP} is

$$\theta^*_{MAP} = \text{argmax}_\theta P(D|\theta)P(\theta).$$

Since $P(D)$ is independent of θ, it is treated as normalizing constant, and the scoring function is simply the product of the likelihood of the data given the parameter vector θ and the prior $P(\theta)$. When the prior distribution is a Dirichlet distribution, which is a conjugate prior, the posterior distribution $P(\theta|D)$ can be easily computed in closed form.

Learning the structure G of the Bayesian network from data is a very challenging problem. The most common approach to discovering the structure of Bayesian networks from data is to define a space of graph models to consider, and then set up a scoring function that evaluates how well a model explains the available data. Then, an optimization algorithm is used to search for the highest-scoring model. The scoring function is the logarithm of the posterior probability of the network structure given the data

$$\text{Score}(G; D) = \log P(G|D) = \log P(D|G) + \log P(G),$$

where $P(D|G) = \int_\theta P(D|G, \theta)P(\theta|G)\,d\theta$. We average over all parameters θ associated with a graph structure G.

Learning a Bayesian network that provably maximizes the above scoring function is NP-hard [6]. Thus, learning optimal Bayesian networks for high-throughput data sets is computationally infeasible.

20.4 Algorithms for Learning Bayesian Networks

There are three main challenges in designing learning algorithms for Bayesian networks. First, the number of potential networks in n variables is superexponential in n. The first challenge, therefore, is to choose an appropriate subset of variables to include in the model. The second challenge is to devise and use good approximation algorithms for guiding search toward biologically plausible solutions consistent with the data.

The second property that makes learning networks difficult is the very small number, M, of samples. Any error associated with each sample is significant, and could lead to erroneous network structures being learnt. Further, when the number of available samples is limited, the data is not sufficient to uniquely identify a structure. In fact, there may be an exponential number of networks with the same score with respect to the available data. Enumerating them is itself infeasible. Extracting common structural properties of a set of high scoring networks, which is a form of model averaging, is usually employed for learning the graph structure of a domain. The third challenge is therefore to devise and use robust methodologies to identify particular network structures.

Another consequence of the small number of samples is that nodes can reliably have at most two or three parents. There is simply insufficient data from which to reliably learn the conditional probability distribution of any nodes with more parents. The natural representations for many biological networks would contain many variables with more parents, so this is a severe limitation that raises challenging issues for determining the biological meaning and validity of the computed networks.

The remainder of this section will address in detail each of these challenges.

20.4.1 Node Selection

In ab initio construction of gene regulatory networks, a starter set of differentially expressed genes obtained from a preprocessing phase (such as by clustering or correlational analyses followed by thresholding on p values) is used [13, 15, 28]. A particular danger of the ab initio approach is that it may select several highly correlated variables. Because there are so few samples, this is inappropriate, since the learnt network will then more likely correspond to noise in the data than to a functional relationship between the genes involved. Nevertheless, while learning Bayesian networks we clearly expect some correlations, so how can we select an appropriate subset of genes from the thousands of potential candidates in a typical high-throughput experiment? One approach is to consider variables that occur on specific pathways of interest, as in [9].

Tools such as Cytoscape [30] and GenMAPP [7] make this selection easy to perform.

20.4.2 Computational Complexity

Since learning optimal Bayesian networks from data is NP-hard, most networks of practical interest are much too large for exact methods to be feasible. Thus considerable research is devoted to finding good approximations to optimal networks. Even so, many of these approximation methods are themselves computationally infeasible for problems involving several thousand genes.

20.4.2.1 Greedy Hill-Climbing Algorithm

A standard algorithm for finding an approximately optimal network is to start with a candidate network (such as the network with no edges), and consider a set of potential modifications, such as the addition, removal, or reversal of an edge between nodes (subject to the acyclic constraint). The scoring function, $P(G|D)$, is evaluated for every modified network. The highest-scoring modified network becomes the current candidate, and the process is repeated until no modified network scores higher than the current candidate. A well-known limitation of this algorithm is that it may become trapped in a local maximum, so it is usual to restart the hill-climbing process a number of times from random permutations of the best candidate, and to keep the network that scores highest overall.

The major computational cost of this algorithm is evaluating the scoring function for each potential candidate network. However, the overall score is composed of the scores for each node given its parents in the network. Many of these node configurations will be shared by many of the networks considered, so the computation can be made more efficient by caching the scores for these nodes. Even so, computing the score for each node, given its parents, for all combinations of parents considered by the algorithm is the major computational expense.

20.4.2.2 Sparse Candidate Algorithm

To reduce the computational expense of learning an approximately optimal Bayesian network containing a few hundred variables, Friedman et al. [13] introduced the *sparse candidate algorithm*, in which the potential parents of a node in the network are initially limited to the k nodes with which it is most highly correlated. Any such nodes that do not appear as parents in the learned network are replaced by the next most highly correlated nodes, and the entire process is repeated. If k is much less than the number n of nodes, the total search space is reduced and, more importantly, far fewer parent configurations must be evaluated for each variable (at most 2^k instead of 2^n). This approximation algorithm was used in [12] to reconstruct portions of the yeast cell cycle from expression data obtained at different points in the cell cycle. Each measurement was treated as an independent sample, and an additional node representing the cell cycle phase was introduced as a mandatory root node in the network. Using no prior biological knowledge or constraints, the method identified several important subnetworks of interactions.

20.4.3 Identifying Robust Network Features

Although gene expression microarrays measure the expression levels of many thousands of genes simultaneously, a typical study includes at most a few hundred different samples, which is far too few to reliably reconstruct a unique network model. In fact, it is not unusual for an exponential number of different networks on a given set of variables to have very similar high scores! To circumvent this fundamental limitation on the amount of data needed to learn network structures with high confidence, it is often more appropriate to learn the probabilities of specific network features, such as edges. Specifically, the probability of a network feature f given the data D is obtained by summing the probabilities of all graphs in which the feature occurs: $\sum_G P(G|D)f(G)$ where $f(G)$ is 1 if the feature is present in graph G, or 0 if not. Note that the resulting set of network features is not necessarily a Bayesian network; for instance, an edge between two commonly connected variables need not always, or even predominately, occur in the same direction.

A simple approach for estimating this probability is to learn a large number of approximately optimal, but different, networks from the data, and then count those network features (such as edges between variables) that are common to these high-scoring networks.

Friedman and Koller [11] describe an efficient Bayesian approach for estimating the probability of network features across all high-scoring networks. They introduce a total order between nodes: only nodes that occur before a node can be parents of that node. They show that the probability of a network feature due to all graph structures consistent with a specific fixed order of variables can be computed efficiently. The total probability of each network feature is then computed by using Markov chain Monte Carlo (MCMC) to integrate over all possible orders. MCMC over the space of orders instead of directly over the space of Bayesian networks converges to the stationary distribution of the Markov chain much faster, since the space of orders is much smaller and much less peaked than the space of Bayesian networks. Friedman and Koller showed that MCMC over orders converges at least 10 times faster than MCMC over Bayesian networks (some of which did not converge within the limits on the number of iterations). Koivisto and Sood [19] modify this approach by using an efficient exponential algorithm to sum over all possible orders, which is computationally feasible for networks of up to about 30 nodes.

A significant issue with both approaches is that the robust features identified are not necessarily biological in origin. As mentioned above, gene expression data typically contains many highly correlated genes. We "identified" significant gene interactions amongst a set of moderately correlated candidate genes by extracting those edges common to hundreds of high-scoring Bayesian networks learnt from the discretized gene expression data using the sparse candidate algorithm. However, when we modified the discretization method, the set of edges obtained changed drastically. Since many of the genes were reasonably correlated, we believe that many of the edges common to the high-scoring networks are merely artifacts of the discretization.

To overcome this problem it is not sufficient merely to require that the genes included in the network not occur in the same cluster, since typical clustering methods exclude all but the most highly correlated genes to reduce the number of false positives identified. Consequently, many of the excluded genes are still sufficiently correlated to cause problems. This is a significant issue for applying these methods to genetic pathways, since genes within the same (or even a closely related) pathway are expected to be highly correlated.

20.4.4 Incorporating Known Biological Information

A complementary approach for overcoming the problems created by the small number of samples is to incorporate known biological information into the network learning process, such as by incrementally adding additional genes into the network using existing knowledge about gene interactions. Segal et al. [29] have combined gene expression data and promoter sequence data to identify transcriptional modules in *Saccharomyces cerevisiae*. Bar-Joseph et al. [4] combined genome-wide location data with the gene expression data to obtain insights into regulatory networks for the same organism.

Another pathway-centric line of work is exemplified by that of Mamitsuka and Okuno [21]. They observe that current metabolic interaction maps imply many possible metabolic pathways, only some of which are biologically active. By synthesizing genetic pathways from the interactions described in these metabolic interaction maps and evaluating their likelihood using existing protein class information and gene expression microarray data, they were able to identify specific biologically active pathways.

Koivisto and Sood [19] describe an extension of their feature estimation algorithm that allows biological information to constrain the possible variable orders, thus making exact structure discovery feasible for larger networks.

Sachs et al. [27] incorporated interventional data into their network learning algorithm. By directly perturbing the phosphorylation states of measured molecules, they were able to infer more strongly whether one molecule was upstream, downstream, or neither of other molecules with which it was correlated.

20.4.5 Biological Relevance and Validation

It is tempting to think that Bayesian networks can naturally represent the modularity found in biological pathways, with the parent–child relationship implying causality. For instance, Sachs et al. [27] used the directionality of parent–child relationships to encode event cascades in signaling networks. A common misgiving is that feedback loops in pathways cannot be represented by acyclic Bayesian networks, but a temporal extension called dynamic Bayesian networks [33] enables the loop to be represented by unrolling it over time.

In practice, however, the interpretation of a network structure derived by computational methods is not trivial. The parent–child relationship in a derived network need not be causal. Even if causal, an edge between variables in a Bayesian network does not imply a direct biological mechanism. There may be a number of intermediate variables between the linked variables that have not been included in the network being modeled. Studies that recreate a known network, perhaps with some new interactions, from high-throughput data, are easily interpretable. It remains a challenge to understand the biological significance of a network learnt de novo from biological data, especially gene expression data for which the only realistic prospect is to learn network features.

20.5 Example: Learning Robust Features from Data

To illustrate the learning of robust network features from data, we will learn the likely links in a Bayesian network for a subset of the publicly available prostate cancer data obtained by Singh et al. [31]. This data set consists of 102 Affymetrix U95Av2 gene expression arrays from prostate samples (50 normals and 52 tumors). The Affymetrix CEL files were processed using Bioconductor to obtain numeric gene expression values for over 12,000 genes.

All gene expression values were individually discretized into three values (low, medium, and high) by determining the two cutoff points that would maximize a weighted average of the gene's self-information (I_s) and its mutual information (I_m) with the sample classification, specifically $0.425I_s + I_m$. The weight of 0.425 was chosen empirically because it appears to balance the tendency to create small discretization ranges that are probably overfitting the data, with the creation of ranges with a uniform number of members.

From this database of discretized genes, we selected probe sets indicative of 13 genes known to be associated with glutathione metabolism. Reduced glutathione (GSH) is an important cellular tripeptide that plays a vital role in the degradation of toxic cellular compounds. GSTM5, GSTP1, GGTL4, and GGTLA1 catalyze the conjugation of GSH with toxic cellular compounds and its subsequent decomposition. Reformation of GSH from its oxidized form involves GSR, GPX4, IDH1, and IDH2, while GSS, GCLC, and GCLM are responsible for the de novo synthesis of GSH from its three constituent peptides. The de novo synthesis rate is controlled by GCLC, whose expression is determined by transcription factors KEAP1 and NFE2L2.

We learnt 500 different high-scoring Bayesian networks from this discretized data using the sparse candidate algorithm with a limit of at most three parents per node. Duplicate networks were excluded by storing generated networks in a database, and excluding previously encountered networks from the search space. The scores of the high-scoring networks were recorded and checked to verify there was no trend.

The network shown in Figure 20.2 was obtained by recording an edge between nodes if there was an edge between those nodes – in either direction – in at least 60% of the high-scoring networks. The most frequently occurring edges occur in more than 99% of the networks and are thick black, and get progressively lighter with reduced frequency (90% black, 80% dark gray, 70% medium gray, 60% light gray). Edges between positively correlated nodes are terminated with a solid arrow if the edge occurs in the same direction at least 90% of the time, with an open arrow if the edge occurs in the same direction between 60 and 90% of the time, or nothing if neither direction is dominant. Edges between inversely correlated nodes are terminated with a solid box (at least 90% directionality), an open box (between 60 and 90%), or a bar (less than 60%). Edges between nodes without a simple linear correlation are terminated in a solid star (and all occur in the same direction at least 90% of the time).

Deriving a biological explanation of these links is challenging. However, by employing what is known about the biological interactions between these genes and their products, we can interpret the significance of the edges that occur in this network, and thereby gain an understanding of the types of biological inferences that could be made from networks of this kind.

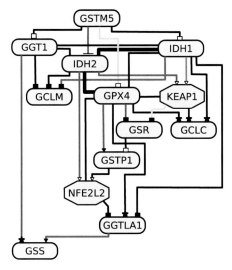

Fig. 20.2. Frequent edge network between 13 genes involved in glutathione synthesis, reclamation, and conjugation. Edges denote commonly occurring edges in 500 high-scoring Bayesian networks learnt from the data, with edge color corresponding to edge frequency, and edge termination denoting positive, negative, or nonmonotonic correlations, as detailed in the text.

From this network, it is apparent that the levels of IDH1, IDH2, and GPX4, which are all involved in the conversion of oxidized glutathione to GSH, are highly correlated. The absence of arrows on the edges between these nodes suggests that this data is insufficient to separate the nodes in this clique. Node GGT1 is also closely correlated with IDH1 and IDH2.

Interestingly, GSR, which catalyzes conversion of oxidized glutathione to GSH, is inversely correlated with GPX4 (and IDH1, IDH2). The two genes that mediate conjugation of GSH with toxins, GSTP1 and GSTM5, occur in different parts of this network, with GSTP1 correlated to GPX4 and GSTM5 inversely correlated with the whole clique of IDH1, IDH2, GPX4, and GGT1.

In the de novo synthesis of GSH, the final, but not rate limiting, step is catalyzed by GSS, whose expression depends most closely on that of GGT1 and GGTLA1, which both occur in the downstream degradation of GSH after its conjugation with toxins.

The rate-limiting step in the de novo synthesis of GSH is controlled by a dimer of the GCLC and GCLM proteins, with GCLC expression controlling the rate. GCLC is expressed when the NFE2L2 protein migrates from the cytoplasm to the nucleus, and this migration is triggered by KEAP1 expression. Thus, KEAP1 expression is the effective regulator of GCLC expression, and so it is reasonable that the figure shows KEAP1 and not NFE2L2 as a parent of GCLC. The edges from the parents of GCLC to GCLC terminate in a star because GCLC expression is highest for medium levels of each parent. High-levels of KEAP1 also correlate with reduced conversion of oxidized glutathione into GSH via GSR. Consequently, for the highest-levels of KEAP1 expression, the levels of GSH would be low since it is being neither synthesized nor reclaimed.

As exemplified by the relations between KEAP1, NFE2L2, and GCLC, the edges in this diagram do not (necessarily) represent direct biological interactions at the protein–protein, protein–DNA, or DNA–DNA levels, but represent a higher level of effective interactions. For instance, expression of GSS, a key gene in GSH synthesis, is highly correlated with its downstream degradation by GGT1 and GGTLA1, even though there is no direct biological interaction. Thus, interaction networks learnt via Bayesian networks show promise for modeling the effective high-level mechanisms that control the underlying molecular interaction pathways.

20.6 Conclusion

This chapter has surveyed computational learning methods for elucidating Bayesian network models, or at least robust features of such models, from high-throughput experimental measurements, such as gene expression data. The challenges imposed by the large number of variables but the small number of sample points were described, and a variety of computational strategies for addressing these challenges were outlined. To date, Bayesian networks have been successfully inferred for microarray data from yeast and for flow cytometry data from human immune system cells, but not for gene expression data from mammalian or oncological sources. Computational inference of Bayesian network structures from high-throughput data is difficult, but new computational methods are making it feasible to automatically deduce robust interactions between variables. The application of these methods to high-throughput biological data sets will help us to understand the nature of the altered biological interactions that lead to and occur in many diseases.

Bibliography

[1] C. ABATE-SHEN AND M. M. SHEN, Molecular genetics of prostate cancer, *Genes Dev.*, 14 (2000), 2410–2434.
[2] V. J. ASSIKIS, K. A. DO, S. WEN, X. WANG, J. H. CHO-VEGA, S. BRISBAY, R. LOPEZ, C. J. LOGOTHETIS, P. TRONCOSO, C. N. PAPANDREOU, AND T. J. MCDONNELL, Clinical and biomarker correlates of androgen-independent, locally

aggressive prostate cancer with limited metastatic potential, *Clin. Cancer Res.*, 10 (2004), 6770–6778.

[3] A.-L. BARABASI AND Z. N. OLTVAI, Network biology: Understanding the cell's functional organization, *Nat. Rev. Genet.*, 5 (2004), 101–112.

[4] Z. BAR-JOSEPH, G. K. GERBER, T. I. LEE, N. J. RINALDI, J. Y. YOO, F. ROBERT, D. B. GORDON, E. FRAENKEL, T. S. JAAKKOLA, R. A. YOUNG, AND D. K. GIFFORD, Computational discovery of gene modules and regulatory networks, *Nat. Biotechnol.*, 21 (2003), 1337–1342.

[5] J. H. CHO-VEGA, P. TRONCOSO, K.-A. DO, C. RAGO, X. WANG, S. TSAVACHIDIS, L. J. MEDEIROS, K. SPURGERS, C. LOGOTHETIS, AND T. J. MCDONNELL, Combined laser capture microdissection and serial analysis of gene expression from human tissue samples, *Mod. Pathol.*, 18 (2005), 577–584.

[6] G. COOPER AND E. HERSKOVITZ, A bayesian method for the induction of probabilistic networks from data, *Mach. Learn.*, 9 (1992), 309–347.

[7] K. D. DAHLQUIST, N. SALOMONIS, K. VRANIZAN, S. C. LAWLOR, AND B. R. CONKLIN, Genmapp, a new tool for viewing and analyzing microarray data on biological pathways, *Nat. Genet.*, 31 (2002), 19–20.

[8] S. M. DHANASEKARAN, D. G. R. R. BARRETTE, R. SHAH, S. VARAMBALLY, K. KURACHI, K. PIENTA, AND A. M. CHINNAIYAN, Delineation of prognostic biomarkers in prostate cancer, *Nature*, 412 (2001), 822–826.

[9] S. DRAGHICI, P. KHATRI, R. P. MARTINS, G. C. OSTERMEIER, AND S. A. KRAWETZ, Global functional profiling of gene expression, *Genomics*, 81 (2003), 98–104.

[10] L. E. EDER, J. BEKTIC, G. BAARTSCH, AND H. KLOCKER, Genes differentially expressed in prostate cancer, *BJU Int.*, 93 (2004), 1151–1155.

[11] N. FRIEDMAN AND D. KOLLER, Being Bayesian about network structure: A Bayesian approach to structure discovery in Bayesian networks, *Mach. Learn.*, 50 (2003), 95–126.

[12] N. FRIEDMAN, M. LINIAL, I. NACHMAN, AND D. PE'ER, Using Bayesian networks to analyze expression data, *J. Comput. Biol.*, 7 (2000), 601–620.

[13] N. FRIEDMAN, I. NACHMAN, AND D. PE'ER, Learning Bayesian network structure from massive datasets: The "sparse candidate" algorithm, in *Proc. Fifteenth Conference on Uncertainty in Artificial Intelligence (UAI '99)*, H. Dubios and K. Laskey, eds., Morgan Kaufmann, San Francisco, 1999, pp. 206–215.

[14] J. R. GRAFF, Emerging targets in the akt pathway for the treatment of androgen-independent prostatic adenocarcinoma, *Expert Opin. Ther. Targets*, 6 (2002), 103–113.

[15] A. HARTEMINK, D. K. GIFFORD, AND T. JAAKOLA, Using graphical models and genomic expression data to statistically validate models of genetic regulatory networks, in *Proceedings of the 6th Pacific Symposium on Biocomputing*, 2001, pp. 422–33.

[16] R. HENRIQUE AND C. JERONIMO, Molecular detection of prostate cancer: A role for GSTP1 hypermethylation, *Eur. Urol.*, 46 (2004), 660–669.

[17] T. IDEKER AND D. LAUFFENBERGER, Building with a scaffold: Emerging strategies for high to low-level cellular modeling, *Trends Biotechnol.*, 21 (2003).

[18] H. D. JONG, Modeling and simulation of genetic regulatory systems: A literature review, *J. Comput. Biol.*, 9 (2002), 67–103.

[19] M. KOIVISTO AND K. SOOD, Exact Bayesian structure discovery in Bayesian networks, *J. Mach. Learn. Res.*, 5 (2004), 549–573.

[20] P. K. MAJUMDER, P. G. FEBBO, R. BIKOFF, R. BERGER, Q. XUE, L. M. MCMAHON, J. MANOLA, J. BRUGAROLAS, T. J. MCDONNELL, T. R. GOLUB,

M. LODA, H. A. LANE, AND W. R. SELLERS, mtor inhibition reverses
Akt-dependent prostate intraepithelial neoplasia through regulation of apoptotic
and HIF-1-dependent pathways, *Nat. Med.*, 10 (2004), 594–601.

[21] H. MAMITSUKA AND Y. OKUNO, A hierarchical mixture of Markov models for
finding biologically active metabolic paths using gene expression and protein
classes, in *Proc. 2004 IEEE Computational Systems Bioinformatics Conference*,
IEEE, 2004, pp. 341–352.

[22] J. PEARL, *Probabilistic reasoning in intelligent systems*, Morgan Kauffman, San
Francisco, 1988.

[23] L. L. PISTERS, C. A. PETTAWAY, P. TRONCOSO, T. J. MCDONNELL, L. C.
STEPHENS, C. G. WOOD, K.-A. DO, S. M. BRISBAY, X. WANG, E. A. HOSSAN,
R. B. EVANS, C. SOTO, M. G. JACOBSON, K. PARKER, J. A. MERRITT, M. S.
STEINER, AND C. J. LOGOTHETIS, Evidence that transfer of functional p53 protein
results in increased apoptosis in prostate cancer, *Clin. Cancer Res.*, 10 (2004),
2587–2593.

[24] D. R. RHODES, T. R. BARRETTE, M. A. RUBIN, D. GHOSH, AND A. M.
CHINNAIYAN, Meta-analysis of miroarrays: Interstudy valication of gene
expression profiles reveals pathway dysregulation in prostate cancer, *Cancer
Res.*, 62 (2002), 4427–4433.

[25] C. J. ROSSER, M. TANAKA, L. L. PISTERS, N. TANAKA, L. B. LEVY, D. C.
HOOVER, H. B. GROSSMAN, T. J. MCDONNELL, D. A. KUBAN, AND R. E. MEYN,
Adenoviral-mediated pten transgene expression sensitizes bcl-2-expressing
prostate cancer cells to radiation, *Cancer Gene Ther.*, 11 (2004), 273–279.

[26] E. RUIJTER, C. VAN DE KAA, G. MILLER, D. RUITER, F. DEBRUYNE, AND J.
SCHALKEN, Molecular genetics and epidemiology of prostate carcinoma, *Endocr.
Rev.*, 20 (1999), pp. 22–45.

[27] K. SACHS, O. PEREZ, D. PE'ER, D. A. LAUFFENBURGER, AND G. P. NOLAN,
Causal protein-signaling networks derived from multiparameter single-cell data,
Science, 308 (2005), 523–529.

[28] E. SEGAL, N. FRIEDMAN, D. KOLLER, AND A. REGEV, A module map showing
conditional activity of expression modules in cancer, *Nat. Genet.*, 36 (2004),
1090–1098.

[29] E. SEGAL, R. YELENSKY, AND D. KOLLER, Genome-wide discovery of
transcriptional modules from DNA sequence and gene expression,
Bioinformatics, 19 (2003), i273–i282.

[30] P. SHANNON, A. MARKIEL, O. OZIER, N. S. BALIGA, J. T. WANG, D. RAMAGE,
N. AMIN, B. SCHWIKOWSKI, AND T. IDEKER, Cytoscape: A software environment
for integrated models of biomolecular interaction networks, *Genome Res.*, 13
(2003), 2498–2504.

[31] D. SINGH, P. G. FEBBO, K. RISS, D. G. JACKSON, J. MANOLA, C. LADD,
P. TAMAYO, A. A. RENSHAW, A. V. D'AMICO, J. P. RICHIE, E. S. LANDER,
M. LODA, P. W. KANTOFF, T. R. GOLUB, AND W. R. SELLERS, Gene expression
correlates of clinical prostate cancer behavior, *Cancer Cell*, 1 (2002), 203–209.

[32] K. B. SPURGERS, K. R. COOMBES, R. E. MEYN, D. L. GOLD, C. J. LOGOTHETIS,
T. J. JOHNSON, AND T. J. MCDONNELL, A comprehensive assessment of
p53-responsive genes following adenoviral-p53 gene transfer in bcl-2-expressing
prostate cancer cells, *Oncogene*, 23 (2004), 1712–1723.

[33] M. ZOU AND S. D. CONZEN, A new dynamic Bayesian network (dbn) approach
for identifying gene regulatory networks from time course microarray data,
Bioinformatics, 21 (2005), 71–79.

21

Bayesian Networks and Informative Priors: Transcriptional Regulatory Network Models

ALEXANDER J. HARTEMINK

Duke University

Abstract

We discuss the use of Bayesian networks as robust probabilistic models of the multivariate statistical dependencies among interacting variables in transcriptional regulatory networks. We explain how principled scores can be computed to compare network models with one another in terms of their ability to explain observed data simply. With principled scores, we can automatically learn static or dynamic network models that provide simple explanations for a variety of high-throughput data. We make a case for, and demonstrate the utility of, informative priors over network structures and parameters: informative priors can be used to incorporate different kinds of data into the learning process, and also to guide the learning process toward network models that exhibit greater biological plausibility. Results from both simulated and experimental data illustrate the benefits of this modeling framework.

21.1 Introduction

Proteins are the primary molecular workhorses of the cell, playing significant roles in metabolism, biosynthesis and degradation, transport, homeostasis, structure and scaffolding, motility, sensing, signaling and signal transduction, replication, and repair. However, one of the most intriguing roles for proteins is that of transcriptional regulation: control of precisely which genes are being transcribed into RNA at any given time. Since ribosomes subsequently translate most of this RNA into protein, proteins are in large part responsible for regulating their own existence. Although much has been learned about the large network of molecular interactions that regulate transcription, it would probably be fair to say that far more still remains to be learned.

Discovering and understanding the operation of large transcriptional regulatory networks is clearly an important problem in both molecular and synthetic biology. Progress has been accelerated by the advent of high-density DNA microarrays, which can be used to profile levels of RNA expression across the entire genome. When this expression data started becoming available after 1996, the first generation of methods for analyzing it were data-driven, initially unsupervised (e.g., clustering, correlation, and visualization) and later also supervised (e.g., classification). While these kinds of data-driven methods are useful in uncovering interesting patterns in the data, they typically provide little traction for explaining the biological mechanisms that give rise to these patterns. To overcome this limitation, model-driven methods for analyzing RNA expression data began to be developed.

The suggestion that probabilistic graphical models – and Bayesian networks in particular – might serve as an appropriate framework for representing transcriptional regulatory networks and learning models of their structure in the presence of noisy high-throughput RNA expression data was made independently in 1999 at least twice (and, in all likelihood, more than twice): by Murphy and Mian in an unpublished technical report [23], and by Hartemink and colleagues in an invited talk [11]. The first publications demonstrating the utility of this approach seem to be the independent work of Friedman et al. [8] and Hartemink et al. [14], shortly thereafter. These papers share a common theme beyond the choice of Bayesian network models: both realized that there was not enough available expression data to accurately learn large networks (a fact that has later been demonstrated repeatedly through simulation studies [18, 34]). Friedman and colleagues responded by focusing on network features that occur with high frequency in a bootstrap analysis, while Hartemink and colleagues restricted their attention to small sets of network models and investigated the utility of biologically relevant informative parameter priors.

However, RNA expression data is not the only high-throughput data available for providing insight into transcriptional regulatory networks: DNA sequence, protein-DNA binding, and protein–protein interaction data are also available. Protein-DNA binding can be assayed in vitro using a protein binding microarray (PBM) [22] or in vivo using chromatin immunoprecipitation followed by microarray (ChIP-chip; sometimes called transcription factor binding location analysis, or location analysis for short) [26]. Protein-protein interactions can be queried experimentally using techniques like yeast two-hybrid (Y2H) or affinity purification followed by mass spectrometry (AP-MS). Incorporating evidence from multiple kinds of data can often overcome the limitations of any one kind of data, because data collected using different technologies usually offer different perspectives on a problem; jointly analyzing such data in a single framework enables a consensus perspective to emerge. In addition, analysis of many kinds of data together is likely to produce more accurate results since noise characteristics and biases of the various technologies should be largely independent.

Many have recognized the value in jointly analyzing disparate kinds of biological data. Marcotte and colleagues made substantial early progress in refining our understanding of protein-protein interactions by integrating multiple kinds of data (see, e.g., [21]), while Ideker and colleagues used both RNA and protein expression data in predicting the effects of perturbations on regulatory networks [19]. Our work in 2001 [12] and early 2002 [15] introduced two new concepts: first, using various kinds of data to derive informative structure priors for guiding Bayesian inference, an idea later extended by Nariai et al. [24] to protein-protein interaction data; and second, combining RNA expression data with protein-DNA binding data, an idea which has been the basis of many later developments in the field (see, e.g., [2, 28] and [32] (this volume)).

After a brief introduction to Bayesian networks and Bayesian network inference (see also [4] (this volume), which provides a more lengthy introduction), we summarize our work on the use of informative priors for learning Bayesian models of transcriptional regulatory networks. We also present examples of the application of this approach to both simulated and actual experimental data.

21.2 Bayesian Networks and Bayesian Network Inference

Imagine a set of N random variables $X = \{X_i\}_{i=1}^{N}$ and consider how these variables may depend on one another. At one end of the spectrum, the variables may be completely independent; at the other end of the spectrum, they may be completely interdependent, which is to say that no two random variables are independent of one another, even conditioned on a subset of the other variables. *Bayesian networks* are a class of models for representing and reasoning about sets of random variables with conditional dependence relationships within this full range of possibilities – from complete independence to complete interdependence.

A Bayesian network (BN) is a graphical model: it uses a graph to represent information about the conditional independencies among random variables. In our context of modeling transcriptional regulatory networks, variables might represent RNA concentrations, protein concentrations, protein modifications or complexes, metabolites or other small molecules, experimental conditions, genotypic information, or conclusions such as diagnosis or prognosis. Variables can be discrete or continuous. To simplify exposition, we consider only discrete variables for the remainder of this chapter. Each variable is thus in one of a finite set of states, and the number of states used to model a variable represents a tradeoff between on the one hand, capturing a variable's behavior with sufficient precision, and on the other hand, retaining an ability to interpret what the states of the variable mean, as well as managing the computational and statistical complexity of learning models over variables with large numbers of states.

Each directed edge in the graph represents a conditional dependency between a pair of random variables; more precisely, the absence of a directed edge between two vertices represents a conditional independency between the corresponding pair of random variables. These conditional independencies are all summarized by the so-called *Markov property*: variables are conditionally independent of their nondescendants given their parents. The fewer edges a model has, the more constrained the model is. Thus, a graph over completely independent random variables is empty, while a graph over completely interdependent random variables is complete. In practice, we seek sparser (simpler) models because they are able to explain "indirect" dependencies through more "direct" dependencies mediated by other variables.

In characterizing the conditional dependencies among a set of random variables, not only does a BN provide a qualitative description in the form of a graph, but it also provides a quantitative description. Following from the Markov property, the joint probability distribution over the space of variables can be factored into a product over variables, where each term is a probability distribution for that variable conditioned on the set of its parent variables:

$$\Pr(X) \equiv \Pr(X_1, \ldots, X_N) = \prod_{i=1}^{N} \Pr(X_i \mid \mathbf{Pa}(X_i)). \tag{21.1}$$

We will denote by θ the parameters that collectively characterize the conditional probability distributions on the right-hand side of (21.1).

Because variables can have many parents, BNs are not limited to pairwise interactions between genes, but rather can describe arbitrary combinatorial control of transcriptional regulation; this is particularly straightforward when working with discrete variables. Also, due to their probabilistic nature, BNs are robust in the face of both noisy data and imperfectly specified transcriptional regulatory networks.

21.2.1 Dynamic Bayesian Networks

A dynamic Bayesian network (DBN) [9] extends the notion of a BN to model the stochastic evolution of a set of random variables over time; the structure of a DBN thus describes the qualitative nature of the dependencies that exist between variables in a temporal process. We use $X_i[t]$ to denote the random variable X_i at time t and the set $X[t]$ is defined analogously. Here, the evolution of the temporal process is assumed to occur over discrete time points indexed by the variable $t \in \{1, \ldots, T\}$, although continuous time DBNs also exist [25]. Under such an assumption, we have $T \times N$ interacting random variables where previously we had N. The resultant joint probability distribution is

$$\mathsf{Pr}(X[1], \ldots, X[T]) = \prod_{t=1}^{T} \left[\prod_{i=1}^{N} \mathsf{Pr}(X_i[t] \mid \mathbf{Pa}(X_i[t])) \right]. \qquad (21.2)$$

To simplify the situation, we make two further assumptions. First, we assume that each variable depends only on variables that temporally precede it. This fairly innocuous assumption still allows us to model natural cyclic phenomena like feedback loops, but guarantees that the underlying graph will be acyclic. It also greatly simplifies the computational complexity of learning. As one example, if we were to further restrict variables in our network to have at most k parents, we could find the globally optimal network in polynomial time: $O(N^{k+1})$. Second, we assume the process is a stationary first-order Markov process, which means that $\mathsf{Pr}(X[t] \mid X[t-1], \ldots, X[1], t) = \mathsf{Pr}(X[t] \mid X[t-1])$. Given these two assumptions, the variables in $\mathbf{Pa}(X_i[t])$ are a subset of $X[t-1]$. The underlying acyclic graph with $T \times N$ vertices can now be compactly represented by a (possibly cyclic) graph with N vertices, where an edge from X_i to X_j indicates that $X_j[t]$ depends on $X_i[t-1]$.

21.2.2 Scoring Models with the Bayesian Scoring Metric

To learn a network model from observed data, we want to maximize some scoring function that describes the ability of a network to explain the observed data simply. In the case of BNs, we can employ the Bayesian scoring metric (BSM). The scores produced by the BSM permit us to rank alternative models, and the score difference for any two models leads to a direct significance measure for determining how strongly one should be preferred over the other. According to the BSM, the score of a model is defined as the logarithm of the probability of the model being correct given the observed data. Formally,

$$\mathsf{BSM}(S) = \log \mathsf{Pr}(S \mid D) = \log \mathsf{Pr}(S) + \log \mathsf{Pr}(D \mid S) + c, \qquad (21.3)$$

where the first term in the last expression is the log prior distribution of the model structure S, the second term is the log (marginal) likelihood of the observed data D given S, and c is a constant that does not depend on S and can thus be safely ignored when comparing structures on the basis of their scores.

The marginal likelihood term can be expanded as

$$\mathsf{Pr}(D \mid S) = \int\limits_{\theta} \mathsf{Pr}(D, \theta \mid S) \, d\theta = \int\limits_{\theta} \mathsf{Pr}(D \mid \theta, S) \, \mathsf{Pr}(\theta \mid S) \, d\theta, \qquad (21.4)$$

and is analytically tractable when the data are complete and the variables in the network are discrete [16], as we assume here. Marginalizing in this way introduces an inherent penalty for model complexity, thereby balancing a model's ability to explain observed data with its ability to do so simply. Consequently, it guards against overfitting models to data when data are limited.

21.2.3 Learning Networks: Model Selection and Averaging

Finding the highest-scoring model under the BSM for a given set of data is known to be NP-complete in the general case [5] (although see the discussion of DBNs above). As a result, in the general case, we resort to heuristic search strategies to find good models. Commonly used strategies include greedy hill-climbing, greedy random, genetic algorithms, Metropolis, and simulated annealing. We have implemented each of these search strategies and have observed that in our own context, simulated annealing seems to find the highest-scoring models, although in many cases greedy methods identify the same models in much less time. The temperature schedule we employ allows for "reannealing" after the temperature becomes sufficiently low.

We need not select only a single maximum a posteriori model. A more principled Bayesian approach is to compute probabilities of features of interest by averaging over the posterior model distribution. Using model averaging in this way reduces the risk of overfitting the data by considering a multitude of models when computing probabilities of features of interest. For example, if we are interested in determining whether the data D support the inclusion of an edge from variable X_i to variable X_j, we compute

$$\mathsf{Pr}(\mathcal{E}_{ij} \mid D) = \sum_{S} \mathsf{Pr}(\mathcal{E}_{ij} \mid D, S) \cdot \mathsf{Pr}(S \mid D) = \sum_{S} 1_{ij}(S) \cdot e^{\mathsf{BSM}(S)},$$

where $\mathcal{E}_{ij}$ is a binary random variable representing the existence of an edge from X_i to X_j, and $1_{ij}(S)$ is an indicator function that is 1 if and only if S has an edge from X_i to X_j. However, this sum is difficult to compute because the number of structures S is enormous. Fortunately, it is possible to approximate this sum by sampling, or since the vast bulk of its mass lies among the highest-scoring models, to further approximate by restricting our attention to the highest-scoring models we encounter in our search. We then compute an appropriately normalized version of the last expression using only these models.

21.2.4 Prior Establishment

In a Bayesian setting, we need to establish prior distributions both over parameters θ and over network structures S. In a discrete BN satisfying reasonable assumptions, the prior over parameters must be a product-of-Dirichlet distribution [17]. If prior information about parameters is available, this can be captured in the form of an equivalent prior network [17]. Otherwise, an uninformative prior is frequently employed. In either case, an "equivalent sample size" needs to be specified, which is a measure of how confident we are in the prior relative to the quantity of data.

An especially common choice for the prior over structures is to assume that it is uniform; in this case, the corresponding term in (21.3) can be safely ignored since it is the same for all structures. In the rare instance where an informative prior is chosen, it is typically hand-constructed by domain experts [16]. Here, we summarize a novel approach for automatically constructing informative priors over network structures based on evidence provided by other kinds of data.

21.3 Adding Informative Structure Priors

To complement RNA expression data, we can extend our BN framework to include data describing the genome-wide DNA binding locations of protein transcription factors. If a transcription factor is reported to bind DNA upstream of a particular gene, it provides evidence that the factor is involved in the regulation of that gene. We can incorporate this evidence when scoring our BN models by modifying the prior distribution over structures. The Bayesian methodology has a natural provision for incorporating prior information into its scoring metric; in practice, determining appropriate weights for diverse sources of information poses a significant challenge.

We can incorporate an informative structure prior in two ways. First, we can adopt what we call a "hard" prior, which is uniform except that it gives zero probability to structures that do not satisfy constraints specifying which edges are required to be present and which are required to be absent. We can implement this prior by restricting our search algorithms to move only through the space of valid network structures. While this means we search in a smaller space, it is inconsistent with the notion that high-throughput data are generally quite noisy. Second, and alternatively, we can adopt what we call a "soft" prior, with varying but positive weights on all networks, down-weighting rather than excluding structures that do not satisfy the constraints. In such a setting, protein-DNA binding location data provides evidence as to whether a regulatory relationship exists, and the more significant the location data (lower the p value), the more likely the edge is to be included. As a consequence, this prior is subtler and more robust; nevertheless, it remains factorable in the context of a DBN, enabling computationally efficient local search. In fact, we can learn a DBN model using a soft informative structure prior in essentially the same amount of time as with an uninformative uniform prior. We describe this in more detail in the following sections.

21.3.1 Probability of an Edge Being Present

Transcription factor binding location data provides (noisy) evidence regarding the existence of regulatory relationships between a transcription factor and each of the genes in the genome. This evidence is reported as a p value, and the probability of an edge being present in the true regulatory network is inversely related to this p value: the smaller the p value, the more likely the edge is to exist in the true structure. In previously published work [3], we provide a detailed derivation of a function for mapping p values to corresponding probabilities of edges being present in structure S, but here we simply state the results. Let β denote $\Pr(\mathcal{E}_{ij})$, the prior probability that an edge exists from X_i to X_j, which we take to be constant for all i and j. Using Bayes' rule, we can show that the probability of $\mathcal{E}_{ij}$ after observing the corresponding p value is

$$\Pr_{\lambda}(\mathcal{E}_{ij} \mid \mathcal{P}_{ij} = p) = \frac{\lambda\, e^{-\lambda p} \beta}{\lambda\, e^{-\lambda p} \beta + (1 - e^{-\lambda})(1 - \beta)}, \qquad (21.5)$$

where λ is a parameter controlling the amount of confidence we place in the reported p values as accurate indicators of binding and nonbinding. Some insight into the role of λ can be gained by considering the value p^* obtained by solving the equation $\Pr_{\lambda}(\mathcal{E}_{ij} \mid \mathcal{P}_{ij} = p^*) = 1/2$, which yields

$$p^* = \frac{-1}{\lambda} \log \left[\frac{(1 - e^{-\lambda})(1 - \beta)}{\lambda \beta} \right]. \qquad (21.6)$$

For any fixed value of λ, an edge from X_i to X_j is more likely to be present than absent if the corresponding p value is below this critical value p^* (and vice versa). As we increase the value of λ, the value of p^* decreases and we become more stringent about how low a p value must be before we consider it as prior evidence for edge presence. Conversely, as λ decreases, p^* increases and we become less stringent; indeed, in the limit as $\lambda \to 0$, we have that $\Pr_{\lambda}(\mathcal{E}_{ij} \mid \mathcal{P}_{ij} = p) \to \beta$ independent of p, revealing that if we have no confidence in the location data, the probability of $\mathcal{E}_{ij}$ is the same value β both before and after seeing the corresponding p value, as expected. Thus, λ acts as a tunable parameter indicating the degree of confidence in the evidence provided by the location data; this allows us to model our belief about the noise level inherent in the location data and correspondingly, the amount of weight its evidence should be given.

One approach to suitably weighing the evidence of the location data would be to select a single value for λ, either through parameter estimation or by some heuristic like finding the value of λ that corresponds to a certain "magic" value for p^*, such as 0.001. Instead, we adopt a Bayesian approach that places a prior on λ and then marginalizes over it. The net effect of marginalization is an edge probability that is a smoother function of the reported p values than without marginalization.

21.3.2 Prior Probability of a Structure

The prior probability of a structure $\mathsf{Pr}(S)$ is proportional to the following product over the edges in S:

$$\prod_{\{ij:\ 1_{ij}(S)=1\}} \left[\frac{\mathsf{Pr}(\mathcal{E}_{ij} \mid \mathcal{P}_{ij} = p)}{1 - \mathsf{Pr}(\mathcal{E}_{ij} \mid \mathcal{P}_{ij} = p)} \right]. \tag{21.7}$$

The normalizing constant can be safely ignored since it is the same for all structures. Analogous to the likelihood calculations, the calculations required for updating the structure prior under a local change to S are computationally efficient because the structure prior factors over the edges in S, as shown in (21.7). In particular, we need not recompute the entire prior from scratch with each local change.

Note that in the absence of location data pertaining to a particular edge, we simply use the probability $\mathsf{Pr}(\mathcal{E}_{ij}) = \beta$ for that edge. Our informative prior is thus a natural generalization of traditional priors: in the absence of any location data whatsoever, the prior probability of a network structure is exponential in the number of edges in the graph, with edges favored if we choose $\beta > 0.5$ and edges penalized if we choose $\beta < 0.5$. In the special case where $\beta = 0.5$, the prior over structures is uniform.

21.4 Applications of Informative Structure Priors

In this section, we present two examples of how BN models and informative structure priors can be used to elucidate transcriptional regulatory networks in the yeast *Saccharomyces cerevisiae*. We examine networks responsible for controlling the expression of various genes that code for proteins involved in pheromone response and in cell cycle regulation. With respect to the former, the protein Ste12 is the ultimate target of the pheromone response signaling pathway and binds DNA as a transcriptional activator for a number of other genes. Transcription factor binding location data indicates which intergenic regions in the yeast genome are bound by Ste12, both in the presence and absence of pheromone [26]. With respect to the latter, a number of known cell cycle transcription factors have also been profiled by location analysis [20, 29].

To demonstrate the full range of methods discussed above, in the first example we use a model averaging approach with a hard informative structure prior to learn a static BN model, while in the second example we use a model selection approach with a soft informative structure prior to learn a dynamic BN model.

21.4.1 Pheromone Response: Static Network, Model Averaging

In the case of pheromone response, we used a set of 320 samples of unsynchronized *S. cerevisiae* populations of various wild-type and mutant strains grown under a variety of environmental conditions including exposure to different nutritive media as well as exposure to stresses like heat, oxidative species, excessive acidity, and excessive alkalinity. Genome-wide RNA expression data for each of these 320 observations were collected using four low-density 50 μm Affymetrix Ye6100 GeneChips per observation (roughly a quarter of the genome can be measured on each chip). The reported "average difference" values from these 1,280 Affymetrix GeneChips were normalized using maximum a posteriori normalization methods based on exogenous spiked controls [13].

From the 6,135 genes of the *S. cerevisiae* genome, 32 were selected either on the basis of their participation in the pheromone response signaling cascade or as being known to affect other aspects of mating response in yeast. The normalized levels of RNA expression for these 32 genes were log-transformed and discretized using discretization level coalescence methods that incrementally reduce the number of discretization levels for each gene while preserving as much total mutual information between genes as possible [12]. In this case, each gene was discretized to have four levels of discretization while preserving over 98% of the original total mutual information between pairs of genes [12]. In addition to the 32 variables representing levels of RNA expression, an additional variable named mating_type was considered. The variable mating_type represents the mating type of the various haploid strains of yeast used in the 320 observations and can take one of two values, corresponding to the MATa and MATα mating types of yeast, respectively.

21.4.1.1 Results Using Experimental Data

We used simulated annealing to visit high-scoring regions of the model posterior and present the results of two of those runs here. In the first run, we traversed the model space with a uniform structure prior. In the second run, we incorporated a hard informative structure prior using available location data by requiring edges from STE12 to FUS1, FUS3, AGA1, and FAR1 which had p values less than 0.001.

After gathering the 500 highest-scoring models that were visited during each run of the search algorithm, we computed the probability of edges being present using model averaging, as discussed above. Thus, the estimated probability of an edge can be exactly 1 if (and only if) the edge appears in all 500 highest-scoring models.

We then compiled a composite network for each run that consists of all edges with estimated posterior probability over 0.5. These networks are shown in Figure 21.1. Nodes have been augmented with color to indicate groups of variables known in the literature to have some commonality with one another. Edges have also been augmented with color: solid black edges have posterior probability of 1, solid blue edges have probability between 1 and 0.99, dashed blue edges have probability between 0.99 and 0.75, and dotted blue edges have probability between 0.75 and 0.5. The strength of an edge does not indicate how *significantly* a parent node contributes to the ability to explain the child node but rather an approximate measure of how *likely* a parent node is to contribute to the ability to explain the child node.

In both of the networks presented in Figure 21.1, we observe a number of interesting properties. In each case, the `mating_type` variable is at the root of the graph, and contributes to the ability to predict the state of a large number of variables, which is to be expected. The links are generally quite strong indicating that their presence was fairly consistent among the 500 highest-scoring models. Almost all the links between `mating_type` and genes known to be expressed only in MATa or MATα strains occur with posterior probability above 0.99. Moreover, in both networks there exists a directly connected subgraph consisting of genes expressed only in MATa cells (magenta) and a directly connected subgraph consisting of genes expressed only in MATα cells (red). In each case the subgraph has the `mating_type` variable as a direct ancestor with strong predictive power, as expected.

The heterotrimeric G-protein complex components GPA1, STE4, and STE18 (green) form a directly connected component with the informative prior but only GPA1 and STE18 are connected with the uniform prior. Indeed, even the link between GPA1 and STE4 with the informative prior is fairly weak. On the other hand, SWI1 and SNF2 (aqua) are weakly adjacent with a uniform

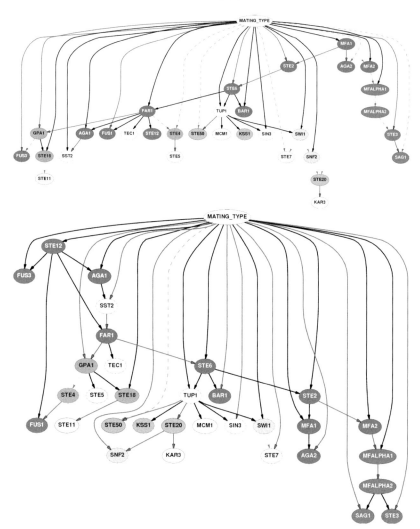

Fig. 21.1. Bayesian network models learned by model averaging over the 500 highest-scoring models visited during the simulated annealing search runs with a uniform prior and hard informative prior, respectively. Edges are included in the figure if and only if their posterior probability exceeds 0.5. Node and edge color descriptions are included in the text. (See color plate 21.1.)

prior, but not adjacent with an informative prior, though in both cases they are close descendants of TUP1. STE11 and STE5, two of the core elements of the primary signaling cascade complex (yellow), are seen as descendants of G-protein complex genes, indicating statistical dependence that may be the result of common or serial regulatory control. STE7 occurs elsewhere, however.

Auxiliary signaling cascade genes (orange) are always descendants of TUP1, sometimes directly and sometimes more indirectly, but STE50 and KSS1 are siblings in both cases. In general, the auxiliary cascade elements do not tend to cluster with the core elements, suggesting that the regulation of their transcript levels may occur by a different mechanism than those of the genes in the core signal transduction complex.

In both networks, TUP1 appears with a large number of children, consistent with its role as a general repressor of RNA polymerase II transcription. Both networks have MCM1 and SIN3 as children of TUP1; Tup1 and Mcm1 are known to interact in the cell [10] and this result that the level of Tup1 is helpful in predicting the level of Mcm1 suggests a possible regulatory relationship between the two. FAR1 is a parent of TEC1 and GPA1 in both networks. Far1, Tec1, and Gpa1 are all known to be cell-cycle-regulated and all three are classified as being transcribed during early G_1 phase [6]. This result suggests that Far1 may play a role in regulating the expression of Tec1 and Gpa1, providing a possible mechanism for their previously observed G_1 phase coexpression.

Though it is produced at higher levels in MATa cells, it is known that Aga1 is produced in both MATa and MATα cells [27]. The networks are each consistent with this knowledge, including a frequent predictive edge from `mating_type` to AGA1, but not clustering AGA1 with other mating type specific genes (magenta and red) as it is likely regulated differently. In both networks, AGA1 and SST2 are adjacent, consistent with the fact that the two are expressed very similarly, both peaking at the M/G_1 phase of the cell cycle [31].

21.4.2 Cell Cycle: Dynamic Network, Model Selection

Turning our attention now to the cell cycle, we earlier assumed that the stochastic dynamics of variables in a DBN arise from a stationary process. This poses a bit of a problem in the case of the cell cycle since we may have a different underlying transcriptional regulatory network during each phase of the cycle. To overcome this problem, we can employ an additional variable ϕ that can be used by the model to explain how each variable's regulators depend on the cell cycle phase, allowing us to model a different stationary process within each phase. The phase variable ϕ is multinomial and the number of states is simply the number of phases we choose to model as having distinct regulatory networks. If we can label each of the time points with the appropriate phase, the inference problem remains an instance of learning network structure from complete data. We prefer this option to the alternative of learning a hidden phase variable because in our context, the quantity of available cell cycle expression data is quite limited; besides, the state of ϕ changes smoothly and predictably, so labeling each time point with the appropriate phase is straightforward. A

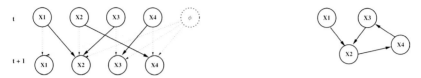

Fig. 21.2. Simplified schematic of a first-order Markov DBN model of the cell cycle. On the left, variables X_1 through X_4 are shown both at time t and $t + 1$; variable ϕ represents the cell cycle phase; dashed edges are stipulated to be present whereas solid edges are recovered by the learning algorithm. On the right, a compact representation of the same DBN model in which the cycle between X_4, X_3, and X_2 is apparent.

simplified schematic of such a DBN model of the cell cycle is depicted in Figure 21.2.

In the context of the cell cycle, we conducted tests with both simulated and actual experimental data. We used a synthetic cell cycle model to evaluate the accuracy of our algorithm and determine the relative utility of different quantities of available RNA expression data. The synthetic cell cycle model involves 100 genes and a completely different regulatory network operates in each of the three modeled phases of the cycle. The 100 genes include synthetic transcription factors, only some of which are involved in the cell cycle, and only some of which have simulated location data available. The target genes of the transcription factors are sometimes activated and sometimes repressed; some are under cell cycle control, but many are not. In addition, we include a number of additional genes whose expression is random and not regulated by genes in the model. The simulated expression data are generated using the (stochastic) Boolean Glass gene model [7]. The expression data are discretized into two states because the generating model is Boolean. Noisy p values for the simulated location data associated with a subset of the regulators are generated with noise models of varying intensity.

For experimental data, we use publicly available cell cycle RNA expression data [31] and transcription factor binding location data [20]. The expression data consist of 69 time points collected over eight cell cycles. Since these belong to different phases, the resultant number of time points in each phase is quite small. As a consequence, we choose to use only three states for the phase variable, by splitting the shortest phase G_2 in half and lumping the halves with the adjacent phases. Thus, the three states of our phase variable correspond roughly to G_1, $S + G_2$, and $G_2 + M$. We assign a phase label for each time point by examining the behavior of characteristic genes known to be regulated during specific phases [31]. This is done separately for each of the four synchronization protocols in the data set (alpha, cdc15, cdc28, and elu). We then select a set of 25 genes to model in our network, of which 10 are known transcription factors for which we have available location data. The only important cell cycle transcription factor missing from this set for which we have location data is FKH2; we are not able to use it in our analysis because RNA expression levels are missing for many of the time points. The remaining 15 genes in our set are selected on the basis of their known regulation by one or more of these 10 transcription factors. The experimental expression data are discretized into three states using interval discretization [12].

Because space is quite limited here, we provide only a brief description of the basic structure of each of our experiments. The discretized data in each case are used to compute the marginal likelihood component of the **BSM**. The soft informative prior component is computed using (21.7), where individual edge probabilities are computed from the location data p values using (21.5) with λ marginalized out. The parameter λ is marginalized uniformly in the interval $[\lambda_L, \lambda_H]$, with $\lambda_L = 1$ to avoid problems near zero ($\lambda_L = 1$ corresponds to $p^* = 0.459$) and $\lambda_H = 10{,}000$ to avoid problems near infinity ($\lambda_H = 10{,}000$ corresponds to $p^* = 0.001$). We set $\beta = 0.5$ so that edges for which we have no location data are equally likely to be present or absent in the graph; as a consequence, without location data, edge presence in the graph depends on expression data alone. The output of our DBN inference algorithm is the network structure with the highest **BSM** score among all those visited by the heuristic search during its execution.

21.4.2.1 Results Using Simulated Data

We repeatedly conduct the following three experiments: score network structures with expression data alone, ignoring the log prior component in (21.3); score network structures with location data alone, ignoring the log marginal likelihood component in (21.3); and score network structures with both expression and location data. We use these experiments to evaluate the effects of location data with different noise characteristics, expression data of varying quantity, and different choices for β.

Each of our experiments is conducted on five independently generated synthetic data sets and results are averaged over those five data sets. Figure 21.3 offers a representative result. The vertical axis measures the (average) total number of errors: the sum of false positives and false negatives in the learned network. As expected, the total number of errors drops sharply as the amount of available expression data increases. The figure demonstrates that our joint learning algorithm consistently reduces the total number of false positives and false negatives learned when compared to the error rate obtained using either expression or location data alone. Also, observe that the availability of location data means that we require typically only half as much expression data to

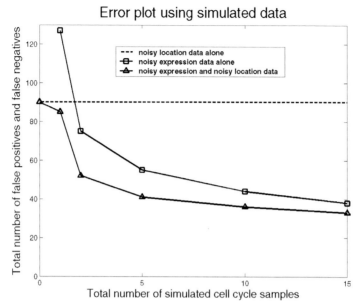

Fig. 21.3. Total number of errors while learning a synthetic cell cycle network using (noisy simulated) expression and location data, separately and with both types of data together. The graph shows the effect of increasing the number of cell cycles worth of expression data, both with and without location data. The dashed horizontal line represents learning using location data alone.

achieve the same error rate as would be achieved with expression data alone, suggesting that the availability of location data can be used to compensate for small quantities of expression data.

21.4.2.2 Results Using Experimental Data

We next apply our soft informative prior in learning networks describing the regulation of transcription during the cell cycle in yeast. As with the simulated data, we learn network structures using expression data alone, using location data alone, and jointly from both expression and location data. In the latter case, we compare our soft informative prior to our hard informative prior with a cutoff of $p = 0.001$ [15].

As an evaluation criterion (which is more difficult in this context than in the synthetic network context), we create a "gold standard" network consisting of the set of edges that are known to exist from one of the 10 transcription factors with both expression and location data to any one of the other genes in our set; we do not count edges from the other 15 genes when comparing with our gold standard since it would be difficult to determine whether recovered edges are

Table 21.1. *Comparison of the Highest-Scoring Networks Found in Four Different Experiments with the Gold Standard Network*

Experiment	TP	TN	FP	FN
Expression data only	7	181	20	32
Location data only	25	184	17	14
Expression and location data (hard prior)	23	187	19	11
Expression and location data (soft prior)	28	189	12	11

Note: As discussed in the text, the gold standard contains edges from only the 10 variables for which both location and expression data are available.

true or false positives, and whether omitted edges are true or false negatives. The gold standard comes from a compiled list of evidence in the literature and from the Saccharomyces Genome Database (http://www.yeastgenome.org), but we have tried to ensure that it depends on neither the specific expression data nor the specific location data used in these experiments. Note also that the gold standard is likely not the true underlying regulatory network, but rather is the best we can do given the current understanding of the yeast cell cycle (a "bronze standard"?).

With these caveats in place, Table 21.1 shows the total number of positives and negatives that are true and false for the networks found in the four experiments, with respect to the gold standard network. We see that the location data by itself does noticeably better than the expression data, suggesting that this particular set of location data are quite insightful or that this particular set of expression data are quite limited in quantity or quality. Despite the relatively poor performance of the expression data when considered in isolation, when we use our soft informative prior to include evidence from the location data along with the expression data, the number of false positives and the number of false negatives are both reduced; in contrast, the hard prior reduces the number of false negatives and increases the number of true negatives, but also increases the number of false positives and reduces the number of true positives. The soft prior uniformly outperforms the other three.

From Table 21.1, we see that combining expression and location data with our soft informative prior results in three fewer false negatives as compared to location data alone. These three are the regulation of SIC1 by ACE2 ($p = 0.010$), of ACE2 by FKH1 ($p = 0.006$), and of CLN2 by SWI4 ($p = 0.005$). These edges are detected because while the evidence of the location data in isolation is below threshold for inclusion, during the joint learning it is reinforced with evidence from expression data. In contrast, consider the regulation of transcription factor FKH1 by the transcription factor MBP1: although this interaction is recovered with expression data alone, it is not included when both location and expression data are used because the corresponding p value of 0.93 is so high that the quantity of expression data is insufficient to overcome the location data evidence against inclusion of the edge. Among the supposed false positives, we observe that both location and expression data provide evidence for the regulation of cyclin PCL2 by the transcription factor SWI6, although this interaction was not reported in the gold standard network. However, SWI6 participates in the SBF complex with SWI4, and SBF is currently believed to regulate the expression of PCL2 [1], reinforcing the notion that our gold standard network is not without flaws.

21.5 Adding Informative Parameter Priors

Thus far, we have discussed the utility of informative priors over structures, but informative priors over parameters are also useful. As with priors over structures, informative priors over parameters can be formulated as a hard prior where parameters that are inconsistent with a set of known constraints are eliminated in advance [14], or as a soft prior where different sets of parameters are relatively up- or down-weighted based on their degree of conformance to the constraints. In the case of a hard prior, the data are not forced to obey the constraints (after all, the data are noisy) but the parameters that characterize the distributions used to model the data are forced to obey these constraints.

What benefit will either of these choices have? The marginal likelihood component of a model's score can be viewed as the average probability of generating the observed data over all possible values of the parameter vector θ. From a sampling perspective, the contribution of the likelihood term to the score can be viewed as a two-level data generation process whereby a realization of θ is selected at random from its prior distribution, and then the probability of generating the observed data is calculated using this realization of θ. The probability of generating the data is averaged over repeated samplings to compute the marginal likelihood. This interpretation reveals that a model will score poorly if there is not a sufficiently large mass of realizations in the complete distribution of θ that are capable of generating the data with sufficiently high probability. On the other hand, if the model is constrained by a prior in the sense that the distribution of θ has more of its mass concentrated on realizations that are capable of generating the data with sufficiently high probability, then the constrained model will score better under the BSM. In short, if the constraint permits the model to avoid unnecessary complexity, then the model's score will increase.

In the case of a hard prior, we simply modify the scoring metric so that the marginal likelihood term is now the average probability of generating the observed data over all possible values of the parameter vector θ that satisfy the constraints [14]. In the case of a soft prior, we adjust the pseudocounts associated with the Dirichlet priors over parameters so that they are not all the same [33].

21.6 Discussion

BNs have certain limitations when used to model transcriptional regulatory networks. The most important of these is the caution with which models must be interpreted. While graphs are highly interpretable structures for representing statistical dependencies, they have the potential to be misleading if interpreted incorrectly. In particular, it is important to distinguish between statistical interaction and physical interaction.

For example, if the data strongly supports the inclusion of an edge between two variables X_i and X_j, that *may* indicate a physical interaction between these two factors in the cell. Alternatively, it is possible that an unmodeled variable Y actually intermediates between X_i and X_j or is a latent common cause of X_i and X_j such that X_i and X_j exhibit statistical dependence but no physical interaction. Caution must be used when interpreting models that may be missing critical explanatory variables. In contrast, if the data strongly supports the exclusion of an edge between two variables X_i and X_j, that *may* indicate no physical interaction between these two factors in the cell. Alternatively, we may not have observed the cell under an appropriate set of conditions where this interaction could have been observed. Incorporating additional complementary sources of data like transcription factor binding location can sometimes clarify the situation.

In general, multiple biological mechanisms may map to the same set of statistical dependencies and thus be hard to distinguish on the basis of statistical tests alone. Moreover, if sufficient data do not exist to observe a system in a number of different configurations, we may not be able to uncover certain dependencies. These two limitations are not specific to this methodology, however, but rather are true for scientific inquiry in general.

Similarly, although the interactions in our dynamic models can be oriented unambiguously (because time cannot flow backwards), that does not necessarily imply that the interactions are causal since we cannot account for cellular interactions that have not been measured, as mentioned above. One of the main hopes of this line of research is that more direct causal information from alternative assays like transcription factor binding location data and protein-protein interaction data will ameliorate this problem when we can include them in the analysis framework in a principled way.

From a computational perspective, BN structure inference should scale fine to networks of hundreds of interacting variables, as we have demonstrated here and elsewhere [30]. The primary factor in its ability to scale is not so much computational as statistical, and not so much with respect to the number of variables but with respect to the number of parents for each variable. As this number increases, larger and larger quantities of data are needed to learn an accurate model [35]. On a related note, while nothing precludes us computationally from modeling a higher-order Markov process in our DBNs, we are often constrained statistically by the limited quantity of available time-series expression data.

Successful elucidation of transcriptional regulatory networks will not likely be a batch learning process. Rather, we will need to increasingly consider learning that is incremental and algorithms that are online. In particular, gathering data sampled even sparsely from the joint probability space over all relevant variables in cellular regulatory networks would require an inordinate amount of data. To overcome this, it will be important to carefully design experiments to learn information about the specific portions of these networks that remain ambiguous. Being able to suggest the next series of experiments to conduct is especially valuable when learning from high-throughput data because the data are often costly to gather. Knowing in advance which are likely to be the most informative experiments to conduct for elucidating biological mechanisms of interest would be quite useful.

This field is known as "active learning" and an existing literature can be applied and extended in this domain. Of special interest is the ability to suggest experiments for collecting not only observational data but also interventional data. In the context of transcriptional regulatory networks, this can be implemented by deleting a gene so that it cannot be expressed, or by constitutively overexpressing a gene from a heterologous promoter. Interventional data needs to be treated differently from observational data in the context of learning, but the framework easily extends to handle interventional data.

Finally, we should offer one last note on the viability of BNs as models of transcriptional regulatory networks in higher eukaryotes. From a biological perspective, regulation in multicellular organisms is quite a bit more complicated owing to extra spatial and temporal complexity, for example in the form of intercellular signaling and differentiation of cell types. From an experimental perspective, collecting data is often more challenging in this context as well because multiple cell types need to be profiled and because there are often technical, financial, or ethical limitations to data collection. However, provided that the models are flexible enough to capture the complexity of these organisms and provided that sufficient data can be collected, there does not seem to be any fundamental limitation of BNs as useful models for representing and elucidating transcriptional regulation in higher eukaryotes.

21.7 Availability of Papers and Banjo Software

This chapter summarizes a large body of work from our research group over the past six years. As such, it borrows heavily from papers written during this period, but offers a broader and more unified perspective on the research program as a whole. We have in some places omitted details that have been published previously; readers interested in greater detail are encouraged to read the original papers.

In addition to the work on BNs as models of transcriptional regulation summarized in this chapter, our group has undertaken research along a number of other directions related to the various topics treated elsewhere in this book. These include analysis of microarray data, analysis of proteomic spectra, modeling of the eukaryotic cell cycle, motif identification, integration of diverse kinds of data, and disease diagnosis and other classification tasks in high-dimensional systems biology. Bayesian statistical formulations and informative priors arise as common themes in all this work. Papers from our group are available from http://www.cs.duke.edu/~amink.

Finally, we have recently developed a software package called Banjo – Bayesian network inference with Java objects – to perform network inference in static and dynamic Bayesian networks of discrete variables. Banjo is designed to be efficient, modular, and extensible. The program and complete source code are available under a noncommercial use license, and commercial licensing opportunities are available as well. For more information, visit http://www. cs.duke.edu/~amink/software/banjo.

21.8 Acknowledgments

I am grateful to my Ph.D. advisors, David Gifford, Tommi Jaakkola, and Rick Young at MIT, for starting me on this path and for continuing to offer advice and shape my thinking. At Duke, Allister Bernard helped me formulate the soft prior over network structures, while Erich Jarvis, V. Anne Smith, and Jing Yu helped develop a simulation framework, which I have not had room to discuss here, that enabled us to improve structure inference algorithms in biological contexts with little data [35]. Jing also helped me formulate the soft monotonicity prior over BN parameters. Jürgen Sladeczek did most of the work in producing our Banjo software package. Finally, I am very thankful for the ideas of many others on this topic, shared either in person or through their writing, including but not limited to David Heckerman, Nir Friedman, Daphne Koller, Greg Cooper, Peter Spirtes, Chris Meek, Max Chickering, Harald Steck, Trey Ideker, Eran Segal, and Satoru Miyano. Finally, I want to thank the editors for inviting this contribution and being patient while I crafted it, especially Marina Vannucci with whom I most frequently interacted.

Bibliography

[1] K. Baetz, J. Moffat, J. Haynes, M. Chang, and B. Andrews. Transcriptional coregulation by the cell integrity MAP kinase Slt2 and the cell cycle regulator Swi4. *Mol. Cell. Biol.*, 21:6515–6528, 2001.

[2] Z. Bar-Joseph, G. Gerber, T. Lee, N. Rinaldi, J. Yoo, F. Robert, B. Gordon, E. Fraenkel, T. S. Jaakkola, R. A. Young, and D. K. Gifford. Computational discovery of gene modules and regulatory networks. *Nat. Biotechnol.*, 21:1337–1341, 2003.

[3] A. Bernard and A. J. Hartemink. Informative structure priors: Joint learning of dynamic regulatory networks from multiple types of data. In *Pac. Symp. Biocomp.*, Vol. 10, pp. 459–470, Jan. 2005.

[4] B. M. Broom and D. Subramanian. Computational methods for learning Bayesian networks from high-throughput biological data. In K.-A. Do, P. Müller, and M. Vannucci, editors, *Bayesian Inference for Gene Expression and Proteomics*, Chapter 20, pp. 385–400. Cambridge University Press, New York, 2006.

[5] D. M. Chickering. Learning Bayesian networks is NP-complete. In D. Fisher and H.-J. Lenz, editors, *Learning from Data: AI and Statistics V*, Chapter 12, pp. 121–130. Springer-Verlag, New York, 1996.

[6] R. J. Cho, M. J. Campbell, E. A. Winzeler, L. Steinmetz, A. Conway, L. Wodicka, T. G. Wolfsberg, A. E. Gabrielian, D. Landsman, D. J. Lockhart, and R. W. Davis. A genome-wide transcriptional analysis of the mitotic cell cycle. *Mol. Cell*, 2:65–73, July 1998.

[7] R. Edwards and L. Glass. Combinatorial explosion in model gene networks. *Chaos*, 10:691–704, Sept. 2000.

[8] N. Friedman, M. Linial, I. Nachman, and D. Pe'er. Using Bayesian networks to analyze expression data. In *RECOMB*, Vol. 4, Apr. 2000.

[9] N. Friedman, K. Murphy, and S. Russell. Learning the structure of dynamic probabilistic networks. In *Proc. Fourteenth UAI*, pp. 139–147. Morgan Kaufmann, San Francisco, 1998.

[10] I. M. Gavin, M. P. Kladde, and R. T. Simpson. Tup1p represses Mcm1p transcriptional activation and chromatin remodeling of an a-cell-specific gene. *Embo J.*, 19:5875–5883, 2000.

[11] A. J. Hartemink. Using HDA data to statistically validate models of genetic regulatory networks in *S. cerevisiae*. EBI conference entitled *Datamining for Bioinformatics: Towards In Silico Biology*, Nov. 1999.

[12] A. J. Hartemink. Principled Computational Methods for the Validation and Discovery of Genetic Regulatory Networks. PhD thesis, Massachussets Institute of Technology, 2001.

[13] A. J. Hartemink, D. K. Gifford, T. S. Jaakkola, and R. A. Young. Maximum likelihood estimation of optimal scaling factors for expression array normalization. In *International Symposium on Biomedical Optics (BiOS 2001)*, pp. 132–140. SPIE, Bellingham, WA, Jan. 2001.

[14] A. J. Hartemink, D. K. Gifford, T. S. Jaakkola, and R. A. Young. Using graphical models and genomic expression data to statistically validate models of genetic regulatory networks. In *Pac. Symp. Biocomp.*, Vol. 6, pp. 422–433, Jan. 2001.

[15] A. J. Hartemink, D. K. Gifford, T. S. Jaakkola, and R. A. Young. Combining location and expression data for principled discovery of genetic regulatory network models. In *Pac. Symp. Biocomp.*, Vol. 7, pp. 437–449, Jan. 2002.

[16] D. Heckerman. A tutorial on learning with Bayesian networks. In M. I. Jordan, editor, *Learning in Graphical Models*, pp. 301–354. Kluwer Academic Publishers, 1998.

[17] D. Heckerman, D. Geiger, and D. M. Chickering. Learning Bayesian networks: The combination of knowledge and statistical data. *Mach. Learn.*, 20:197–243, 1995.

[18] D. Husmeier. Sensitivity and specificity of inferring genetic regulatory interactions from microarray experiments with dynamic Bayesian networks. *Bioinformatics*, 19:2271–2282, 2003.

[19] T. Ideker, V. Thorsson, J. A. Ranish, R. Christmas, J. Buhler, J. K. Eng, R. Bumgarner, D. R. Goodlett, R. Aebersold, and L. Hood. Integrated genomic and proteomic analyses of a systematically perturbed metabolic network. *Science*, 292:929–934, 2001.

[20] T. I. Lee, N. J. Rinaldi, F. Robert, D. T. Odom, Z. Bar-Joseph, G. K. Gerber, N. M. Hannett, C. T. Harbison, C. M. Thompson, I. Simon, J. Zeitlinger, E. G. Jennings, H. L. Murray, D. B. Gordon, B. Ren, J. J. Wyrick, J. B. Tagne, T. L. Volkert, E. Fraenkel, D. K. Gifford, and R. A. Young. Transcriptional regulatory networks in *Saccharomyces cerevisiae. Science*, 298:799–804, 2002.

[21] E. M. Marcotte, M. Pellegrini, M. J. Thompson, T. Yeates, and D. Eisenberg. A combined algorithm for genome-wide prediction of protein function. *Nature*, 402:83–86, 1999.

[22] S. Mukherjee, M. F. Berger, G. Jona, X. S. Wang, D. Muzzey, M. Snyder, R. A. Young, and M. L. Bulyk. Rapid analysis of the DNA binding specificities of transcription factors with DNA microarrays. *Nat. Genet.*, 36:1331–1339, Dec. 2004.

[23] K. Murphy and S. Mian. Modelling gene expression data using dynamic Bayesian networks. Technical Report, University of California at Berkeley, 1999.

[24] N. Nariai, S. Kim, S. Imoto, and S. Miyano. Using protein-protein interactions for refining gene networks estimated from microarray data by Bayesian networks. In *Pac. Symp. Biocomp.*, Vol. 9, pp. 384–395, Jan. 2004.

[25] U. Nodelman, C. R. Shelton, and D. Koller. Learning continuous time Bayesian networks. In *Proc. Nineteenth UAI*, pp. 451–458, 2003.

[26] B. Ren, F. Robert, J. J. Wyrick, O. Aparicio, E. G. Jennings, I. Simon, J. Zeitlinger, J. Schreiber, N. Hannett, E. Kanin, T. L. Volkert, C. J. Wilson, S. P. Bell, and R. A. Young. Genome-wide location and function of DNA-binding proteins. *Science*, 290:2306–2309, Dec. 2000.

[27] A. Roy, C. Lu, D. Marykwas, P. Lipke, and J. Kurjan. The AGA1 product is involved in cell surface attachment of the *Saccharomyces cerevisiae* cell adhesion glycoprotein a-agglutinin. *Mol. Cell. Biol.*, 11:4196–4206, 1991.

[28] E. Segal, R. Yelensky, and D. Koller. Genome-wide discovery of transcriptional modules from DNA sequence and gene expression. *Bioinformatics*, 19:i273–i282, 2003.

[29] I. Simon, J. Barnett, N. Hannett, C. T. Harbison, N. J. Rinaldi, T. L. Volkert, J. J. Wyrick, J. Zeitlinger, D. K. Gifford, T. S. Jaakkola, and R. A. Young. Serial regulation of transcriptional regulators in the yeast cell cycle. *Cell*, 106:697–708, 2001.

[30] V. A. Smith, E. D. Jarvis, and A. J. Hartemink. Evaluating functional network inference using simulations of complex biological systems. *Bioinformatics*, 18(S1):S216–S224, 2002.

[31] P. T. Spellman, G. Sherlock, M. Q. Zhang, V. R. Iyer, K. Anders, M. B. Eisen, P. O. Brown, D. Botstein, and B. Futcher. Comprehensive identification of cell cycle-regulated genes of the yeast *Saccharomyces cerevisiae* by microarray hybridization. *Mol. Biol. Cell*, 9:3273–3297, 1998.

[32] N. Sun and H. Zhao. A misclassification model for inferring transcriptional regulatory networks. In K.-A. Do, P. Müller, and M. Vannucci, editors, *Bayesian Inference for Gene Expression and Proteomics*, Chapter 18, pp. 347–365. Cambridge University Press, New York, 2006.

[33] J. Yu. Developing Bayesian Network Inference Algorithms to Predict Causal Functional Pathways in Biological Systems. PhD thesis, Duke University, May 2005.

[34] J. Yu, A. Smith, P. Wang, A. Hartemink, and E. Jarvis. Using Bayesian network inference algorithms to recover molecular genetic regulatory networks. In *Proc. International Conference on Systems Biology*, Dec. 2002.

[35] J. Yu, A. Smith, P. Wang, A. Hartemink, and E. Jarvis. Advances to Bayesian network inference for generating causal networks from observational biological data. *Bioinformatics*, 20:3594–3603, 2004.

22

Sample Size Choice for Microarray Experiments

PETER MÜLLER

The University of Texas M.D. Anderson Cancer Center

CHRISTIAN ROBERT AND JUDITH ROUSSEAU

CREST, Paris

Abstract

We review Bayesian sample size arguments for microarray experiments, focusing on a decision theoretic approach. We start by introducing a choice based on minimizing expected loss as theoretical ideal. Practical limitations of this approach quickly lead us to consider a compromise solution that combines this idealized solution with a sensitivity argument. The finally proposed approach relies on conditional expected loss, conditional on an assumed true level of differential expression to be discovered. The expression for expected loss can be interpreted as a version of power, thus providing for ease of interpretation and communication

22.1 Introduction

We discuss approaches for a Bayesian sample size argument in microarray experiments. As is the case for most sample size calculations in clinical trials and other biomedical applications the nature of the sample size calculation is to provide the investigator with decision support, and allow an informed sample size choice, rather than providing a black-box method to deliver an optimal sample size.

Several classical approaches for microarray sample size choices have been proposed in the recent literature. Pan et al. (2002) develop a traditional power argument, using a finite mixture of normal sampling model for difference scores in a group comparison microarray experiment. Zien et al. (2002) propose to plot ROC-type curves to show achievable combinations of false-negative and false-positive rates. Mukherjee et al. (2003) use a machine learning perspective. They consider a parametric learning curve for the empirical error rate as a function of the sample size, and proceed to estimate the unknown parameters in the learning curve. Lee and Whitmore (2002) set up an ANOVA model, and reduce the sample size choice to a traditional power analysis in the ANOVA model. Bickel (2003) proposes an approach based on a formal loss function with terms corresponding to a payoff for correct discoveries and a penalty for false discoveries. The loss function is equivalent to the loss L introduced below.

An interesting sequential approach is developed in Fu et al. (2005). After each microarray, or batch of arrays, they compute the posterior predictive probability of misclassification for the next sample. Sampling continues until this probability achieves some prespecified threshold.

In Müller et al. (2004) we develop a Bayesian decision theoretic approach to sample size selection for group comparison microarray experiments. We assume that each array reports expression for n genes. Also, we assume that the sample size choice is about multiple arrays with independent biologic samples recorded on each array (excluding, among others, technical repeats based on the same biologic sample).

Main features of the proposed approach. Before introducing the formal setup and approach we provide a brief summary of the results discussed in more detail later. This will help to motivate and focus the following formal discussion. Let J denote the sample size, that is, the number of microarrays that we recommend to be carried out. In a decision theoretic approach, we define a criterion for the sample size recommendation by stating how much a specific sample size would be worth for a hypothetical outcome y of the experiment, and an assumed hypothetical truth, that is, true values of all relevant parameters θ. This function of decision, data, and parameters is known as the utility function. Alternatively, flipping signs we get the loss function. Of course, at the time of the sample size selection the future data y is not known, and the parameters θ will never be known. One can argue (DeGroot, 1970; Robert, 2001) that a rational decision maker should then choose a sample size based on expected loss, taking the expectation with respect to the relevant probability distribution on parameters and future data. The relevant distribution is the posterior predictive distribution conditional on any data available at the time of making the decision. In the absence of any data this is the prior predictive distribution. Some complications arise when the nature of the decision is sequential. See below.

Figure 22.1 shows expected loss for a microarray sample size selection. The loss function is $L(J, y, \theta) = \text{FD} + c\text{FN} - k \cdot J$, where FD denotes the number of false positives (truly not differentially expressed genes that are flagged), and FN the number of false negatives (truly differentially expressed genes that are not discovered). See Section 22.2.1 for a formal definition of FD and FN. The function includes two tradeoff parameters, c and k. See the following sections for more details about the choice of the loss function, the nature of the expectation, including complications that arise from a sequential

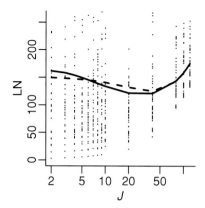

Fig. 22.1. Expected loss as a function of sample size J for a two-group comparison microarray experiment. Evaluating the expectation involves a large scale Monte Carlo simulation. See the text for details. The dots show realized losses for simulated experiments. The solid line plots an estimate of expected loss based on a parametric fit of the dots. The dashed line shows the same using a spline fit. Sample size J is plotted on a logarithmic scale. Note the relatively flat nature of the expected loss, rendering a sample size recommendation difficult.

decision setup, details of the probability model, and the Monte Carlo simulation used to evaluate expected loss. The relatively flat nature of the expected loss hinders a decisive sample size recommendation based on expected loss alone. To be of practical use, the minimum is too sensitive to technical, arbitrary choices of details in the loss function and probability model. We will therefore proceed with a closer look at important features of the expected loss function. In particular, we will consider expected loss conditional on an assumed true level of differential expression for one gene, marginalizing with respect to future data and all other parameters as before. This adds an additional dimension to the plot in Figure 22.1. Let ρ_i denote the assumed true level of differential expression for gene i. We assume that ρ_i is defined such that $\rho_i = 0$ is interpreted as nondifferential expression, and $\rho_i > 0$ as differential expression. We consider expected loss as a function of J and ρ_i. Focusing on only the change in expected utility across J and ρ_i, and dropping the deterministic sampling cost $k \cdot J$, we argue that the plot can be interpreted as a variation of power. Details are discussed in the next section. See Figure 22.2 for an example.

The rest of this chapter is organized as follows. In Section 22.2 we cast sample size choice as a decision problem. In Section 22.2.1 we argue that sample size choice should be considered as a sequential decision problem. Solving the sequential decision problem we start in Section 22.2.2 with the terminal decision of selecting a list of differentially expressed genes, and proceed in Section 22.2.3 to address the sample size problem. In Section 22.3 we develop a Monte Carlo scheme to evaluate expected losses. In Section 22.4 we introduce a specific probability model. Section 22.5 discusses the use of pilot data. Finally, Section 22.6 demonstrates the proposed approach in an example.

22.2 Optimal Sample Size as a Decision Problem

A decision problem is specified by a set of possible actions $d \in D$; a set of relevant unknown quantities, typically parameters θ and data y; a probability model $p_d(\theta, y)$; and a loss function $L(d, y, \theta)$ that formalizes the relative preferences over decisions for assumed hypothetical values of y and θ. The probability model for data and parameters can depend on the decision d. See, for example, Berger (1993) for a general description. In the application to microarray sample size choice the decision d includes the sample size J, the data y are the gene expressions that will be recorded in the J microarray experiments, and θ typically includes indicators for true differential expression for each of the n genes under the biologic conditions of interest.

The optimal decision is the action d^* that minimizes the loss in expectation, $d^* = \arg\min E\{L(d, \theta, y)\}$. The expectation is with respect to the relevant probability model. In so-called nonsequential problems, the relevant probability model is $p_d(\theta, y)$. In general, the calculation of expected utility might involve more steps. As we will argue, this is the case for the sample size problem.

22.2.1 The Decision Problem

Approaching sample size choice as a decision problem it is important to recognize the sequential nature of the decision. In words, optimal sample size is always defined in the context of the intended inference or decision that will be carried out eventually, once all data is collected (terminal decision). Different inference goals might lead to different sample size recommendations. We therefore need to consider the entire sequence of (i) the sample size decision, (ii) the observation of gene expressions for the chosen number of arrays, and (iii) the terminal decision about differentially expressed genes. Let J denote the sample size choice, let n denote the number of genes that are recorded on each of the J arrays, let $y^J = (y_1, \ldots, y_J)$ denote the data for J arrays, and let $\delta = (\delta_1, \ldots, \delta_n)$ denote the terminal decision, with $\delta_i = 1$ if gene i is reported as differentially expressed, and $\delta_i = 0$ otherwise. The problem involves two decisions, $d = (J, \delta)$. The terminal decision δ is made *after* observing the data. We thus condition on y^J, and the expected loss integral is only with respect to the unknown parameters θ. In contrast, the sample size is chosen *before* observing the data. We thus marginalize with respect to both, data y and parameters θ, substituting the optimal terminal decision δ^*. Decision problems with such multistep structures are known as sequential decision problems. The optimal decision δ^* is defined as before, with the expected loss taken w.r.t. the posterior distribution, $\delta^*(y^J) = \arg\min \int L(d, \theta, y) \, dp(\theta \mid y^J)$. We include an argument y^J in the notation for δ^* to highlight the dependence on the observed data. The optimal sample size choice is defined by

$$J^* = \arg\min \int L(\delta^*(y^J), \theta) \; dp_d(\theta, y^J). \tag{22.1}$$

The conditions for J^* and $\delta^*(y^J)$ define an ideal solution, following from first principles about rational decision making (Robert, 2001). In practice, several compromises are made when implementing Bayesian optimal design.

An attractive feature of the proposed approach is that the nature of the optimal decision does not depend on details of the probability model. The only required assumption is that the probability model include indicators $r_i \in \{0, 1\}$ for true differential expression of gene i. Except for this minimal assumption, we can discuss the optimal decision before defining a specific probability model, requiring only a loss function to complete the formal description of the decision problem.

We define a loss function that defines a tradeoff of false negative and false rejection counts. Let $\mathrm{FN} = \sum_i (1 - \delta_i) \, r_i$ denote the number of false negatives, and let $\mathrm{FD} = \sum_i \delta_i (1 - r_i)$ denote the false rejections (discoveries). The counts FN and FD are functions of the parameters r_i and the data y^J, implicitly through $\delta_i(y^J)$. We use the loss function

$$L(J, \delta, \theta, y^J) = \mathrm{FD} + c \, \mathrm{FN}.$$

The loss function does not include a term representing sampling cost. See the discussion below, when we consider the optimal decision sample size choice.

22.2.2 The Terminal Decision δ^*

The decision about the optimal sample size in any experiment is always relative to the intended data analysis after carrying out the experiment. This is formalized in the definition (22.1) by requiring to plug in the optimal rule δ^* about reporting genes as differentially expressed. It is therefore natural to first discuss δ^* before we consider the original sample size question.

Let $\bar{r}_i = Pr(r_i = 1 \mid y^J)$ denote the marginal posterior probability of gene being differentially expressed. It can be easily shown (Müller et al., 2004) that under L the optimal decision δ_i^* is of the form

$$\delta_i^*(y^J) = I(\bar{r}_i > t),$$

that is, flag all genes with marginal posterior probability of differential expression beyond a certain threshold. The threshold is $t = c/(c + 1)$. The optimal rule is very intuitive and similar to a popularly used method to control (frequentist) expected false discovery rate (Benjamini and Hochberg, 1995; Storey, 2003), with the critical difference that the rule is defined as a cutoff for marginal probabilities instead of nominal p values. See also Genovese and Wasserman (2003) for more discussion of Bayesian variations of the Benjamini and Hochberg rule.

22.2.3 Sample Size Choice

We now use the optimal decision δ^* to substitute in definition (22.1). First we note that $L(J, \delta, \theta, y^J)$ does not include any sampling cost. To define an optimal sample size J^* we could add a deterministic sampling cost, say kJ. However, the choice of the tradeoff k is problematic. We therefore prefer to use a goal programming approach, plotting expected loss as a function of J, and allowing the investigator to make an informed choice by, for example, selecting the minimum sample size to achieve expected loss below a certain target.

Doing so we run into an additional complication. Let $\bar{L}(J)$ denote the expected loss

$$\bar{L}(J) = \int L(\delta^*(y^J), \theta) \; dp_d(\theta, y^J). \tag{22.2}$$

For relevant sample sizes the expected loss $\bar{L}(J)$ is far too flat to allow a conclusive sample size choice. In fact, in Müller et al. (2004) we show that the prior expectation of FN, plugging in the optimal rule δ^*, decreases asymptotically as $O_P(\sqrt{\log J / J})$.

The flat nature of the expected loss surface is a typical feature for decision problems in many applications. A common solution to address this problem is to consider sensitivity analysis of the expected loss with respect to some relevant features of the probability model. In particular, we assume that for each gene the probability model includes a parameter $\rho_i \geq 0$ that can be interpreted as level of differential expression, with $\rho_i = 0$ for non-differentially expressed genes. Assuming a gene with true $\rho_i > 0$, we explore the change in expected loss as a function of ρ_i and J. In other words, we consider the integral (22.2), but conditioning on an assumed true value for ρ_i, instead of including it in the integration. Assuming a large number of genes, fixing one ρ_i leaves the inference for all other genes approximately unchanged, impacting the loss function only when the ith gene is (wrongly) not flagged as differentially expressed and adds to FN. Thus, for $\rho_i > 0$, the only effected term in the loss function is the ith term in the definition of FN, that is, $(1 - \delta_i) r_i$. We are led to consider

$$\beta_i(J, \rho_i) \equiv Pr(\delta_i = 1 \mid y^J, \rho_i) = Pr(\bar{r}_i > t \mid y^J, \rho_i). \qquad (22.3)$$

The probability includes the marginalizations over all other genes, and the application of the optimal terminal rule δ^*. Assuming that the probability model is exchangeable over genes, we can drop the index from β_i. The expression $\beta(J, \rho)$ has a convenient interpretation as power, albeit marginalizing over all unknowns except for ρ_i. We refer to $\beta(J, \rho)$ as predictive power.

22.3 Monte Carlo Evaluation of Predictive Power

Evaluation of $\beta(J, \rho)$ is most conveniently carried out by Monte Carlo simulation. Let J_0 and J_1 denote minimum and maximum sample sizes under consideration. We first describe the algorithm in words. Simulate many, say M, possible experiments $(\theta^m, y_{J_1}^m)$, $m = 1, \ldots, M$, simulating responses for a maximum number J_1 of arrays. For a grid of sample sizes, from J_1 down to J_0, compute $\bar{r}_i$ for each gene i, each simulation m, and each sample size J on the grid. Record the triples $(J, \rho_i, \bar{r}_i)$ across m, i, and J. Plot $\delta_i = I(\bar{r}_i > t)$ against J and ρ_i. Finally, fitting a smooth surface through δ_i as a function of (J, ρ_i) we estimate $\beta(J, \rho)$. The algorithm is summarized by the following steps. To simplify notation we drop the i index from $\bar{r}_i$, ρ_i, and δ_i.

(i) Simulate experiments $(\theta^m, y_{J_1}^m) \sim p(\theta) \, p(y_{J_1} \mid \theta)$, $m = 1, \ldots, M$.
(ii) Compute $\bar{r}$ across all genes $i = 1, \ldots, n$, simulations $m = 1, \ldots, M$, and for all sample sizes J on a given grid. Record all triples $(J, \rho, \bar{r})$.
(iii) Let $\delta = I(\bar{r} > t)$ and fit a smooth surface $\hat{\beta}(J, \rho)$ through δ as a function of (J, ρ).

> *Note 1:* Most probability models for microarray data assume that y_j are independent given the parameters θ. This allows easy simulation from the joint probability model.
> *Note 2:* Evaluating posterior probabilities $\bar{r}_i$ usually involves posterior Markov Chain Monte Carlo (MCMC). However, the MCMC requires no burn-in since $p(\theta) p(y^J \mid \theta) = p(y^J) \, p(\theta \mid y^J)$. In words, the prior draw θ generated in step (i) is a draw from the posterior distribution given y^J. It can be used to initialize the posterior MCMC.

The plot of $\hat{\beta}(J, \rho)$ is used for an informed sample choice, in the same way as power curves are used in sample size arguments under a frequentist paradigm.

22.4 The Probability Model

22.4.1 A Hierarchical Mixture of Gamma/Gamma Model

The proposed approach builds on the model introduced in Newton et al. (2001) and Newton and Kendziorski (2003). Let X_{ij} and Y_{ij} denote appropriately normalized intensity measurements for gene i on slide j under the two biologic conditions of interest, that is, $y^J = (X_{ij}, Y_{ij}, \ i = 1, \ldots, n$ and $j = 1, \ldots, J)$. We assume conditionally independent measurements given gene-specific scale parameters $(\theta_{0i}, \theta_{1i})$:

$$X_{ij} \sim \text{Gamma}(a, \theta_{0i}) \quad \text{and} \quad Y_{ij} \sim \text{Gamma}(a, \theta_{1i}).$$

We define a hierarchical prior probability model, including a positive prior probability for a tie between θ_{i0} and θ_{i1}, corresponding to nondifferential expression across the two conditions. We introduce a parameter $r_i \in \{0, 1\}$ as latent indicator for $\theta_{0i} = \theta_{1i}$, and assume

$$\theta_{0i} \sim \text{Gamma}(a_0, \nu)$$

and

$$p(\theta_{1i} \mid r_i, \theta_{0i}) = \begin{cases} I(\theta_{1i} = \theta_{0i}) & \text{if } r_i = 0 \\ \text{Gamma}(a_0, \nu) & \text{if } r_i = 1 \end{cases}$$

with $Pr(r_i = 0) = p_0$. The model is completed with a prior for the parameters $(a, a_0, p) \sim \pi(a, a_0, p)$, and fixed ν. We assume a priori independence and use marginal gamma priors for a_0 and a, and a conjugate beta prior for p. As in Newton et al. (2001), the above model leads to a closed form marginal likelihood after integrating out θ_{1i}, θ_{0i}, but still conditional on $\eta = (p, a, a_0)$. Let $X_i = (X_{ij}, \ j = 1, \ldots, J)$ and $Y_i = (Y_{ij}, \ j = 1, \ldots, J)$. We find

$$p(X_i, Y_i | r_i = 0, \eta) = \left\{ \frac{\Gamma(2Ja + a_0)}{\Gamma(a)^{2J} \Gamma(a_0)} \right\} \frac{(\nu)^{a_0} \left(\prod_j X_{ij} \prod_j Y_{ij} \right)^{a-1}}{\left[\left(\sum_j X_i + \sum_j Y_i + \nu \right) \right]^{2a+a_0}}$$

and

$$p(X_i, Y_i | r_i = 1, \eta) = \left\{ \frac{\Gamma(aJ + a_0)}{\Gamma(a)^J \Gamma(a_0)} \right\}^2 \frac{(\nu\nu)^{a_0} \left(\prod_j X_{ij} \prod_j Y_{ij} \right)^{a-1}}{\left[\left(\sum_j X_{ij} + \nu \right) \left(\sum_j Y_{ij} + \nu \right) \right]^{a+a_0}},$$

and thus the marginal distribution is

$$p(X_i, Y_i | \eta) = p_0 \, p(X_i, Y_i \mid r_i = 0, \eta) + (1 - p_0) \, p(X_i, Y_i \mid r_i = 1, \eta).$$
(22.4)

Availability of the closed form expression for the marginal likelihood greatly simplifies posterior simulation. Marginalizing with respect to the random effects reduces the model to the three-dimensional marginal posterior $p(\eta \mid y) \propto p(\eta) \prod_i p(X_i, Y_i | \eta)$. Conditional on currently imputed values for η we can at any time augment the parameter vector by generating $r_i \sim p(r_i \mid \eta, X_i, Y_i)$ as simple independent Bernoulli draws, if desired.

22.4.2 A Mixture of Gamma/Gamma Model

One limitation of a parametric model like this hierarchical Gamma/Gamma model is the need to fix specific model assumptions. The investigator has to select hyperparameters that reflect the relevant experimental conditions. Also, the investigator has to assume that the sampling distribution for observed gene expressions can adequately be approximated by the assumed model. To mitigate problems related with these requirements we consider a model extension that still maintains the computational simplicity of the basic model, but allows for additional flexibility.

A computationally convenient implementation is a mixture extension of the basic model. In particular, we replace the Gamma distributions for $p(X_{ij}|\theta_{0i})$ and $p(Y_{ij}|\theta_{1i})$ by scale mixtures of Gamma distributions

$$X_{ij} \sim \int Ga(a, \theta_{0i} \, q_{ij}) \, dp(q_{ij}|w, m) \quad \text{and}$$

$$Y_{ij} \sim \int Ga(a, \theta_{1i} \, s_{ij}) \, dp(s_{ij}|w, m),$$
(22.5)

where $p(q \mid w, m)$ is a discrete mixing measure with $P(q = m_k) = w_k$ ($k = 1, \dots, K$). Locations $m = (m_1, \dots, m_K)$ and weights $w = (w_1, \dots, w_K)$ parameterize the mixture. To center the mixture model at the basic model, we fix $m_1 = 1.0$ and assume high prior probability for large weight w_1. We use the same mixture for s_{jk}, $P(s_{jk} = m_h) = w_h$. The model is completed with $m_k \sim Ga(b, b)$, $k > 1$, and a Dirichlet prior $w \sim Dir_K(M \cdot W, W, \dots, W)$. Selecting a large factor M in the Dirichlet prior assigns high prior probability for large w_1, as desired. By assuming a dominating term with $m_1 = 1.0$ and $E(m_k) = 1$, $k > 1$, we allocate large prior probability for the basic model and maintain the interpretation of θ_{0i}/θ_{1i} as level of differential expression.

Model (22.5) replaces the Gamma sampling distribution with a scale mixture of Gamma distributions. This is important in the context of microarray data experiments, where technical details in the data collection process typically introduce noise beyond simple sampling variability due to the biological process. A concern related to microarray data experiments prompts us to introduce a further generalization to allow for occasional slides that are outliers compared to the other arrays in the experiment. This happens for reasons unrelated to the biologic effect of interest but needs to be accounted for in the modeling. We achieve this by adding a second mixture to (22.5)

$$(X_{ij}|q_{ij}, g_j) \sim Ga(a, \theta_{0i}\, g_j\, q_{ij}) \quad \text{and} \quad (Y_{ij}|s_{ij}, g_j) \sim Ga(a, \theta_{1i}\, g_j\, s_{ij}),$$
$$(22.6)$$

with an additional slide-specific scale factor g_j. Paralleling the definition of $p(q_{ij}|w, m)$ we use a finite discrete mixture $P(g_j = m_{gk}) = w_{gk}, k = 1, \ldots, L$, with a Dirichlet prior $(w_{g1}, \ldots m_{gL}) \sim Dir_L(M_g \cdot W_g, W_g, \ldots, W_g)$, $m_{gk} \sim Ga(b_g, b_g)$ for $k > 1$ and $m_{g1} \equiv 1$.

22.4.3 Posterior MCMC

Posterior inference is implemented by MCMC posterior simulation. See, for example, Tierney (1994), for a review of MCMC methods. MCMC simulation proceeds by iterating over the following transition probabilities. We use notation like $[x \mid y, z]$ to indicate that x is being updated, conditional on the known or currently imputed values of y and z. We generically use θ^- to indicate all parameters, except the parameter on the left side of the conditioning bar.

(i) $[q_{ij} \mid \theta^-, X_i]$, for $i = 1, \ldots, n$ and $j = 1, \ldots, J$.
(ii) $[s_{ij} \mid \theta^-, Y_i]$, for $i = 1, \ldots, n$ and $j = 1, \ldots, J$.
(iii) $[g_j \mid \theta^-, X, Y]$, $j = 1, \ldots, J$.
(iv) $[a \mid \theta^-, X, Y]$
(v) $[a_0 \mid \theta^-, X, Y]$
(vi) $[m_h \mid \theta^-, X, Y]$, $h = 1, \ldots, K$
(vii) $[w \mid \theta^-, X, Y]$, $w = (w_1, \ldots, w_K)$
(viii) $[m_g \mid \theta^-, X, Y]$, $g = 1, \ldots, L$
(ix) $[w_g \mid \theta^-, X, Y]$, $w_g = (w_{g1}, \ldots, w_{gL})$.
(x) $[K \mid \theta^-, X, Y]$
(xi) $[L \mid \theta^-, X, Y]$

All but steps x and xi are standard MCMC transition probabilities. Changing K and L we use reversible jump MCMC (Green, 1995). See Richardson and Green (1997) for a description of RJMCMC specifically for mixture models.

Our reversible jump implementation includes a merge move to combine two terms in the current mixture, a matching split move, a birth move, and a matching death move. Details are similar to Richardson and Green (1997), with the mixture of gammas replacing the mixture of normals. Inference is based on a geometric prior on the number of terms K and L in both mixtures.

22.5 Pilot Data

The flexible mixture model allows to use pilot data to learn about details of the sampling distribution. We envision a process where the investigator either uses available data from similar previous experiments, or collects preliminary data to allow estimation of the mixture model parameters before proceeding with the sample size argument. The pilot data might not include samples under both biologic conditions. Pilot data is often available only for control tissue. For such data a reduced version of the model, using only the parts of the model relevant for X_{ij}, is used. This is sufficient to estimate the mixture model parameters.

In summary, we proceed in two stages. In the first stage the pilot data is used to fit the mixture model. Let X_{ij}^o, $j = 1, \ldots, J^o$, denote the pilot data. We will use posterior MCMC simulation to estimate the posterior mean model. This is done once, before starting the optimal design. We then fix the mixture model at the posterior modes $\widehat{K}$ and $\widehat{L}$, and the posterior means $(\bar{w}, \bar{m}, \bar{w}_g, \bar{m}_g) = E(w, m, w_g, m_g \mid X^o, \widehat{K}, \widehat{L})$. We proceed with the optimal sample size approach, using model (22.5) with the fixed mixtures.

22.6 Example

For illustration we consider the data reported in Richmond et al. (1999), and used in Newton et al. (2001). We use the control data as pilot data to plan the sample size for a hypothetical future experiment. Estimating the mixture model we find a posterior mode $\hat{K} = 3$ and $\hat{L} = 2$.

We now fix K and L at the posterior mode, and the remaining mixture parameters (m, w, m_g, w_g) at their conditional posterior means, conditional on $K - 3$ and $L = 2$. We then use the mixture Gamma/Gamma model with fixed mixture parameters to proceed with the Monte Carlo simulation to compute $\beta(J, \rho)$. In the context of the mixture of Gamma/Gamma model we define $\rho_i = \log(\theta_{0i}/\theta_{1i})$, the log ratio of scale parameters for gene i. Figure 22.2 shows the estimated predictive power curves $\beta(J, \rho)$. The left panel shows $\beta(J, \rho)$ for fixed ρ. Aiming for fourfold differential expression, the plot shows the predictive power that can be achieved with increasing sample size. The left panel of Figure 22.2 summarizes the surface $\beta(J, \rho)$ by fixing J at $J = 15$, and

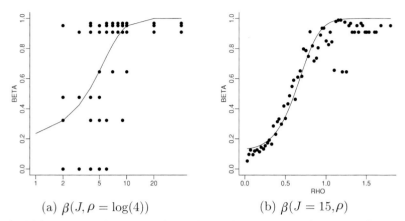

(a) $\beta(J, \rho = \log(4))$ (b) $\beta(J = 15, \rho)$

Fig. 22.2. Power β (labeled BETA in the plot) against sample size for assumed fourfold overexpression, $\rho = \log(4)$ (left), and against ρ for sample size $J = 15$ (right). Power $\beta(J, \rho)$ is defined in (22.3) as the average posterior probability of discovery, conditional on the true level of differential expression $\rho_i = \log(\theta_{0i}/\theta_{1i})$.

plotting predictive power against assumed level of differential expression ρ. For increasing level of ρ the figure shows the predictive power that can be achieved with $J = 15$ arrays.

The points show the simulated true fraction of rejections for J and ρ on a grid. The estimated surface $\beta(J, \rho)$ is based on *all* simulations, across all ρ and J. But the plot only shows the simulations corresponding to the shown slice of the surface.

22.7 Conclusion

We have discussed ideas for a Bayesian decision theoretic sample size argument for microarray experiments. The strength of the approach is the opportunity to use essentially arbitrarily complex probability models. The proposed mixture Gamma/Gamma model is an example. But the argument is valid for any probability model, as long as the model includes latent variables r_i that can be interpreted as indicators for a true effect for gene i, and parameters ρ_i that can be interpreted as strength of the effect. In particular, the probability model could include more complicated designs than two-sample experiments.

Limitations of the proposed approach are the assumed independence across genes, and the implicit 0-1 loss function. More general loss functions could, for example, include a weight proportional to the true ρ_i in the penalty for false negatives. More general models could explicitly allow for networks and dependence.

Bibliography

Benjamini, Y. and Hochberg, Y. (1995), "Controlling the false discovery rate: A practical and powerful approach to multiple testing," *Journal of the Royal Statistical Society, Series B*, 57, 289–300.

Berger, J. O. (1993), *Statistical Decision Theory and Bayesian Analysis*, Springer-Verlag Inc., New York.

Bickel, D. R. (2003), "Selecting an optimal rejection region for multiple testing: A decision-theoretic alternative to FDR control, with an application to microarrays," Technical Report, Medical College of Georgia.

DeGroot, M. (1970), *Optimal Statistical Decisions*, New York: McGraw-Hill.

Fu, W., Dougherty, E., Mallick, B., and Carroll, R. (2005), "How many samples are needed to build a classifier: A general sequential approach," *Bioinformatics*, 21, 63–70.

Genovese, C. and Wasserman, L. (2003), *Bayesian Statistics 7*, Oxford: Oxford University Press, chap. Bayesian and Frequentist Multiple Testing, pp. 145–162.

Green, P. J. (1995), "Reversible jump Markov chain Monte Carlo computation and Bayesian model determination," *Biometrika*, 82, 711–732.

Lee, M.-L. and Whitmore, G. (2002), "Power and sample size for microarray studies," *Statistics in Medicine*, 11, 3543–3570.

Mukherjee, S., Tamayo, P., Rogers, S., Rifkin, R., Engle, A., Campbell, C., Golub, T., and Mesirov, J. (2003), "Estimating dataset size requirements for classifying DNA microarray data," *Journal of Computational Biology*, 10, 119–142.

Müller, P., Parmigiani, G., Robert, C., and Rousseau, J. (2004), "Optimal sample size for multiple testing: The case of gene expression microarrays," *Journal of the American Statistical Association*, 99, 990–1001.

Newton, M. A. and Kendziorski, C. M. (2003), "Parametric empirical Bayes methods for microarrays," in *The Analysis of Gene Expression Data: Methods and Software*, New York: Springer.

Newton, M. A., Kendziorski, C. M., Richmond, C. S., Blattner, F. R., and Tsui, K. W. (2001), "On differential variability of expression ratios: Improving statistical inference about gene expression changes from microarray data," *Journal of Computational Biology*, 8, 37–52.

Pan, W., Lin, J., and Le, C. T. (2002), "How many replicates of arrays are required to detect gene expression changes in microarray experiments? A mixture model approach," *Genome Biology*, 3(5), research0022.1–0022.10.

Richardson, S. and Green, P. (1997), "On Bayesian analysis of mixtures with an unknown number of components," *Journal of the Royal Statistical Society, Series B*, 59, 731–792.

Richmond, C. S., Glasner, J. D., Mau R., Jin, H., and Blattner, F. (1999), "Genome-wide expression profiling in *Escherichia coli* K-12," *Nucleic Acid Research*, 27, 3821–3835.

Robert, C. P. (2001), *The Bayesian Choice: From Decision-Theoretic Foundations to Computational Implementation*, Springer-Verlag Inc.

Storey, J. D. (2003), "The positive false discovery rate: A Bayesian interpretation and the q-value," *The Annals of Statistics*, 31, 2013–2035.

Tierney, L. (1994), "Markov chains for exploring posterior distributions (with Discussion)," *Annals of Statistics*, 22, 1701–1762.

Zien, A., Fluck, J., Zimmer, R., and Lengauer, T. (2002), "Microarrays: How many do you need?" Technical Report, Fraunhofer-Institute for Algorithms and Scientific Computing (SCAI), Sankt Augustin, Germany.

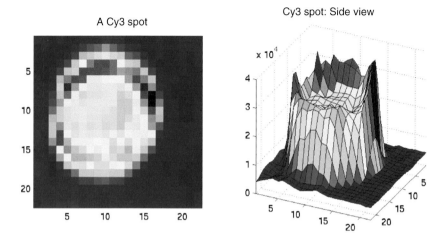

Plate 1.6. Zoom on a single Cy3 spot. The ring shape is visible, indicating uneven hybridization. Further, the side view shows that readings outside the spot are not at zero intensity.

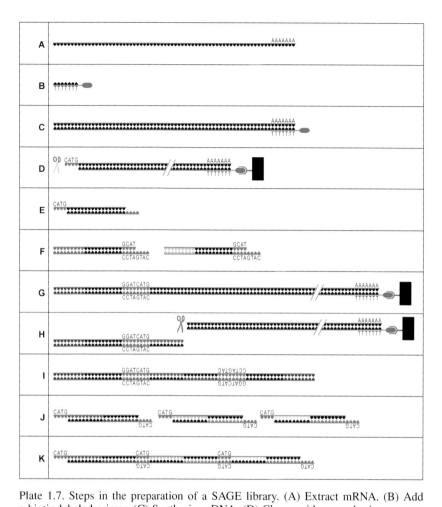

Plate 1.7. Steps in the preparation of a SAGE library. (A) Extract mRNA. (B) Add a biotin-labeled primer. (C) Synthesize cDNA. (D) Cleave with an anchoring enzyme (AE). (E) Discard loose segments. (F) Split cDNA into two pools, and introduce a linker for each. (G) Ligate linker to bound cDNA fragments. (H) Cleave the product with a tagging enzyme, and discard the bound parts. In addition to the linker, the piece remaining contains a 10-base "tag" that can be used to identify the initial mRNA. (I) Ligate the fragments, and use PCR starting from the primers attached to the linkers to amplify. (J) Cleave with the AE again, and discard the pieces bound to the linker. The remaining fragments contain pairs of tags, or "ditags," bracketed by the motif recognized by the AE. (K) Ligate the ditags and sequence the product.

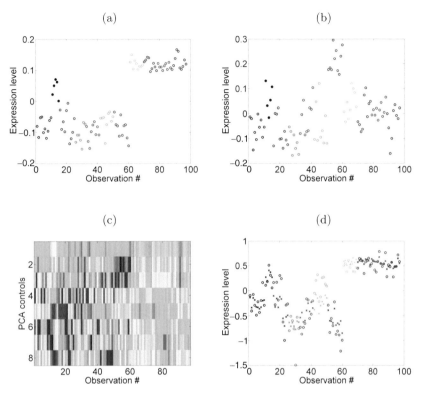

Plate 8.2. First (a) and second (b) principal components in the expression levels across oncogene experiment observations of the set of normalisation control and housekeeping probe sets. The black symbols represent samples in the two control groups (10 initial control samples as open black circles, and 5 later control samples as filled black circles) that were assayed several months apart; the nine oncogene intervention groups are then color-coded for presentation. Frame (c) displays an image intensity plot of the first eight principal components across samples. Frame (d) displays the (centered) expression levels of gene PEA-15 (PED) plotted across samples (circles); superimposed (as crosses) are the (centered) fitted values from the sparse ANOVA/regression model with normalisation control factors.

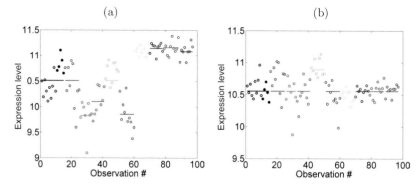

Plate 8.3. Frame (a) displays expression levels of gene PEA-15 (PED) across samples; the horizontal lines superimposed represent the estimated levels of expression within each of the groups in the analysis that ignores the normalisation control factors. Frame (b) displays corrected expression levels from the sparse regression analysis using the control factors; the fitted effects of the control components have been subtracted from the samples displayed, and the horizontal lines superimposed represent the fitted parameters/levels for the intervention effects on expression within each group.

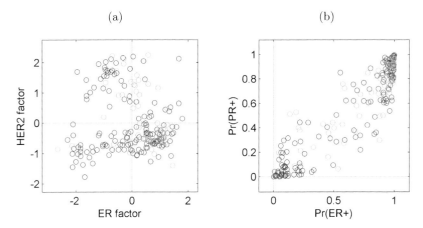

Plate 8.5. Frame (a) is a scatter plot of the fitted values of 2 of the 14 latent factors – factor 1, the "HER2 factor," and factor 2, the primary "ER factor" – in the breast cancer example. The colour coding indicates IHC assay ER+ tumours (red), ER− cases (blue), and intermediate/indeterminate cases (cyan). The plot is concordant with the known association between HER2 and ER; HER2 overexpression generally occurs much more frequently in ER− tumours at a rate of about 30–40%. Frame (b) displays the fitted probabilities from the probit regression model linked to the latent factors as predictors of the IHC binary measures of ER and PR positivity, with colour coding as in frame (a). The positive correlation of ER and PR is evident in these factor-based probabilities, as is the discriminatory role of the estimated factors.

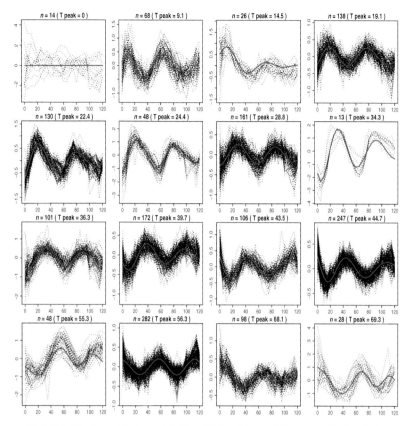

Plate 9.9. Final partitioning with $K = 16$ fixed (note different vertical scales).

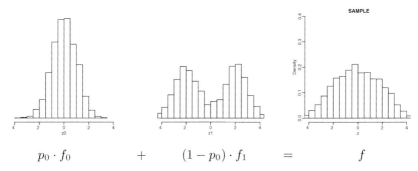

$$p_0 \cdot f_0 \qquad + \qquad (1 - p_0) \cdot f_1 \qquad = \qquad f$$

Plate 12.1. Hypothetical distribution of difference scores for nondifferentially expressed (left, f_0) and differentially expressed genes (center, f_1), and the observed mixture (right, f).

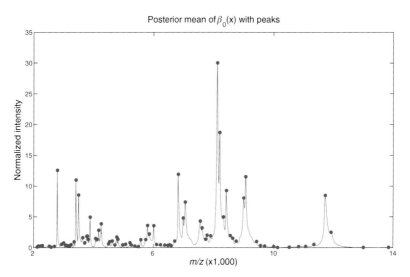

Plate 14.4. Peak detection. Posterior mean for the overall mean spectrum, $\beta_0(t)$, with detected peaks indicated by the dots. A peak is defined to be a location for which its first difference and the first difference immediately preceding it are positive, and the first differences for the two locations immediately following it are negative.

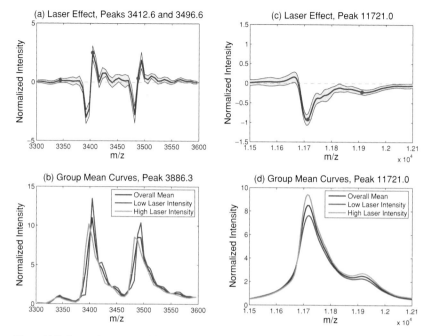

Plate 14.7. Laser intensity effect. Posterior mean laser intensity effect near peaks of interest at (a) 3412.6 and 3496.6 and (c) 11721, along with 95% pointwise posterior credible bands. The red dots indicate the locations of peaks detected in the fitted mean spectrum. Panels (b) and (d) contain the corresponding fitted posterior mean curves for the overall mean and the laser intensity-specific mean spectra in the same two regions. Note that the nonparametrically estimated laser intensity effects are able to adjust for both shifts in location (x-axis, see (a) and (b)), and shifts in intensity (y-axis, see (c) and (d)).

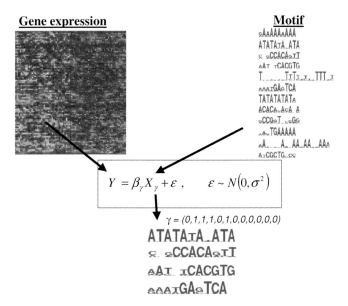

Plate 17.1. Graphical representation of the methodology of Tadesse et al. [21]: Expression levels are regressed on a large list of candidate motif scores. Bayesian variable selection methods are used to locate sets of motifs that best predict changes in gene expression.

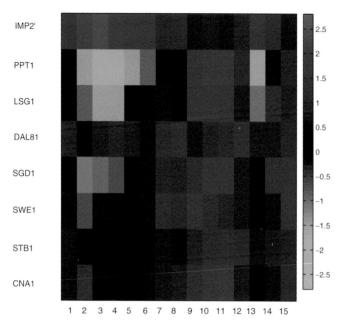

Plate 17.2. Selection of motifs and regulators: Heatmap of the selected regulators over the 15 experiments under consideration.

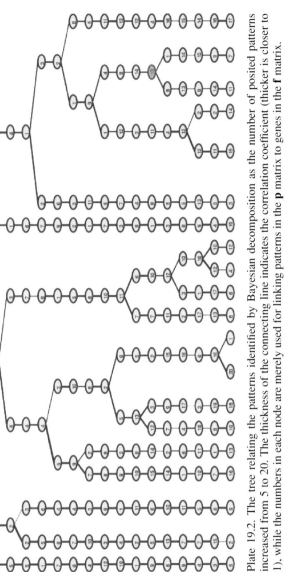

Plate 19.2. The tree relating the patterns identified by Bayesian decomposition as the number of posited patterns increased from 5 to 20. The thickness of the connecting line indicates the correlation coefficient (thicker is closer to 1), while the numbers in each node are merely used for linking patterns in the **p** matrix to genes in the **f** matrix.

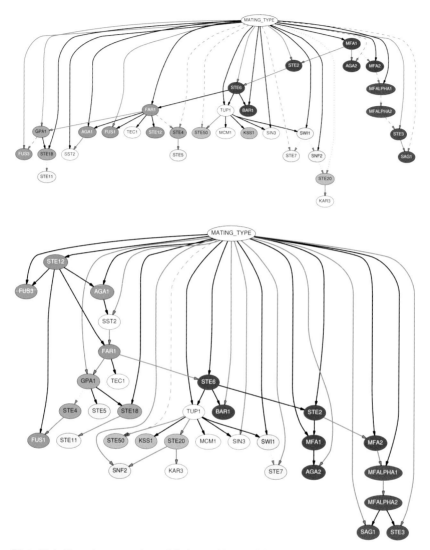

Plate 21.1. Bayesian network models learned by model averaging over the 500 highest-scoring models visited during the simulated annealing search runs with a uniform prior and hard informative prior, respectively. Edges are included in the figure if and only if their posterior probability exceeds 0.5. Node and edge color descriptions are included in the text.

Printed in the United States
by Baker & Taylor Publisher Services